Assistive Products: An Illustrated Guide to Terminology

Gordon C. Krantz, PhD
Margaret A. Christenson, MPH, OTR, FAOTA
Adam Lindquist, BS

The American Occupational Therapy Association Mission Statement:

The mission of the American Occupational Therapy Association is to support a professional community for members, and to develop and preserve the viability and relevance of the profession. The organization serves the interests of its members, represents the profession to the public, and promotes access to occupational therapy services.

Disclaimers

"This publication is designed to provide accurate and authoritative information in regard to the subject matter covered. It is sold or distributed with the understanding that the publisher is not engaged in rendering legal, accounting, or other professional service. If legal advice or other expert assistance is required, the services of a competent professional person should be sought."

—From the Declaration of Principles jointly adopted by the American Bar Association and a Committee of Publishers and Associations.

It is the objective of the American Occupational Therapy Association to be a forum for free expression and interchange of ideas. The opinions and positions expressed by the contributors to this work are their own and not necessarily those of either the editors or the American Occupational Therapy Association.

Frances E. McCarrey, AOTA Director of Nonperiodical Publications
Mary C. Fisk, Managing Editor of Nonperiodical Publications
Paul A. Platosh, Production Editor of Nonperiodical Publications

Printed in the United States of America

ISBN 1-56900-089-1

Table of Contents

ABOUT THE AUTHORS

Margaret A. Christenson, MPH, OTR, FAOTA

Ms. Christenson is president and founder of Lifease, Inc. She also consults with organizations, architects, and interior designers, and with administrators of senior housing, assisted living, and long-term-care facilities concerning the environments used by the elderly. She is a frequent lecturer and seminar leader on adaptations of the living environment to compensate for the changes of aging. She has written several articles on this topic and a book, *Aging in the Designed Environment.* In 1989, she was honored as the Minnesota Occupational Therapist of the Year. She is past chair of the Gerontology Special Interest Section of the American Occupational Therapy Association (AOTA) and was the delegate to the 1995 White House Conference on Aging. She was inducted into the Roster of Fellows of AOTA in 1995.

Gordon C. Krantz, PhD

Dr. Krantz has 47 years of experience in vocational rehabilitation, special education, vocational education, and similar services, and in the design of human service systems, program evaluation, and information systems. He has taken part in a number of national and international conferences, authored several book chapters, was founding editor of the *Vocational Evaluation and Work Adjustment Bulletin,* and published a number of professional papers. He was a (Minnesota) Licensed Consulting Psychologist until his retirement from that field to enter other consulting fields in 1989. In his work with Lifease, Inc., he was responsible for the logic and system design of the EASE programs, and he formulated the generic name terminology used in this publication.

Adam A. Lindquist, BS

Mr. Lindquist is Director of Marketing for Lifease, Inc., where he contributes to the clarity and user interface of the EASE programs, as well as to new product and market development. Mr. Lindquist has over 10 years of experience in market research, marketing strategy, and management for all levels of business. He is a national consultant in the senior living, long-term-care, and rehabilitation industries. Prior to his work on the EASE programs, he was a partner in a marketing communications company specializing in medically related marketing for invasive and noninvasive technology and for health care service delivery businesses.

Lifease, Inc., the company in which the authors have been key employees since 1991, is a Minnesota corporation. The conceptual content of this publication is an outgrowth of the authors' work together there. It is based upon a critical link in the company's EASE programs, that of generic names to designate products in response to clients' functional problems. The EASE programs are a series of computerized decision support tools that first compare the subject person's functional abilities with the functional demands of that person's home environment. The EASE programs then list the options of products, suggestions, and services that can make the environment usable to the person with functional limitations. When a product is chosen, EASE provides specific information on sources and ordering information. The EASE programs originally were designed for use by occupational therapists, particularly those dealing with elderly people, but they also are used with people who have similar functional limitations. Lifease, Inc., is located at 2451 15th Street NW, New Brighton, MN 55112.

Gordon C. Krantz, PhD

Margaret A. Christenson, MPH, OTR, FAOTA

Adam Lindquist, BS

Introduction

The set of illustrations in this publication is based upon a list of generic names of products. These are products that have been found useful to facilitate the home independence of people who have functional limitations. The publication first gives nearly 400 pictures of selected products, followed by the list itself, which has over 5300 items, followed in turn by a glossary.

The products chosen from the list to be illustrated here are those that need a picture in order to most accurately identify and specify them or those that typify a class of items. A publication of this length cannot, of course, illustrate more than a sample of such items.

Illustrations

Drawings are used instead of photographs. Their purpose is to emphasize the functional utility of each product in a simplified way.

The generic name that appears beside each illustration is intended to define that type of product. Like the illustration, the name is generic; a generic name designates all products that are, in practical and functional terms, the same thing. The generic names are not trade names nor are they restricted to items from particular sources.

Scope

The scope covered in this publication is

- products that are physical
- products that compensate for or otherwise get around the effects of the functional limitations of the person, whether or not they were originally designed as assistive technology
- products that are useful in the tasks of independent home living
- products that usually are available in commerce
- products that are used by the subject person rather than by a caregiver.

The list does not include either behavioral adaptations or most features of home construction. These also are important to home independence, but they are a different subject.

The products are mostly "on the market," available for purchase by the lay public. Almost all are available nationally. Some items were left out of the scope of this publication because the authors believe that professional advice is needed when they are selected. Thus, the list of generic names includes the accessories to canes, such as ice tips, but not the various kinds of canes themselves; it has wheelchair accessories, but not wheel chairs.

The products that are illustrated compensate for or circumvent problems in home independence. The guiding ideas are those of functional limitation and of dealing with functional limitation by intervention in the environment and by management of the environment.

Most of the items are of "low technology," in that they tend to be common objects or objects that are simple in design. There are some exceptions, mostly electronic devices.

The products relate to use in the activities of the home. Home recreation and social communicative activities are included within home independence. Community activities, travel off the premises, and activities not concerned with personal independence are not covered. Neither are other arenas of action, such as therapy; a forearm support for a reacher is within the scope of this publication, but a brace as such is not.

Because the products are primarily for direct use by the functionally limited person, items like patient lifts used by caregivers are not pictured.

Limitation

Appearance of a type of product in this publication does not constitute an endorsement by the authors or by the American

Occupational Therapy Association. The items are not claimed to be safe, effective, or specifically useful. Neither does the omission of a type of product imply that it is not appropriate; this is merely a finite list of generic names. All product types illustrated are, or have recently been, actually available in the marketplace.

List of Generic Names

A long list of generic product names, from which the labels of the illustrations were selected, follows the illustrations. That list is so designed that it can be presented in sequence, as is done in the printed version given here, or it can be searched randomly by key word in a computerized base.

So that the generic names can better specify products that meet particular functional needs, a glossary is provided following the list. The glossary defines some of the terms used in the list.

The list of generic names is not to be considered as completed at any given time. It is intentionally open-ended, and it can be added to or its scope can be changed without the need to change its structure. For example, it could be expanded to include products that are useful in broader community activities or in therapy. Its structure (up to four terms per type of product, with the terms in descending order of generality) is designed to be generally applicable to specifying the generic nature of any kind of product. The essential features of the list are that it is generic, that it is independent of any set of trade names or suppliers, and that it is functional in focus.

Acknowledgments

This publication has been prepared with partial support from the American Occupational Therapy Association. Publication is by the American Occupational Therapy Association, which has rights of additional publication. Except for the rights of American Occupational Therapy Association, all other rights are reserved by the authors.

The authors are principals of Lifease, Inc., a Minnesota corporation. Lifease is the publisher of the EASE series of instruments, which are computerized decision support tools that initially were designed for use by occupational therapists to facilitate home independence by older people, and of related instruments. The list of generic product names was developed from the copyrighted data base of EASE, with substantial consultation from related sources.

The list of generic names of products is also available on computer disk from the authors. The list in that medium can be searched by keyword using any common word processor, or it can be searched with the aid of its included search program. Inquiries regarding it and related programs should be made to: Lifease, Inc., 2451 15th St. NW, Suite D, New Brighton, MN 55112, phone (612) 636-6869.

The authors wish to acknowledge the extensive and able consultation furnished by Mary Lee Cherney, OTR, in the initial editing of the list, as well as the programming consultation provided by Paul Christenson, BA, BS.

The drawings were made by Jeff Felson.

Illustrations of Selected Products

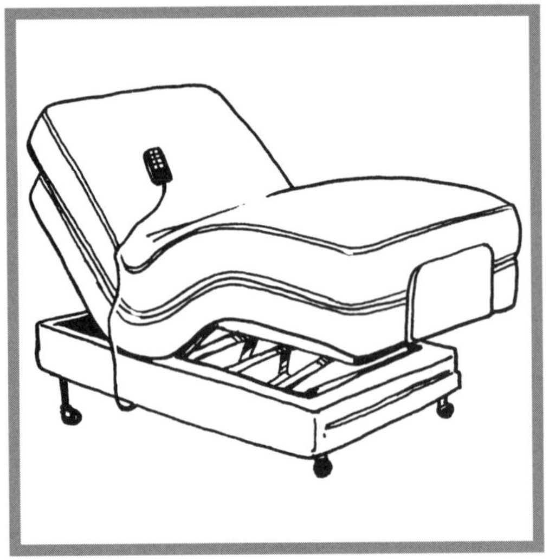

Adjustable bed
Electric & remote control
Raise head and/or flex knees
Dual king size

1

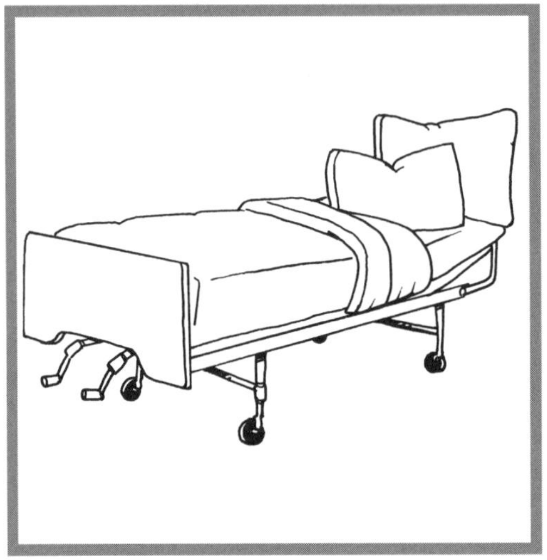

Adjustable bed
Manual crank
Raise head and/or flex knees
Extra long twin size

2

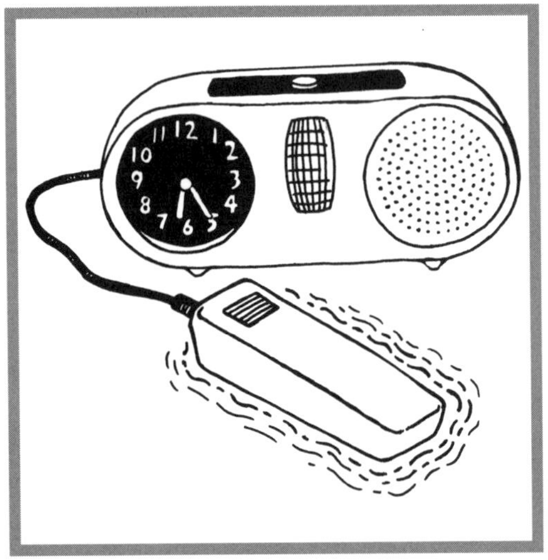

Alarm clock
5 inch dial display
Vibrating & sound
Battery powered

3

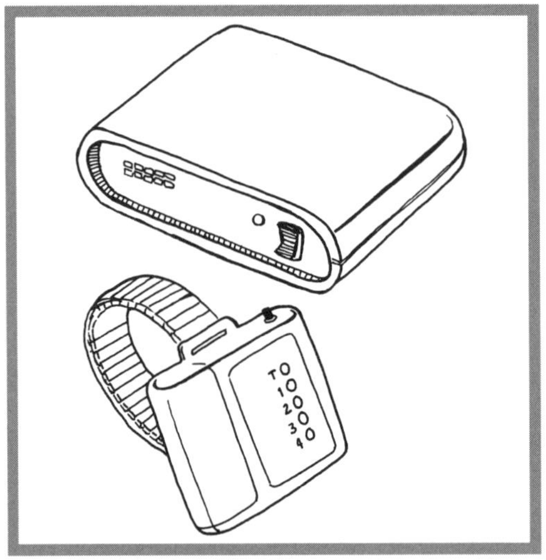

Alerting device
Wrist receiver
Sound activated remote
Send & receive units

4

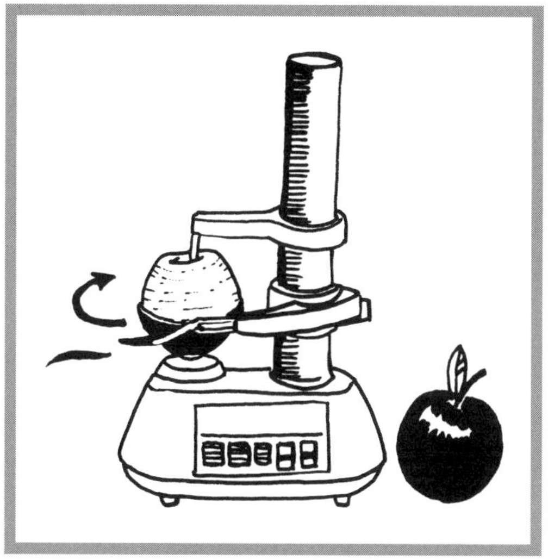

5

Apple peeler
One-hand operated
Removes only the skin
AC powered

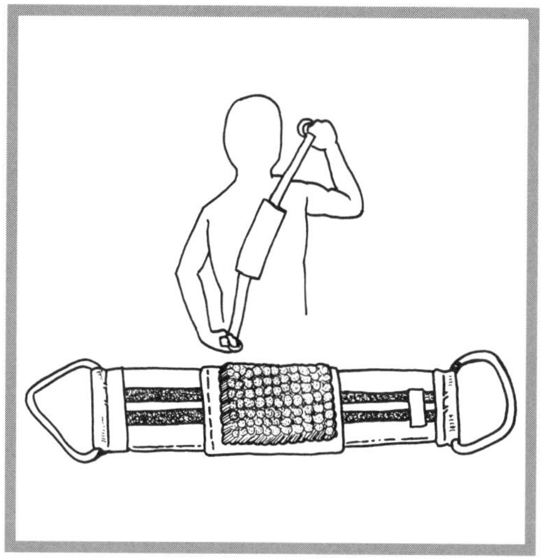

6

Back scrubber
Requires two hands
Webbing loops
Terrycloth

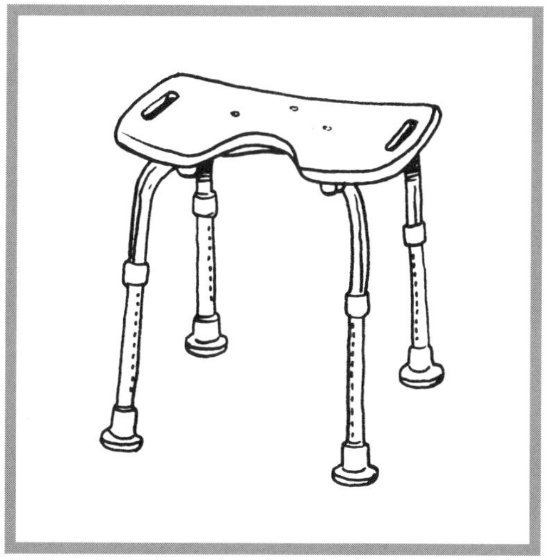

7

Bath bench
Adjustable height
13-19 inch
With hand grips
Drainage holes

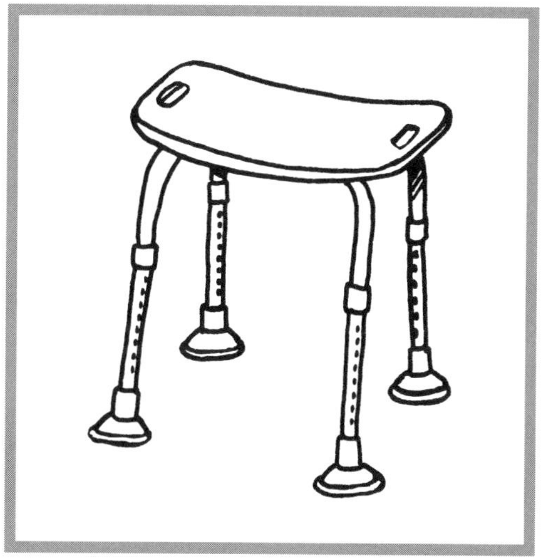

8

Bath bench
Adjustable height
13-20 inch
With hand grips
11 x 19 inch seat

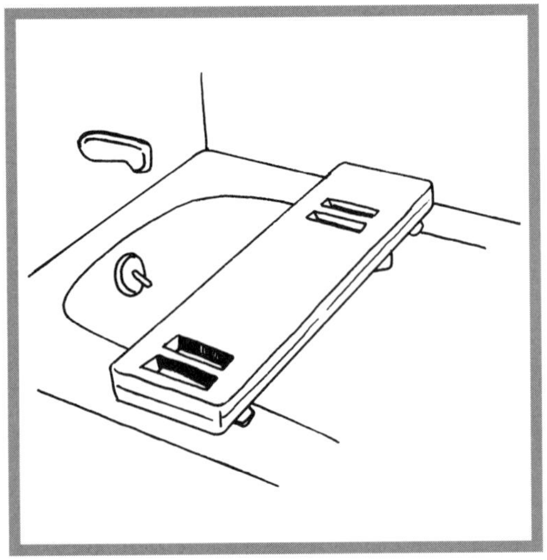

Bath bench
Fixed height
With hand grips
Fits across tub edge

9

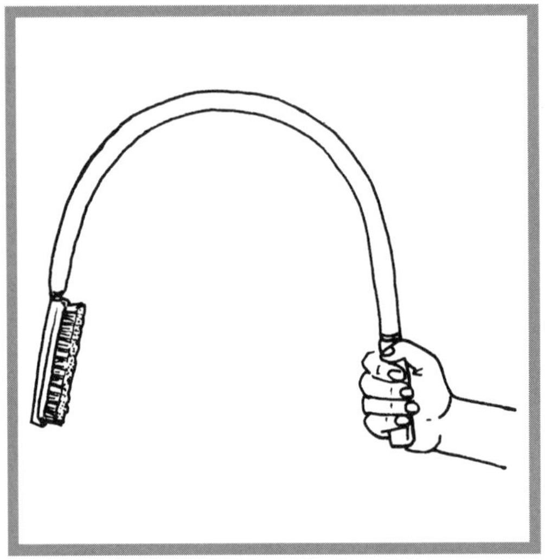

Bath brush
Curved handle
Fixed head

10

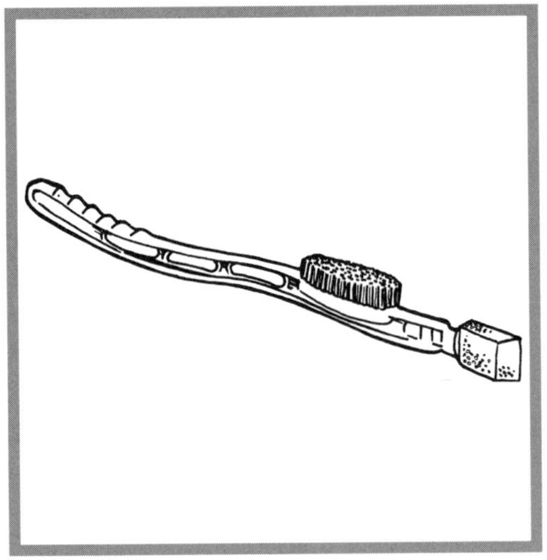

Bath brush
Long handle
Brush on shaft
Small wedge sponge tip

11

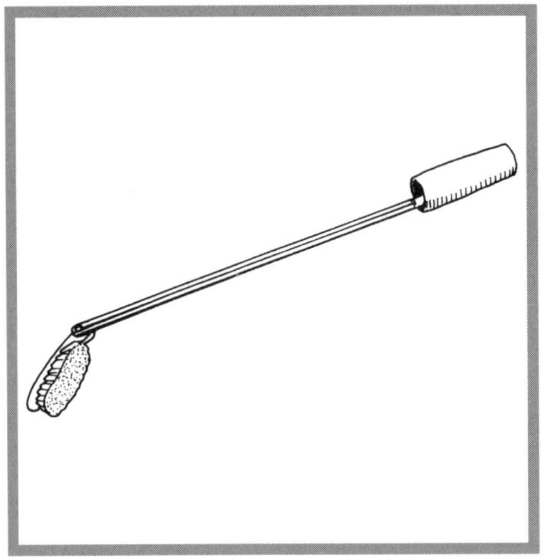

Bath brush
Long handle
Head adjusts to 90 degrees

12

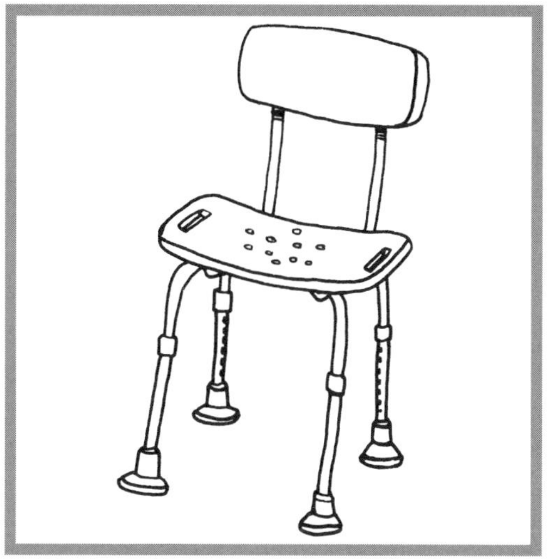

Bath chair
Adjustable height
With hand grips
Drainage holes

13

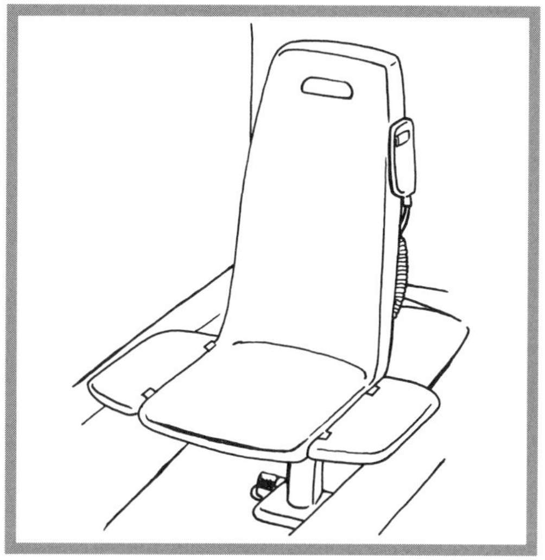

Bath lift
Chair with transfer extensions
Extensions fold into tub
Battery pack powered

14

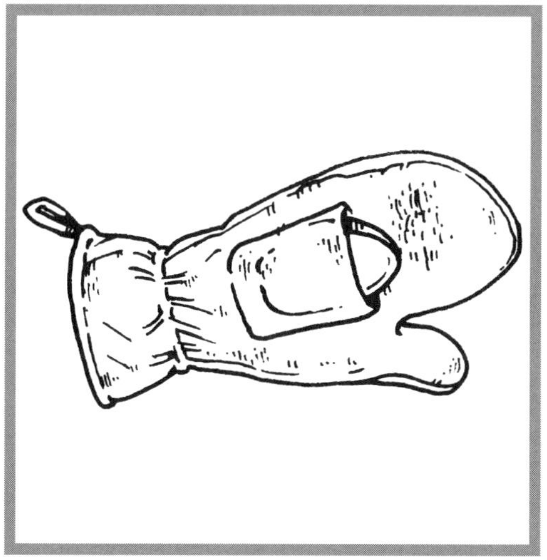

Bath mitt
Hand shaped with thumb
Elastic at wrist
Palm soap pocket

15

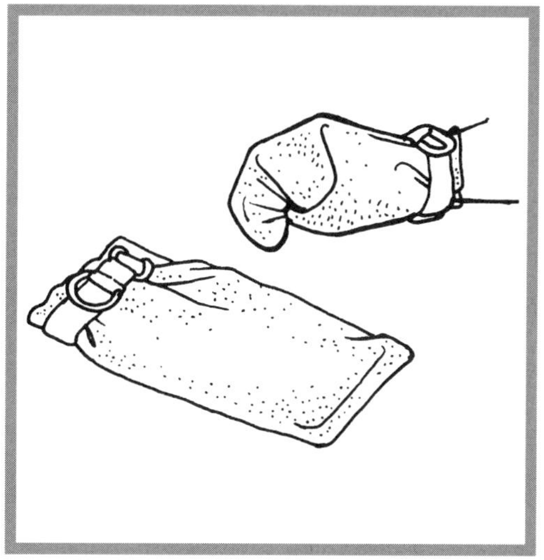

Bath mitt
Large rectangular
Velcro & D-ring closure

16

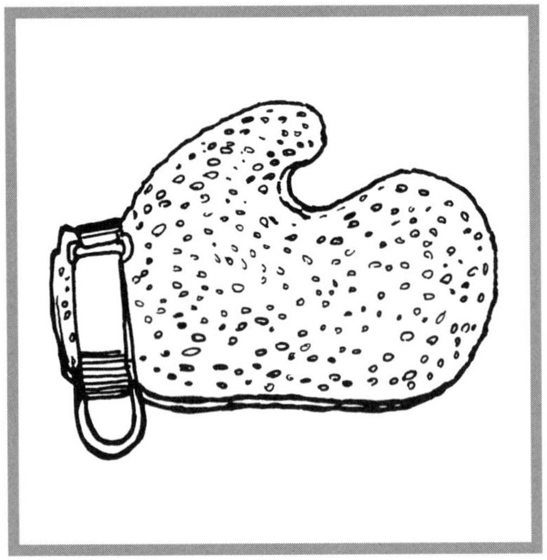

17

Bath mitt/sponge
Hand shaped with thumb
Velcro & D-ring closure

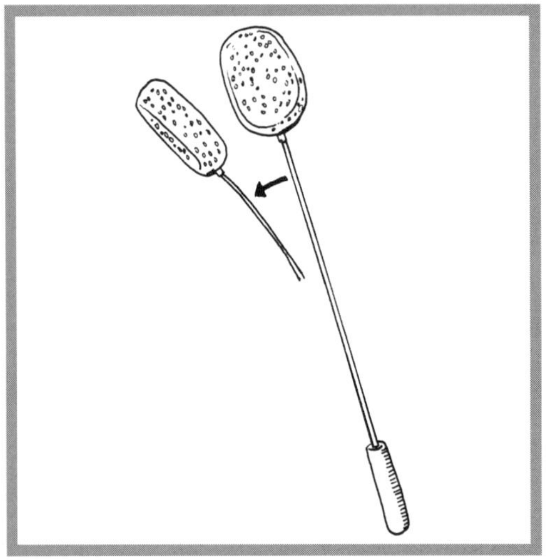

18

Bath sponge with handle
Standard sponge
12 inch bendable handle
Built-up handle

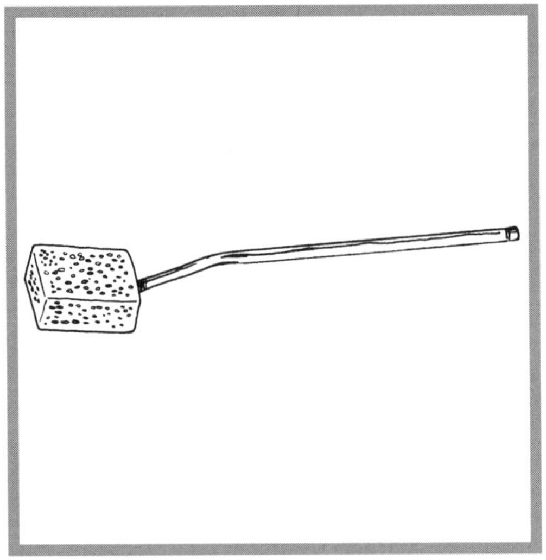

19

Bath sponge with handle
Standard sponge
18 inch handle
Heat-adjustable handle

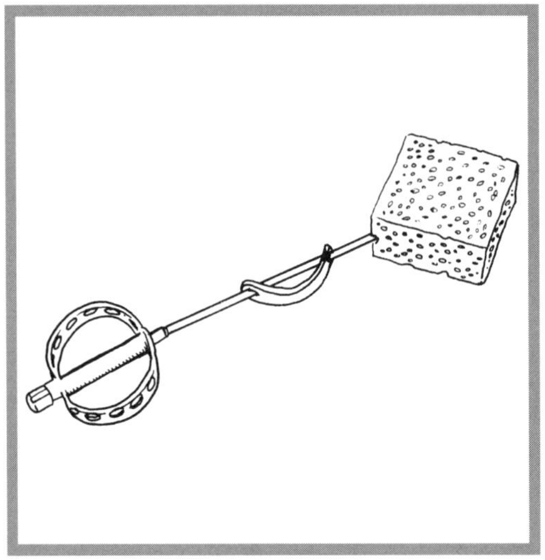

20

Bath sponge with handle
Standard sponge
handle with hand loops

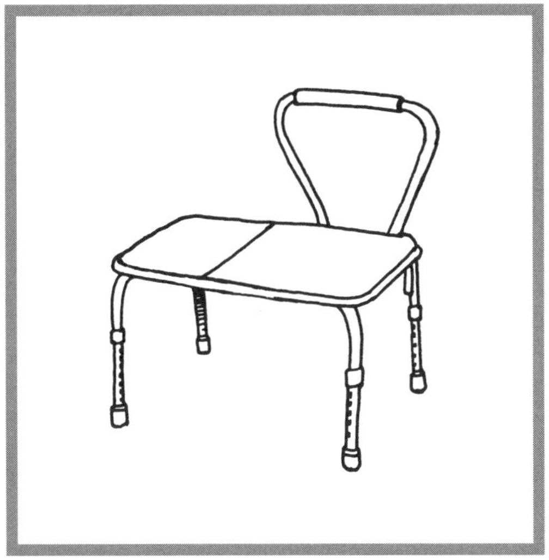

Bath transfer bench
Adjustable height
Extends over tub

21

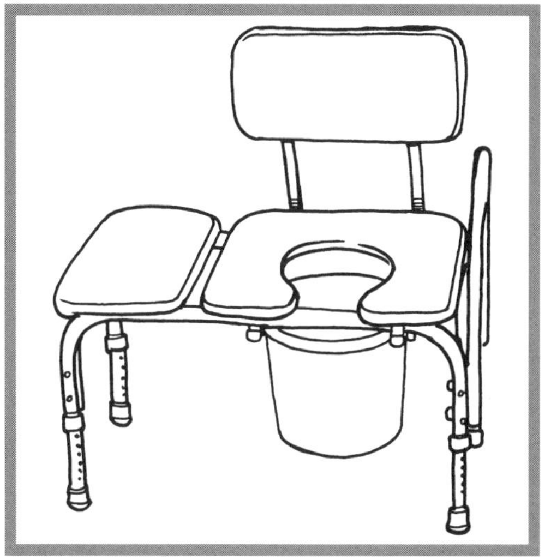

Bath transfer chair
Adjustable height
Backrest &
right-or-left arm

22

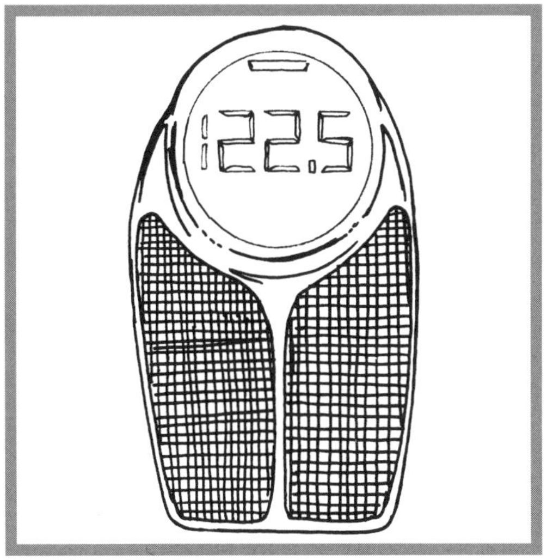

Bathroom scale
2 inch display
numbers
Red LED display
300 pound capacity

23

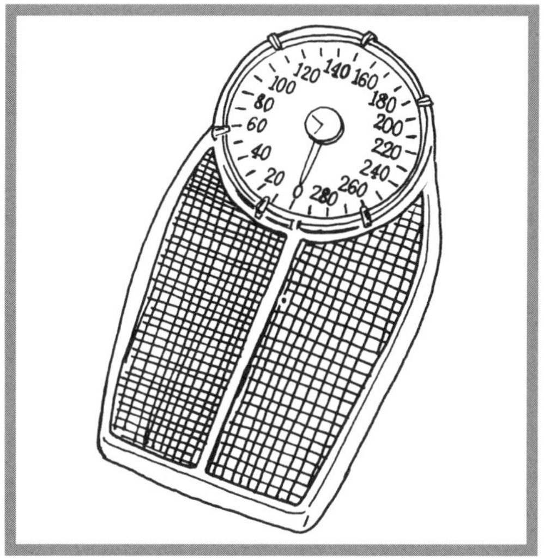

Bathroom scale
Extra large display
Dial display

24

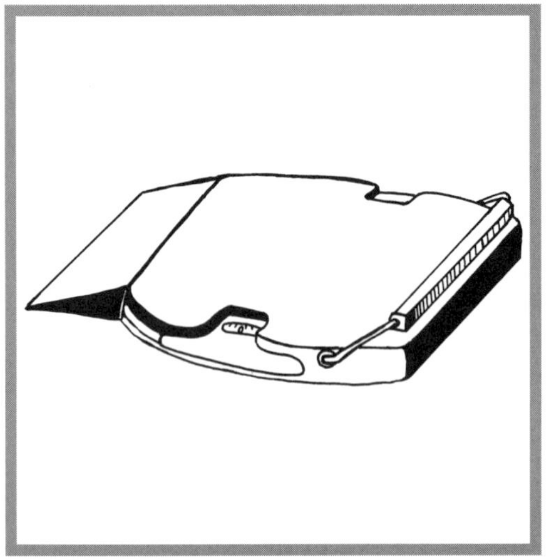

Bathroom scale
With wheelchair platform
Digital display to 580 pounds
Side ramp & guard rail

25

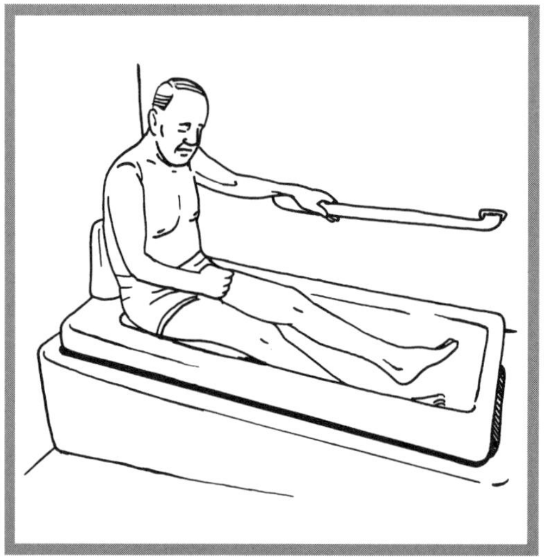

Bathtub insert
Supported on tub rim
Makes tub shallow

26

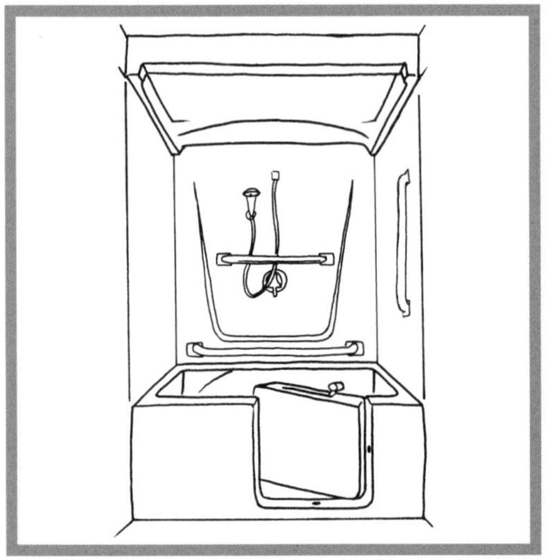

Bathtub with side opening
Door entry
Floor level entry

27

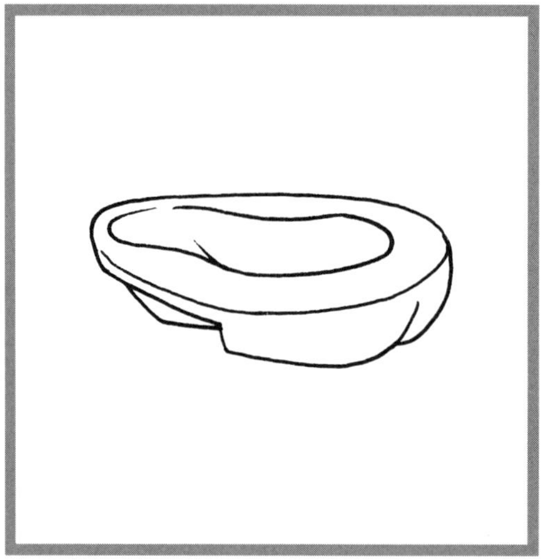

Bed pan
Contoured
Stainless steel
No handles

28

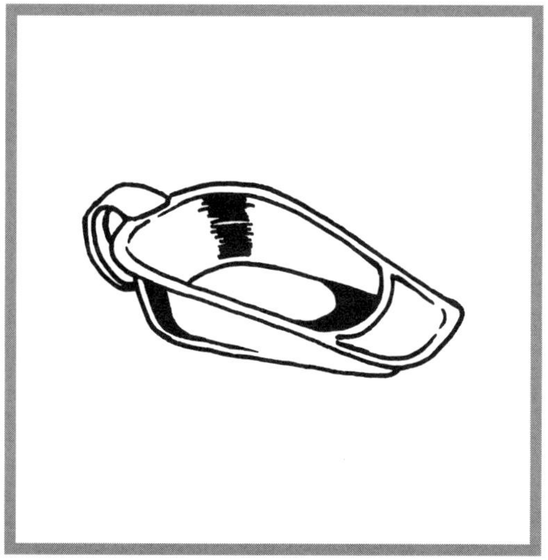

Bed pan
Wedge shape
Plastic
Loop handle

29

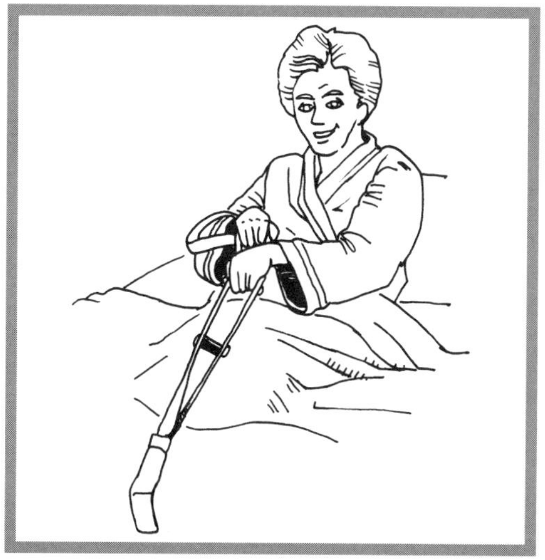

Bed pull-up
Ladder type
4 webbing loops

30

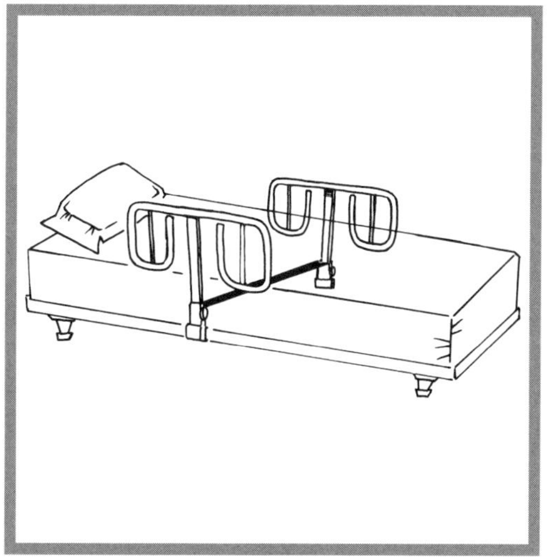

Bed rail half length
Adjusts to fit all beds
15 inch height

31

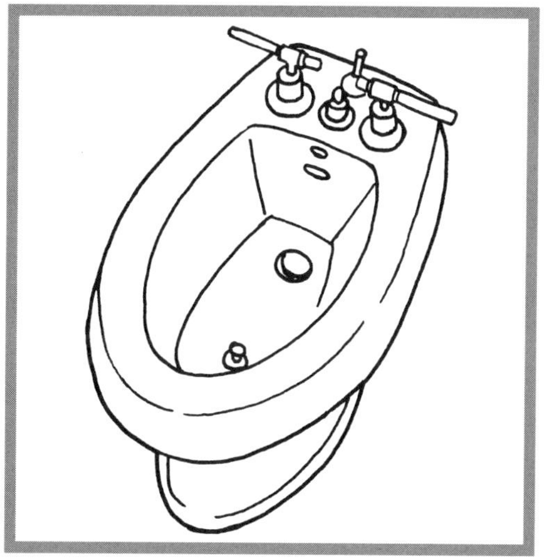

Bidet
Floor mounted
Plumbed

32

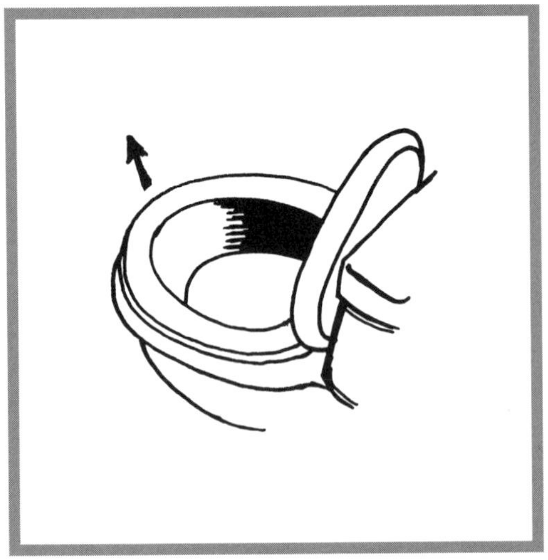

Bidet basin
Basin on toilet rim

33

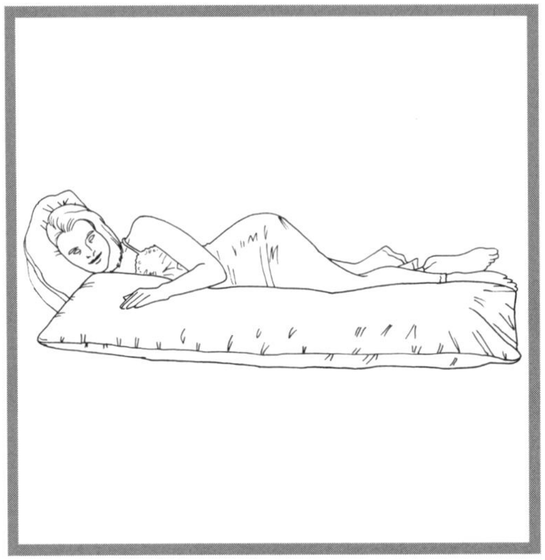

Body pillow
Body length support
Polyester fill

34

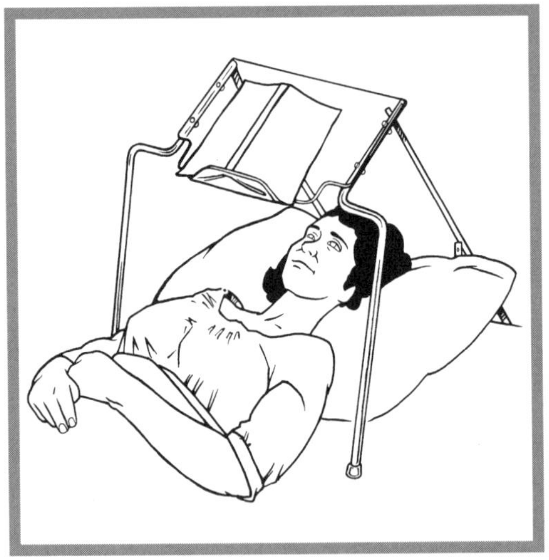

Book holder
Overhead easel
Adjustable
angle/height

35

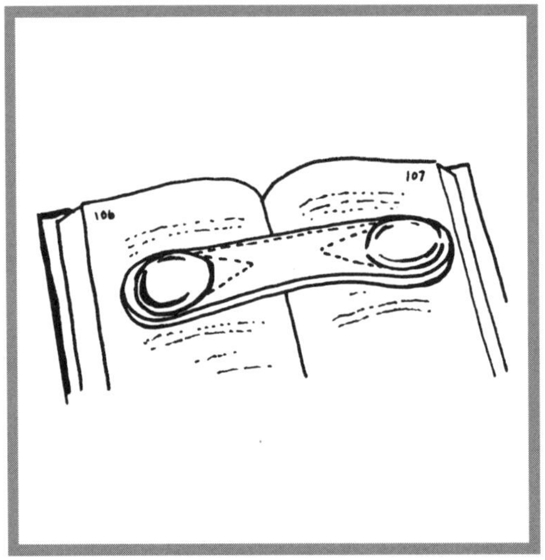

Bookmark
Holds book open
Leather strip

36

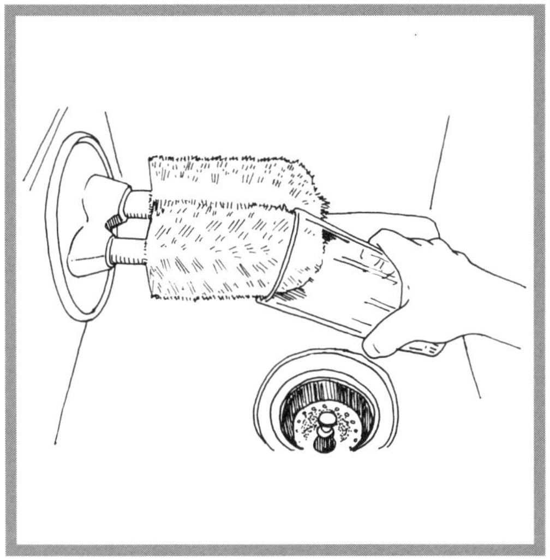

Bottle brush
Double nylon brush
Suction base
6 inch diameter base

37

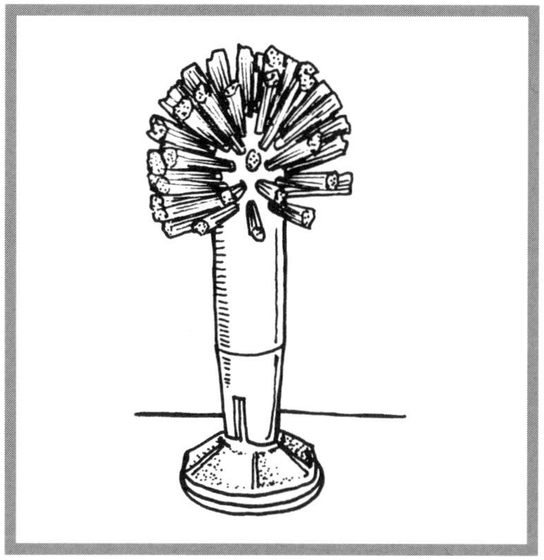

Bottle brush
Nylon brush
Suction base

38

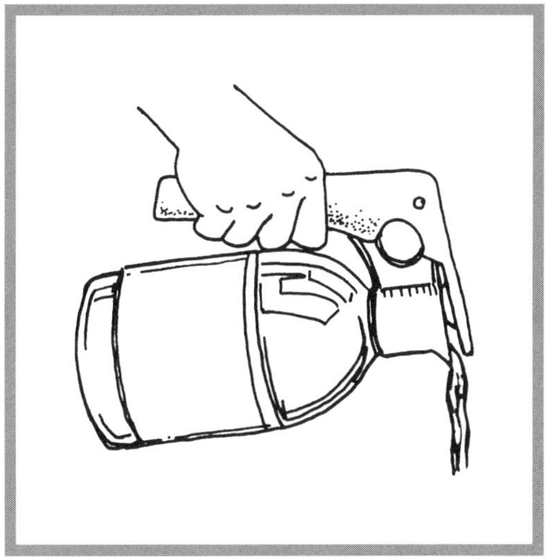

Bottle handle
For 1 or 2 liter bottle
Replaces screw top
Lever opens lid

39

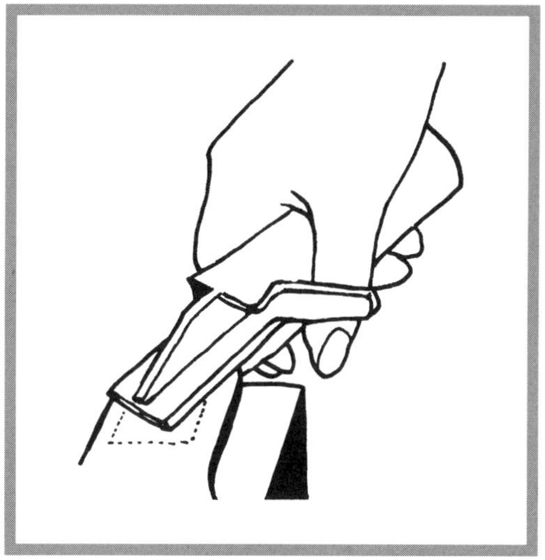

Box top opener
Hand held
Push/turn/lift required
Built-up handle

40

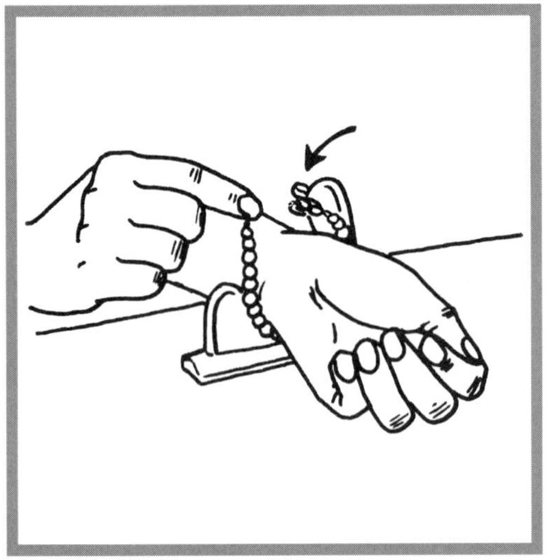

41

Bracelet fastener
One-hand operated
Clips hold bracelet

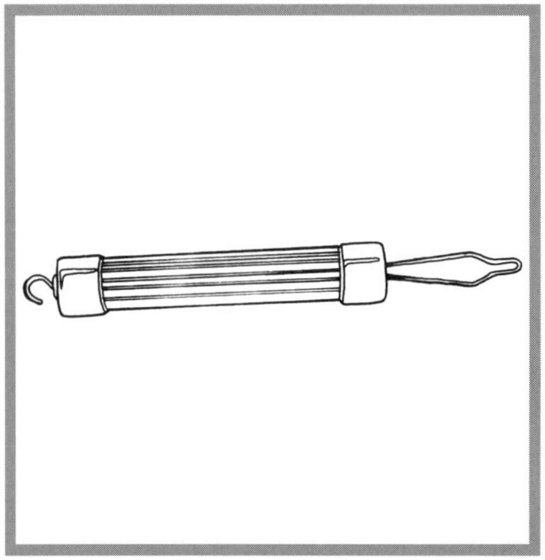

42

Button & zipper aid
Built-up handle
Grooved cylinder handle
Metal loop & zipper hook

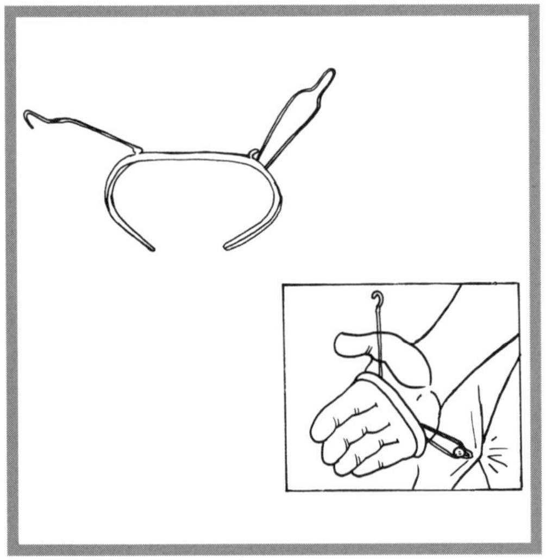

43

Button & zipper aid
Palm clip handle
C-shaped clip
Metal loop & zipper hook

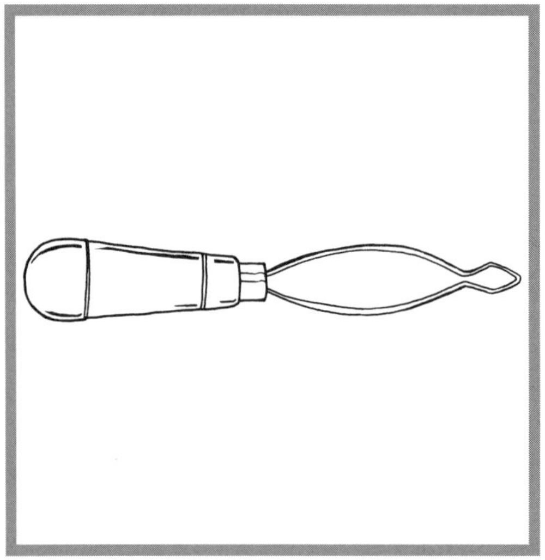

44

Button hook
Knob handle
Wood handle
Metal button loop

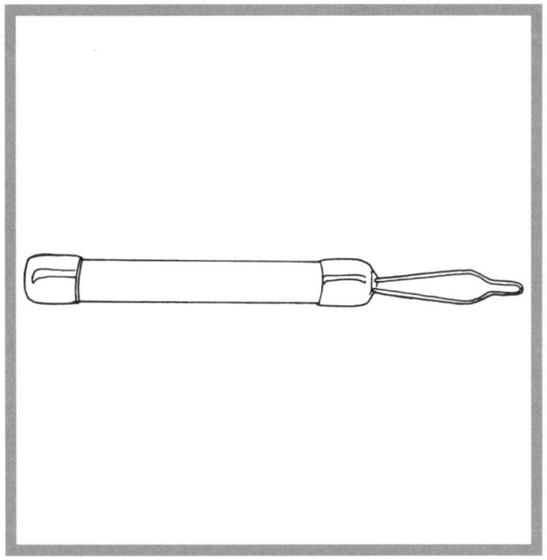

Button hook
Straight handle
Wood handle
Metal button loop

45

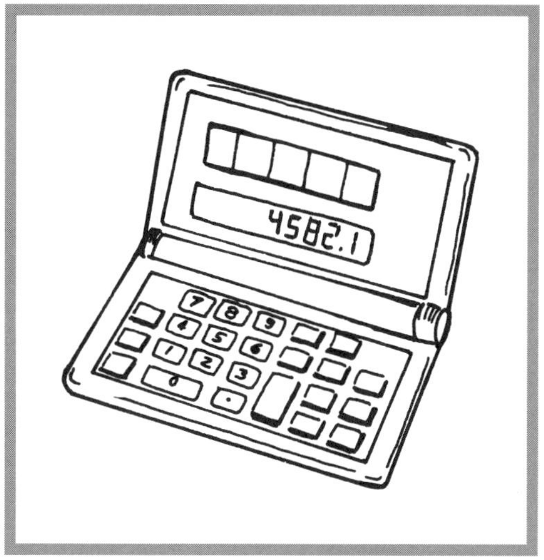

Calculator
Large keys & display
Adjustable display angle
Solar/battery operated

46

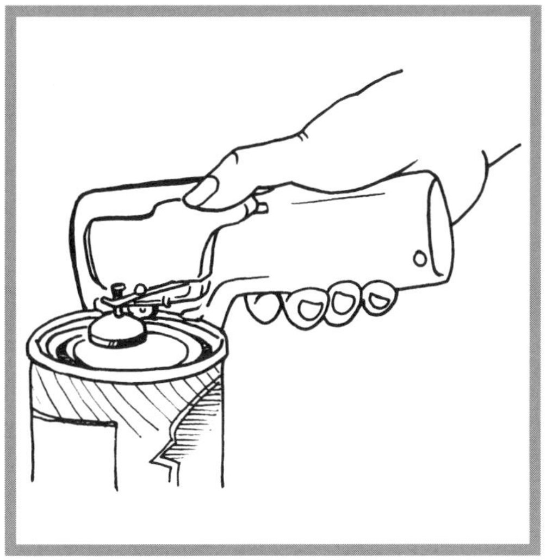

Can opener
One-hand operated/hand held
Right hand thumb press lever
Cordless rechargeable

47

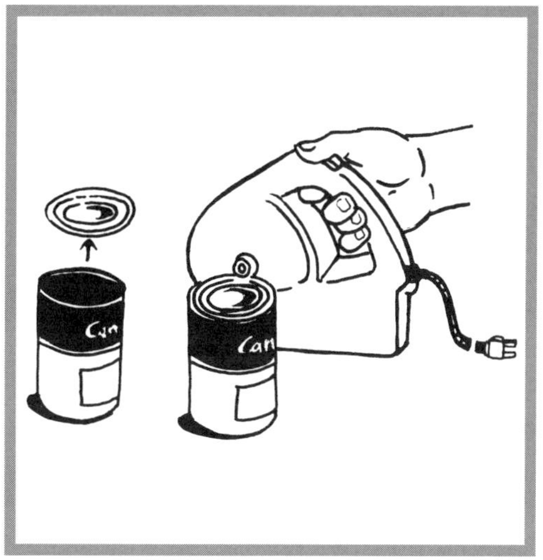

Can opener
One-hand operated/hand held
Uncrimps rim
AC powered

48

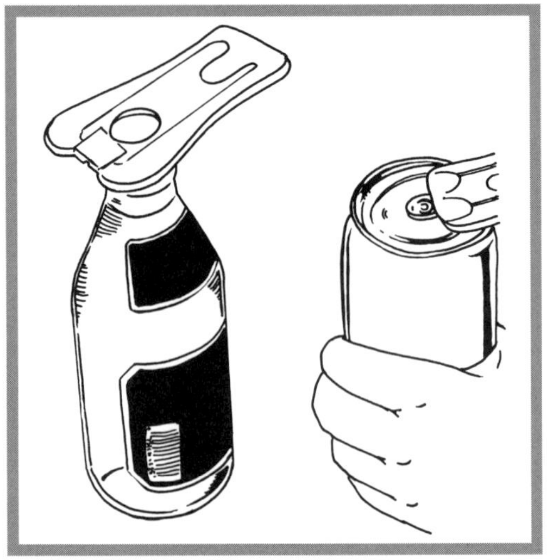

Can tab & twist-cap opener
Two hands needed to operate
For pop/soda bottles and cans

49

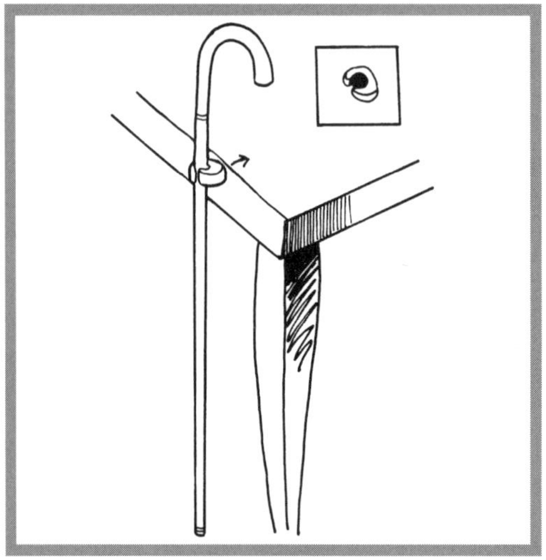

Cane holder
Adjustable clip-on
Hooks cane on table edge

50

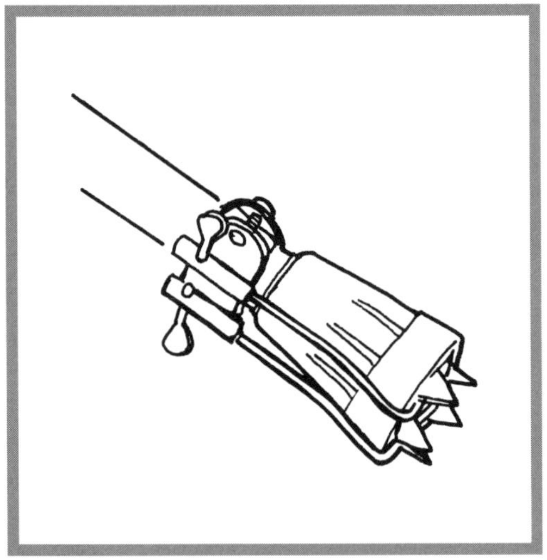

Cane ice tip
4-point
Retractable
Over cane tip

51

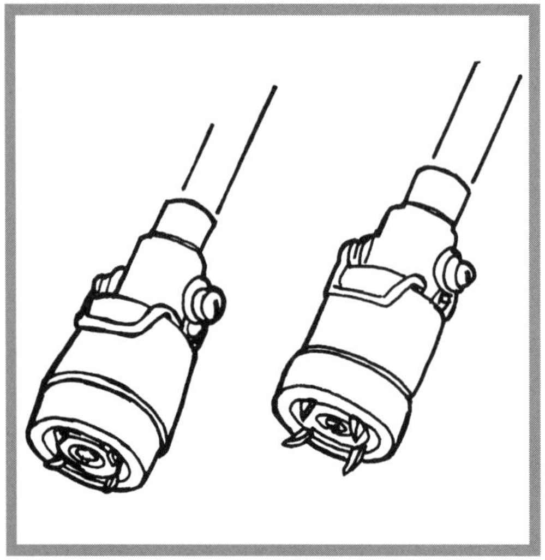

Cane ice tip
4-point
Retractable with wire handle
Replaces cane tip

52

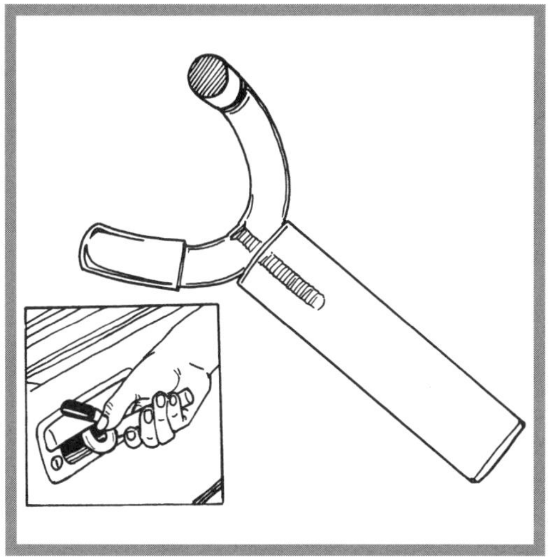

Car door opener
Hand held
For button or pull
Y-shaped

53

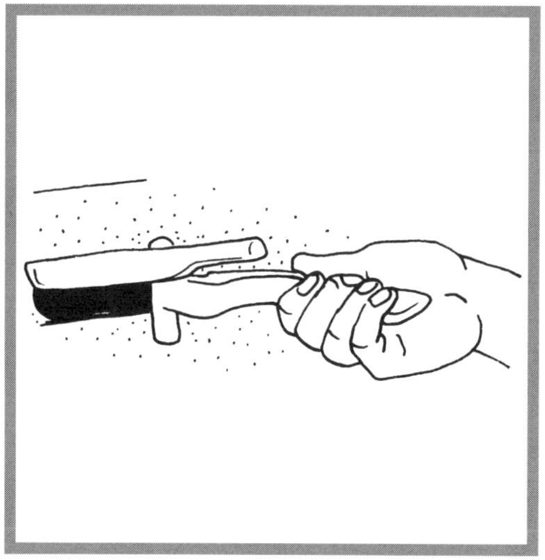

Car door opener
Hand held
For pull-up handle

54

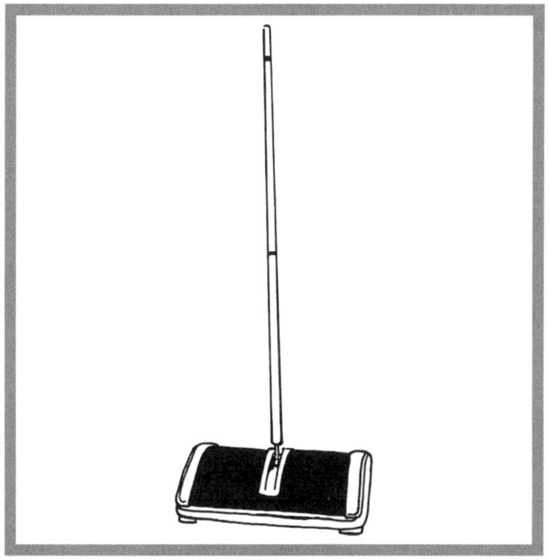

Carpet sweeper
Manual
180 degree arc handle

55

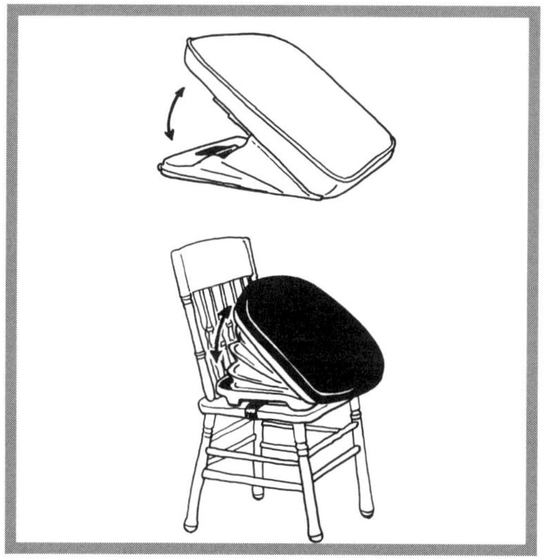

Chair rising aid
Spring loaded seat
Padded

56

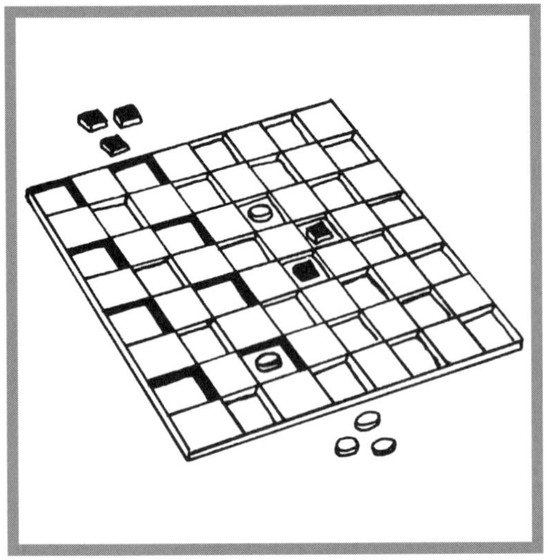

57

Checker set
Tactile & visual
Raised/recessed squares
Red and black checkers

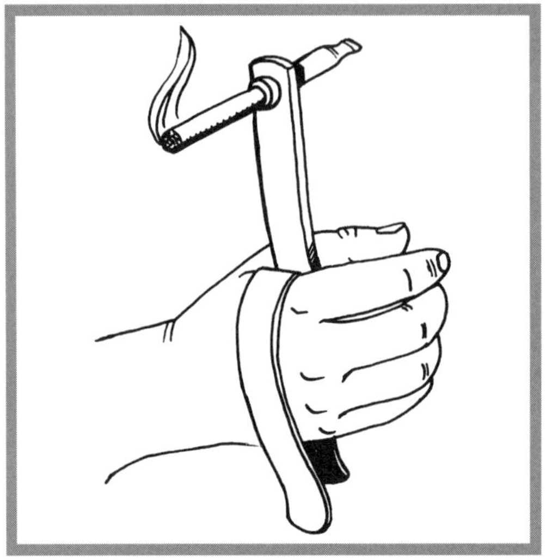

58

Cigarette holder
Adjustable palm clip
Cigarette held by clip

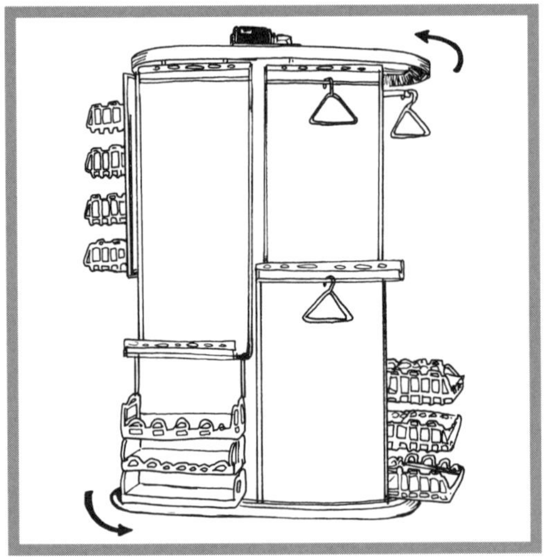

59

Closet carousel
Wire rack system
Motorized rotating

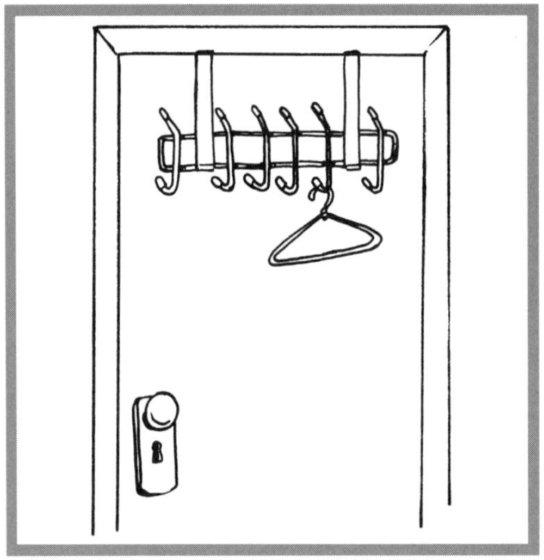

60

Clothes hook rack
Six clothes hooks
Hangs over door

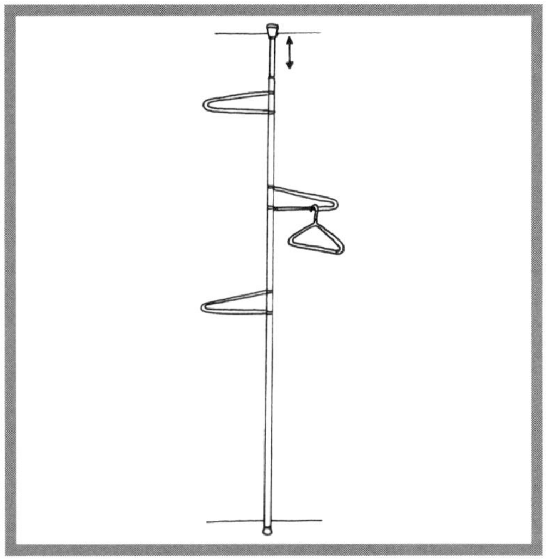

Clothes rod
Three loop type rods
On tension pole
Portable

61

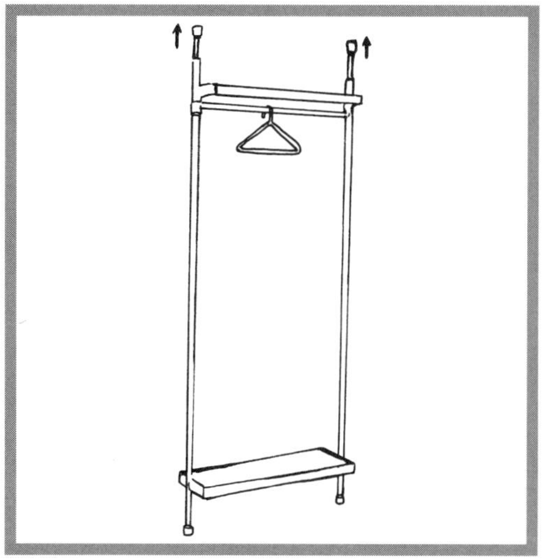

Clothes rod
With shoe shelf
On two tension poles
Portable

62

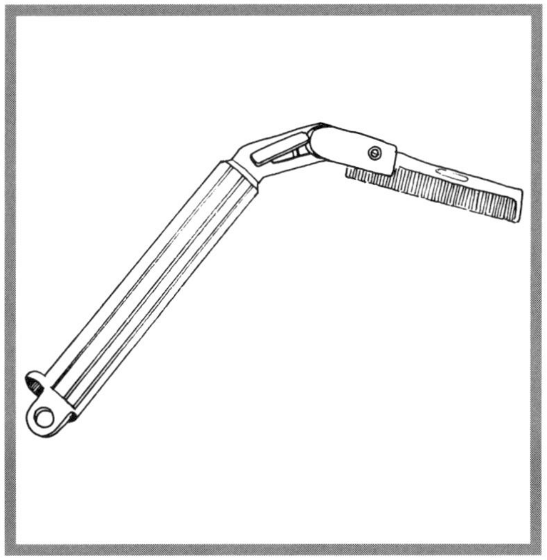

Comb
19 inch handle
Adjustable angle

63

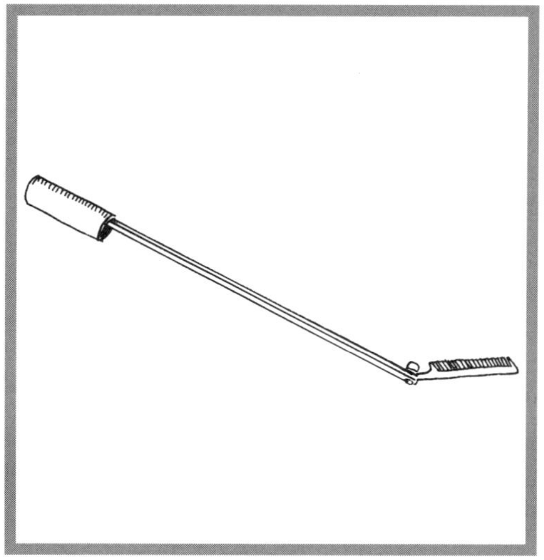

Comb
Long handle
Adjustable angle
Built up handle grip

64

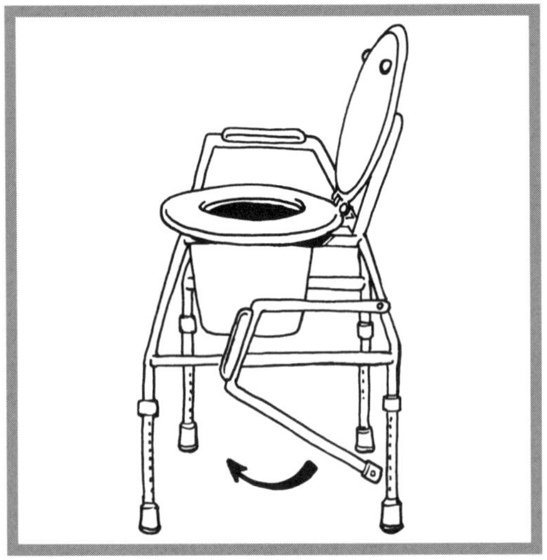

Commode
Adjustable height
Backless with drop arms

65

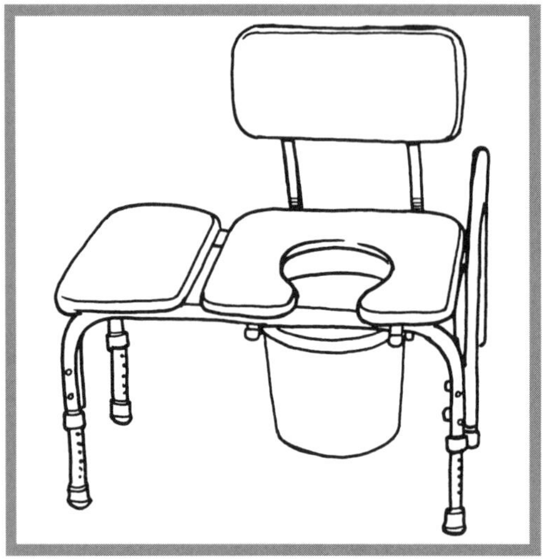

Commode
Adjustable height
With back and arms
With transfer seat on right

66

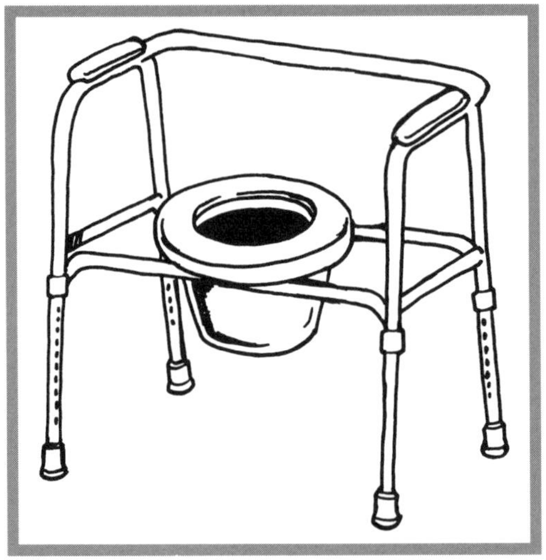

Commode
Adjustable height
With side rails & rail back
No lid

67

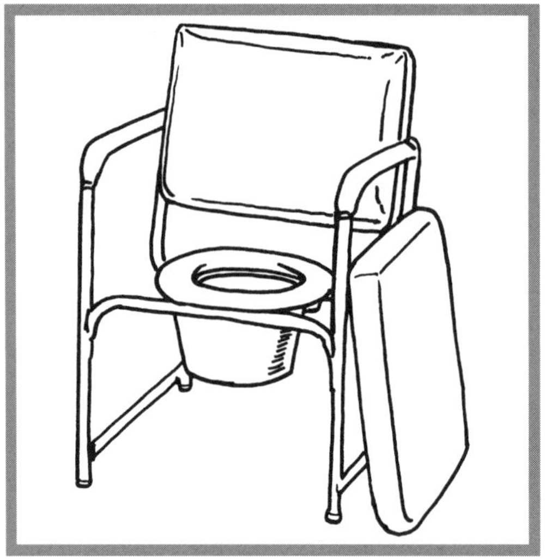

Commode
Fixed height
With back and arms
Chair look-alike

68

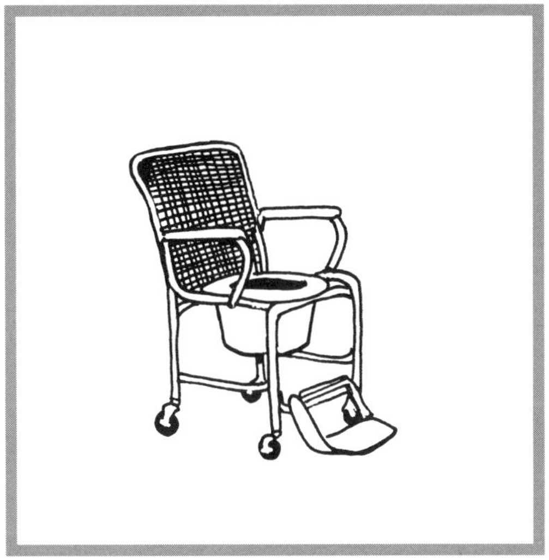

69

Commode
Fixed height
With back and arms

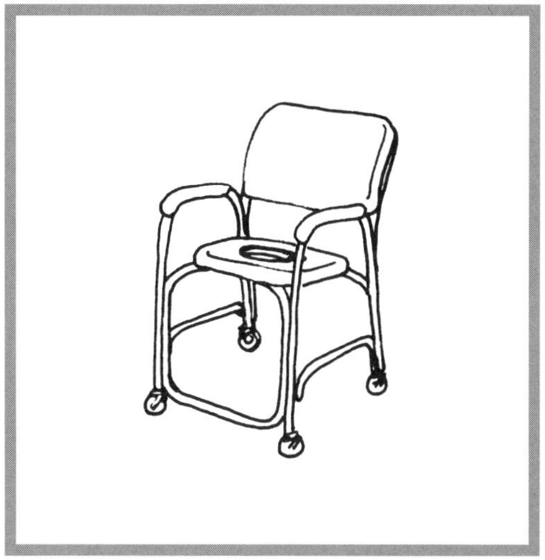

70

Commode
Fixed height
With back and arms
Rolling

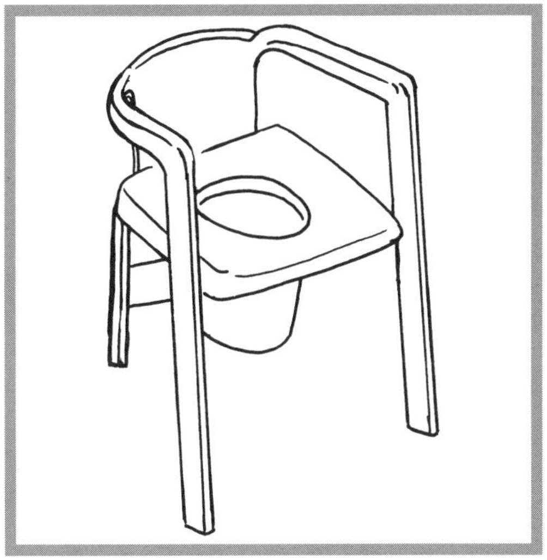

71

Commode/bath chair
Fixed height
Back and arms
Lightweight plastic resin

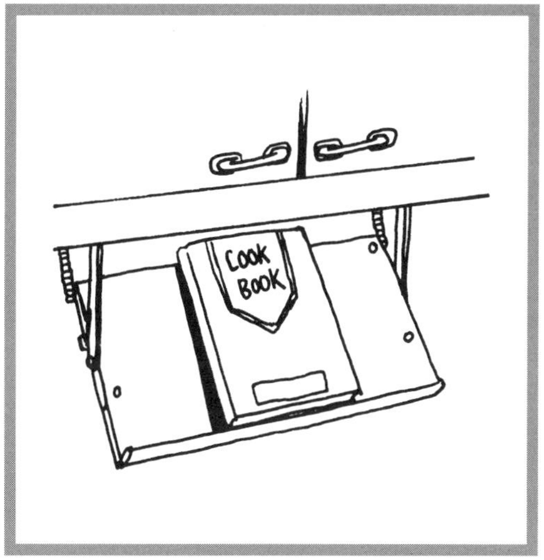

72

Cookbook rack
Under-cabinet mount
Spring hinge mount

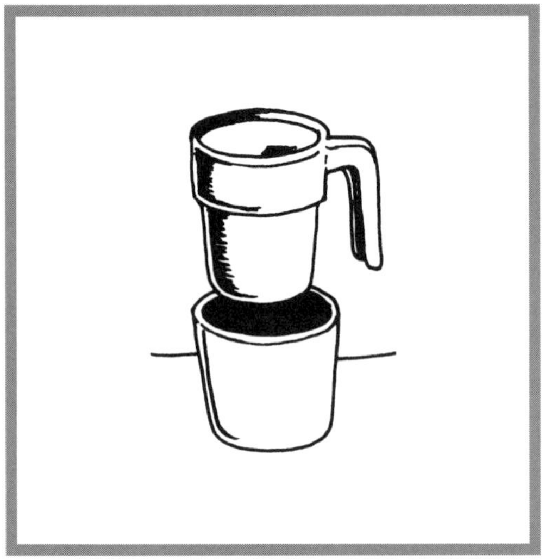

73

Cup holder/handle
Attaches to table
Cup has hook handle
Non-spill lid

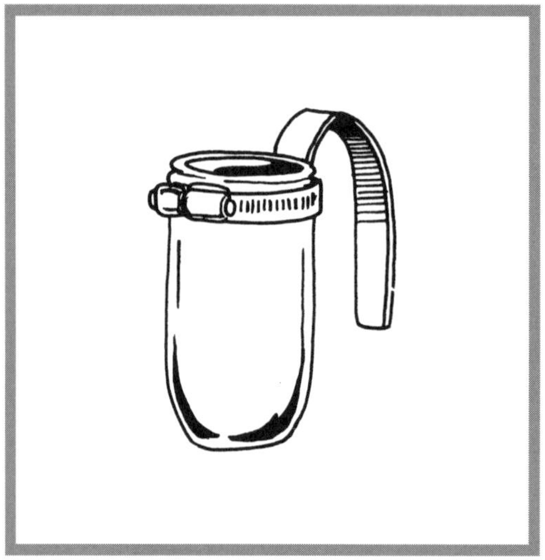

74

Cup holder/handle
Hook handle
Adjustable diameter

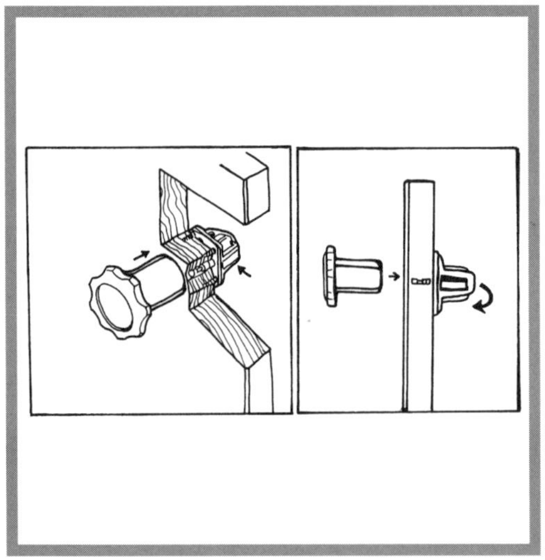

75

Cupboard lock
Magnetic key release

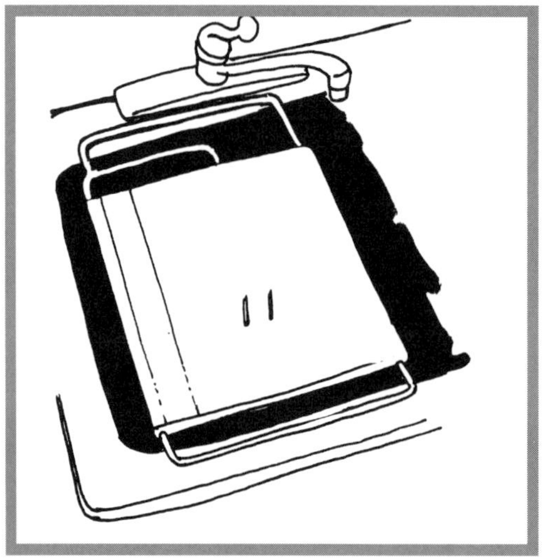

76

Cutting board
With spikes
For over-sink
Flat top

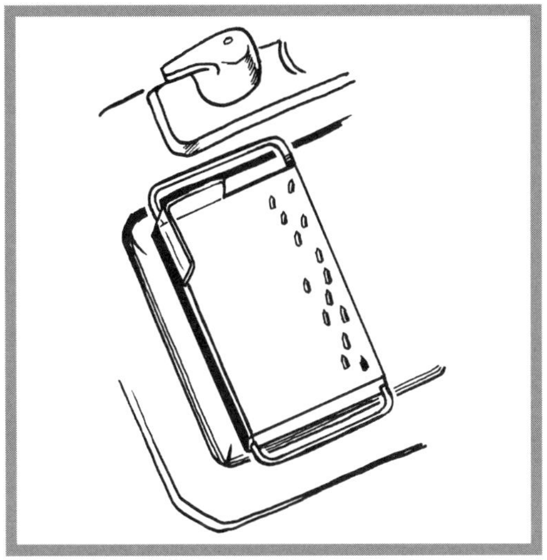

77

Cutting board
With spikes & corner guard
For over-sink
Flat top

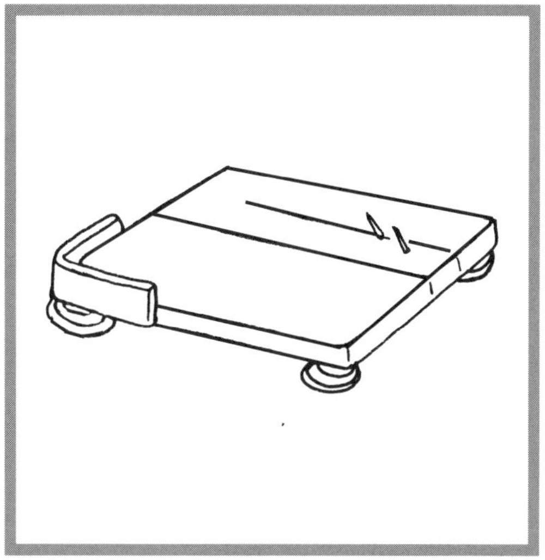

78

Cutting board
With spikes & corner guard
Suction cup base
Flat polyethylene

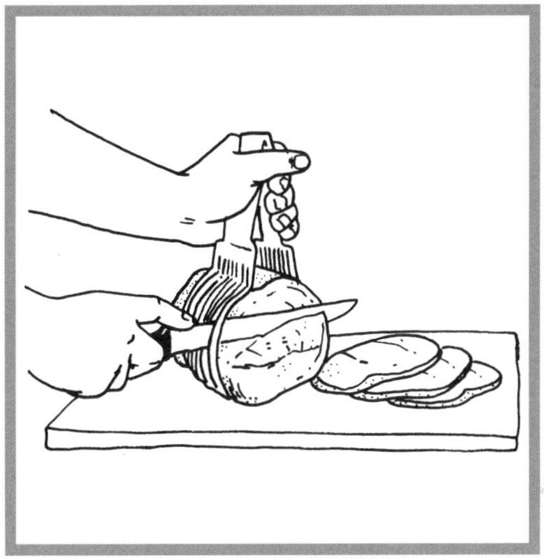

79

Cutting frame
Two hands needed to operate
Gripping jaws/squeeze handles
Steel

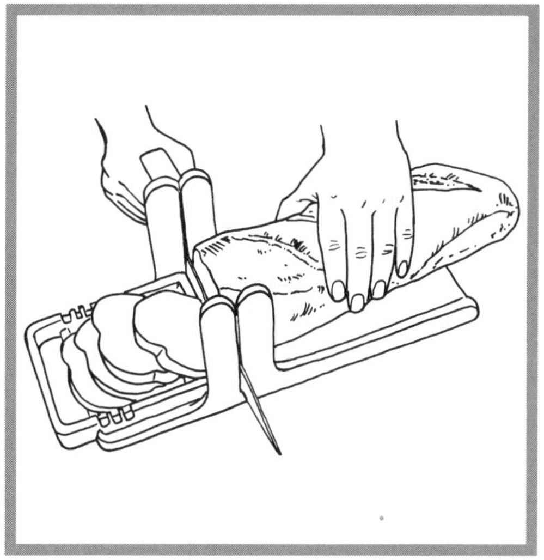

80

Cutting frame/knife
Base with adjustable width
With serrated knife

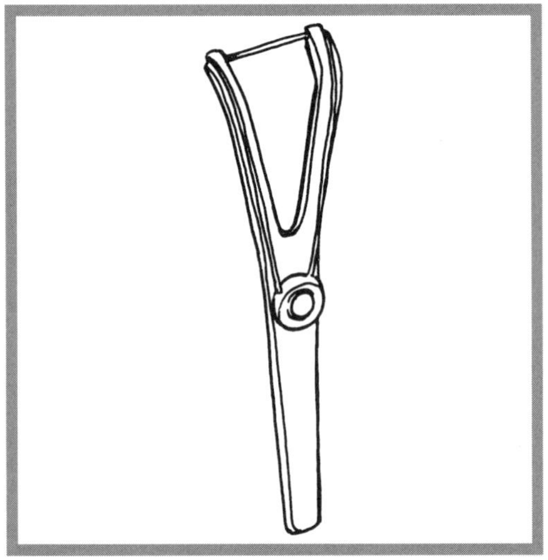

Dental flosser
Hand held
Fork shape
Plastic

81

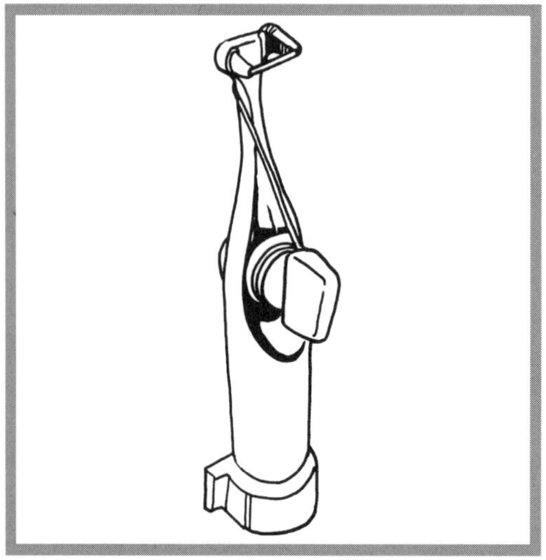

Dental flosser
Stand mounted
With floss spool

82

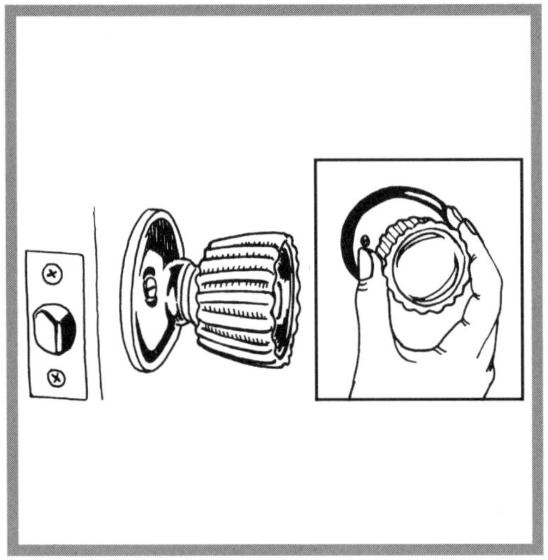

Door knob gripper
Textured grip
Stretches over knob

83

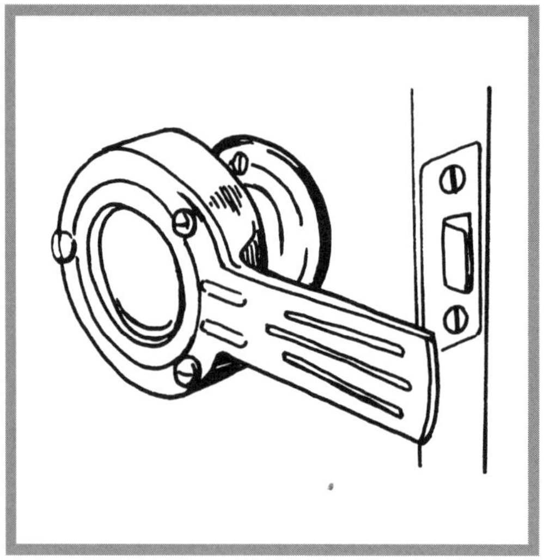

Door knob lever
3 inch lever
Screw fastened
2-1/2 inch diameter knob

84

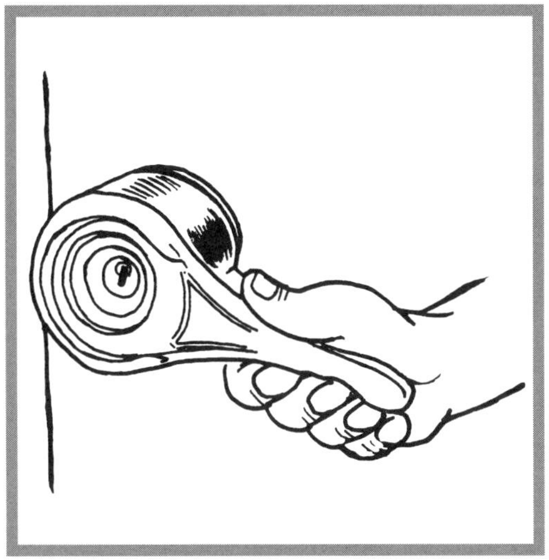

85

Door knob lever
4 inch lever
Grips with gaskets
Fits various knobs

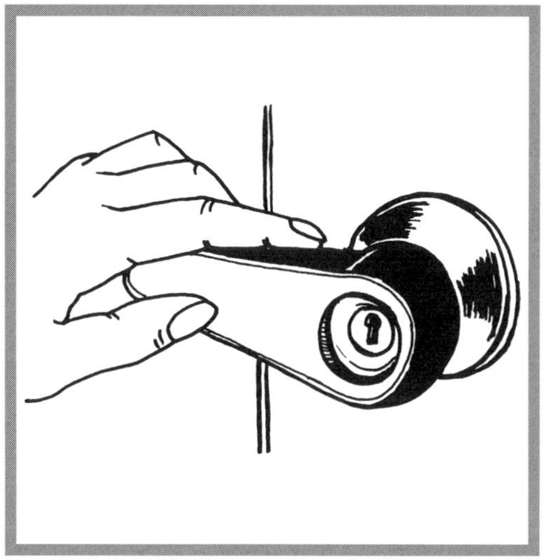

86

Door knob lever
4-1/2 inch lever
Soft rubber slip-on
Fits standard knobs

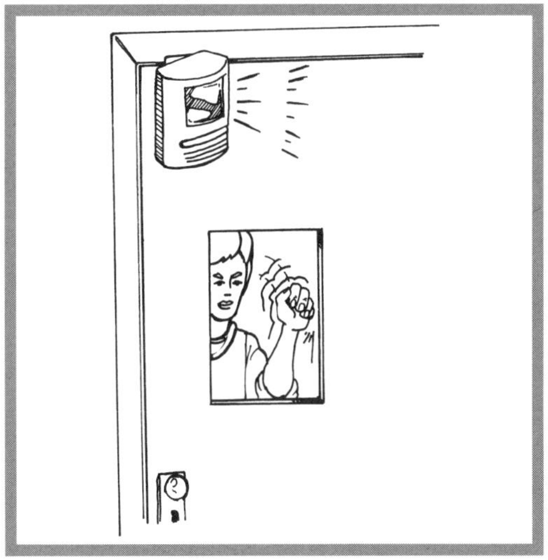

87

Door knock sensor
Knock activated
Flashing light signal

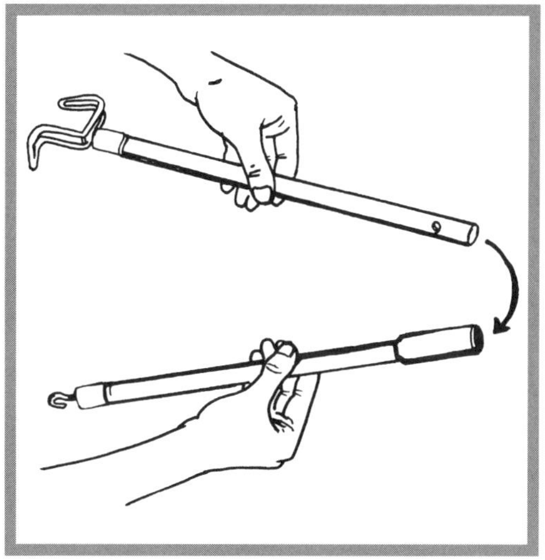

88

Dressing stick
Push-pull hooks
24 inches
Folding

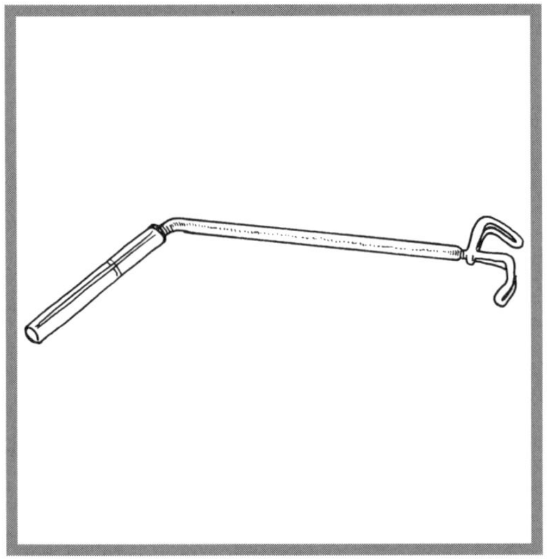

89

Dressing stick
Push-pull hooks
24 inches

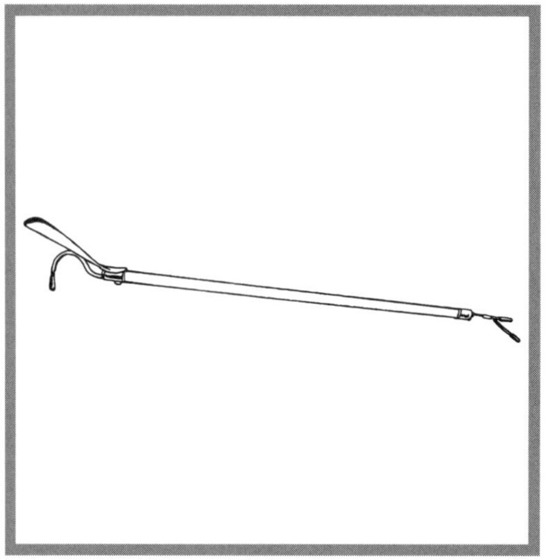

90

Dressing stick
Push-pull hooks
30 inches
With shoehorn end

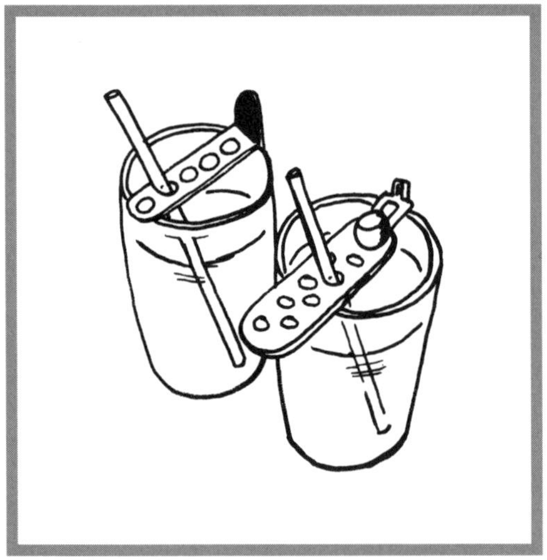

91

Drinking straw holder
Spring clip
For 4 straw sizes
Metal

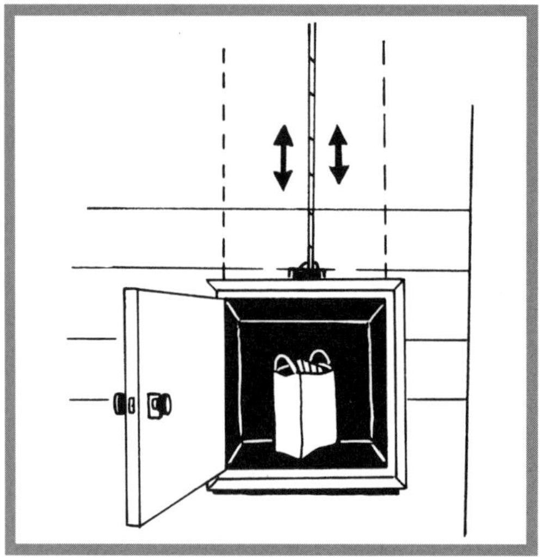

92

Dumbwaiter
Built-in
Various sizes
Swing door

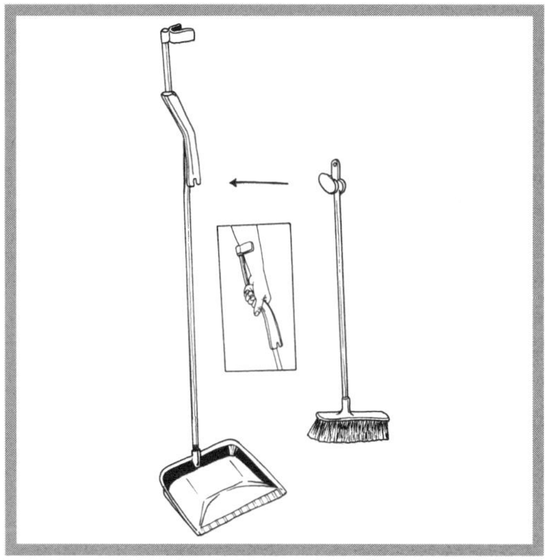

Dustpan/brush set
No-stooping type
33 inch handles
Dustpan with wrist support

93

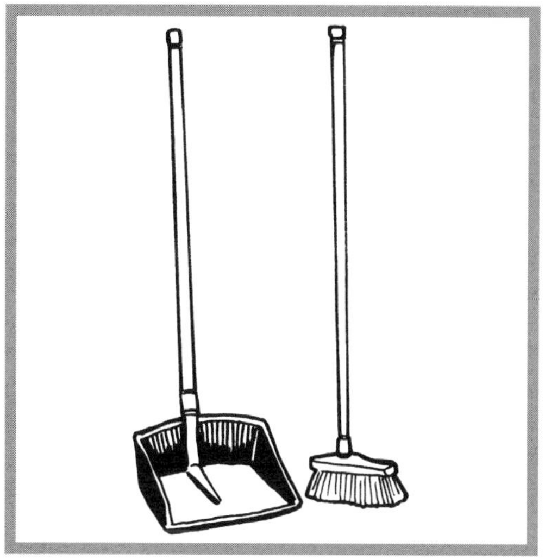

Dustpan/brush set
No-stooping type
36 inch handles

94

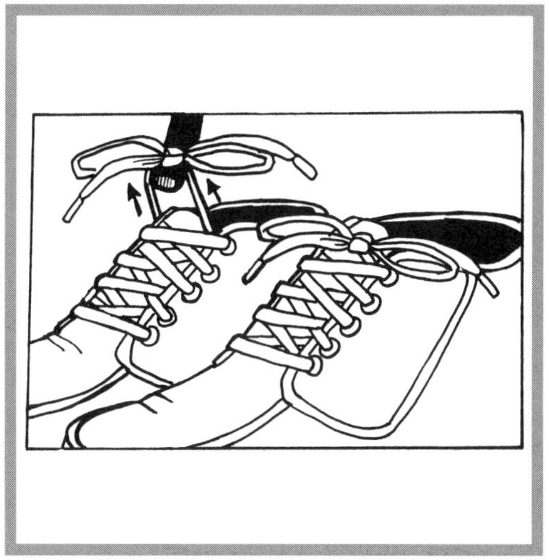

Elastic shoe lace
One-hand operated
No fastener

95

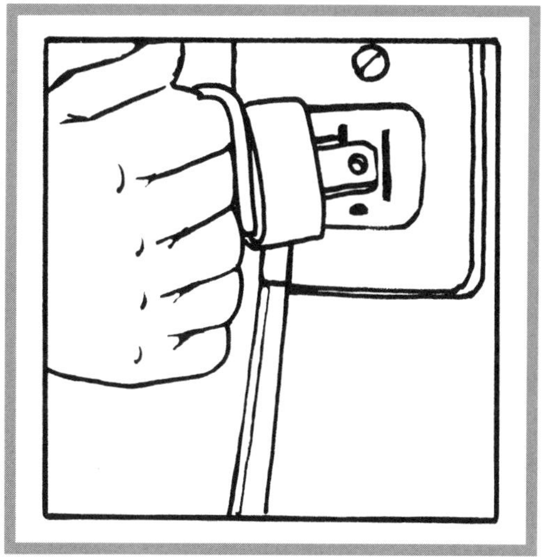

Electric extension cord

Loop handle on plug
Plug built into cord

96

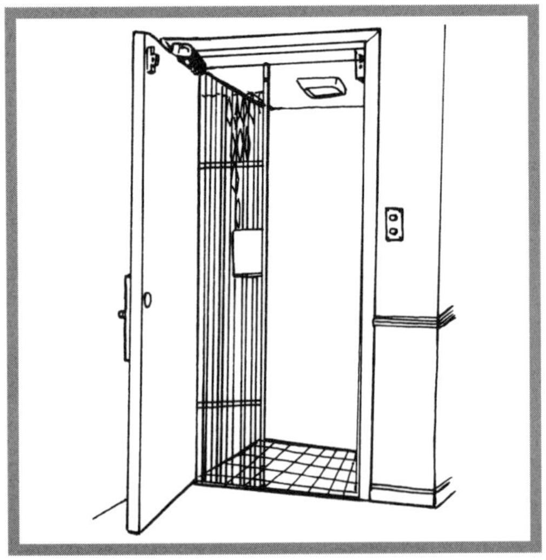

97

Elevator
For wheelchair
Cable mount in-closet

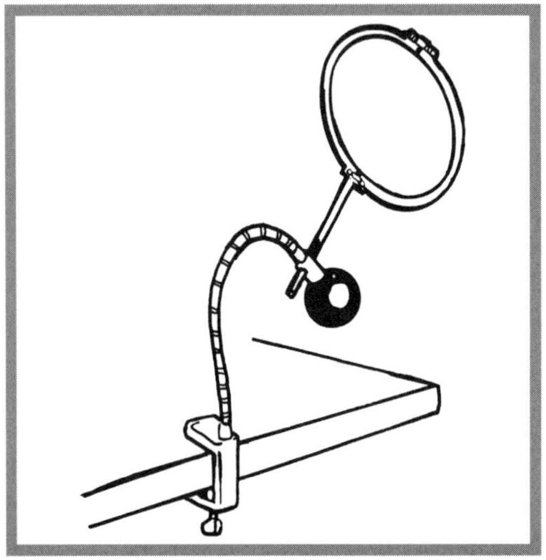

98

Embroidery hoop
One-hand operated
Gooseneck
Clamps to table edge

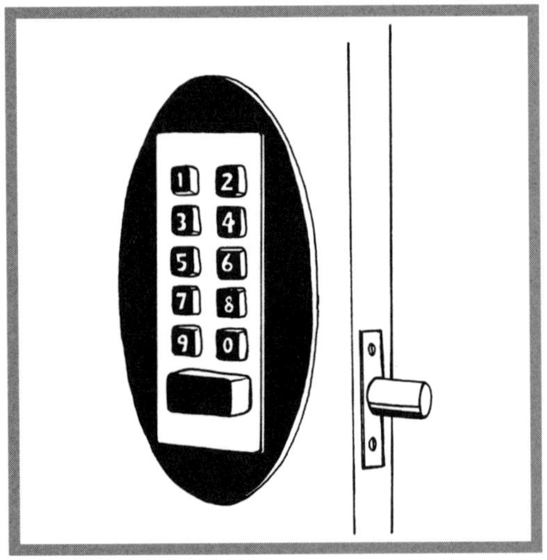

99

Entry system
Keyless
Coded access

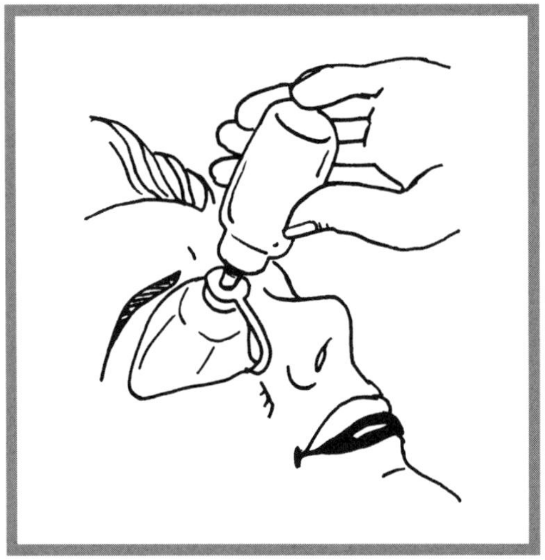

100

Eye drop dispenser
Bottle is squeezed

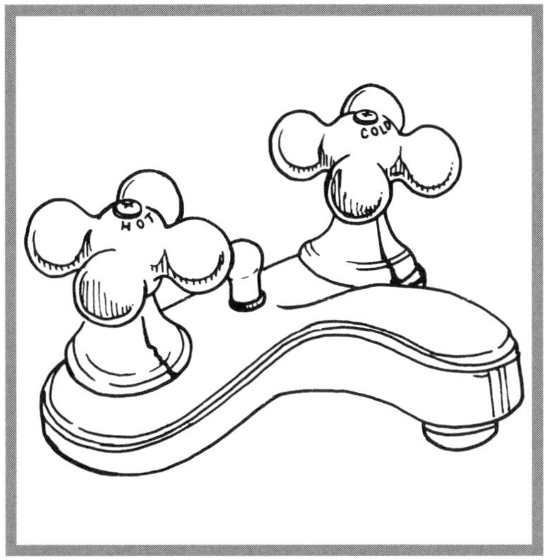

101

Faucet
Crossbar handles
Mixer spout

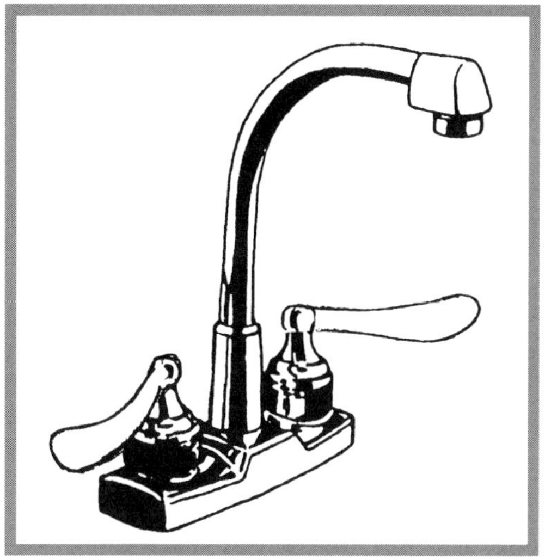

102

Faucet
Lever handles
Mixer spout

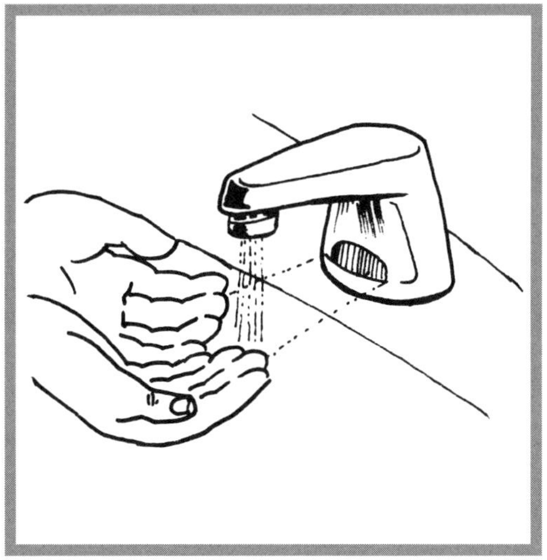

103

Faucet
Motion sensor valve

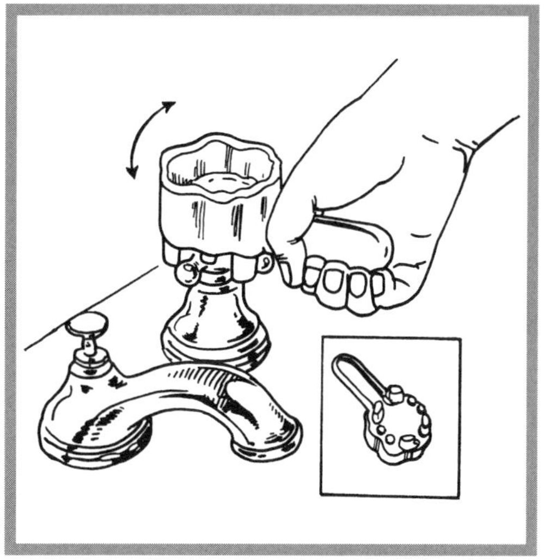

104

Faucet turner
Clamps onto knob faucet grip
Wrench handle

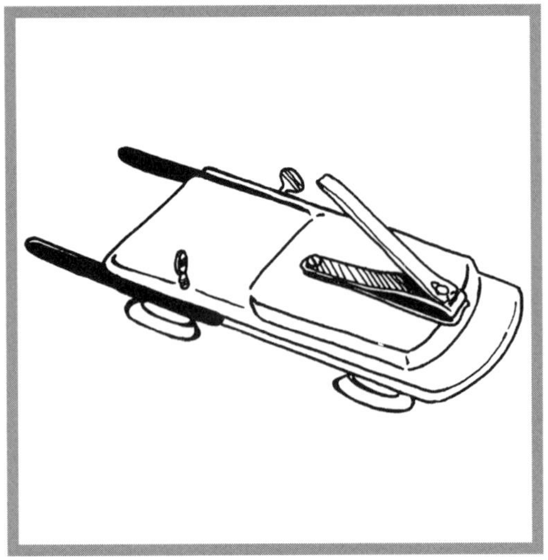

Fingernail clipper
Mounted on base
Large lever operated
With emery board holder

105

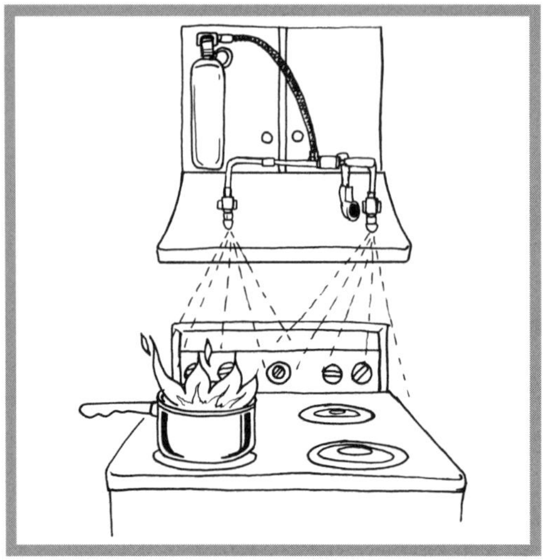

Fire extinguisher
In-range hood
Automatic
Heat sensitive

106

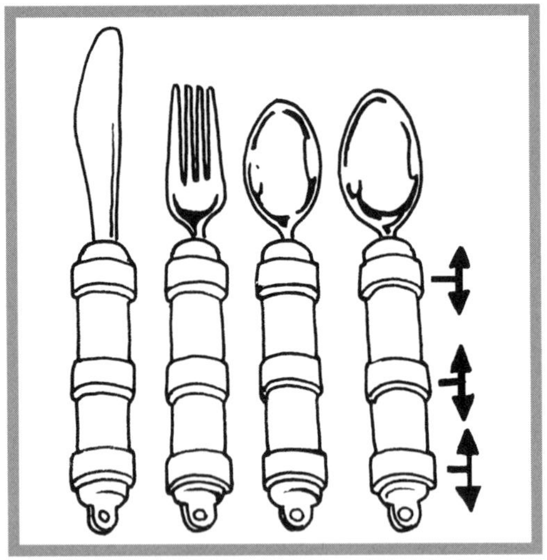

Flatware
Built-up handles
Adjustable finger rings

107

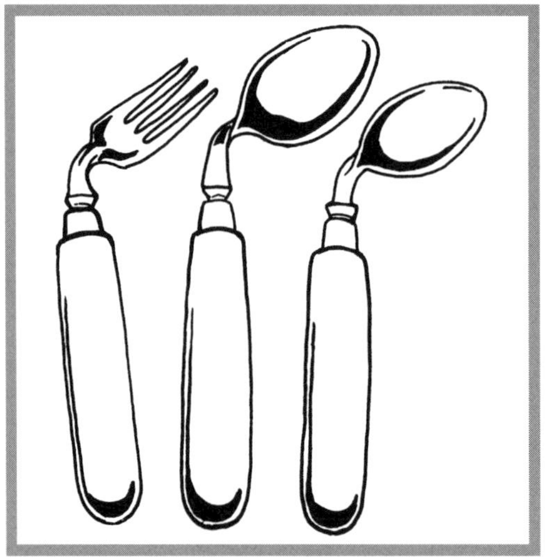

Flatware
Built-up handles
Angled for Left hand use

108

Flatware
Built-up handles
Angled for Right hand use

109

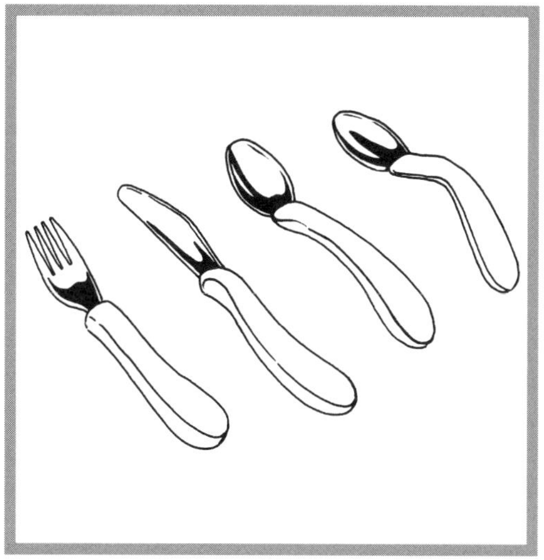

Flatware
Built-up handles
Curved for arthritis
Polypropylene handles

110

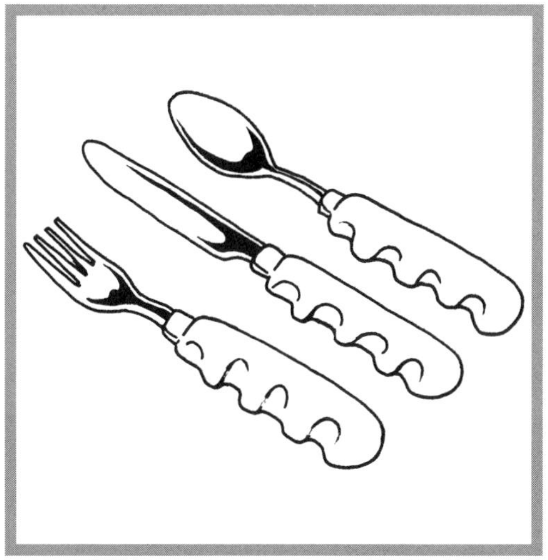

Flatware
Built-up handles
Indented for Right hand use

111

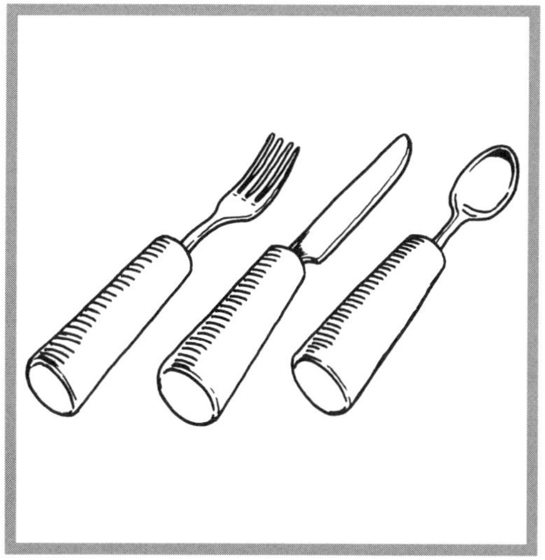

Flatware
Coated tube handles
Standard heads
1 inch diameter

112

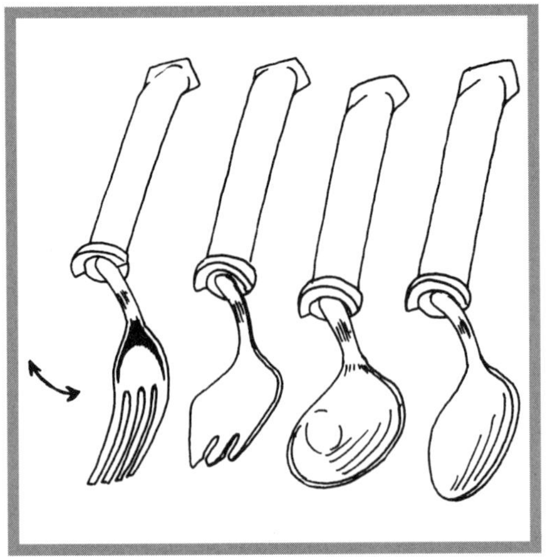

Flatware
Drop head handles
Swivel heads
adjustable stops

113

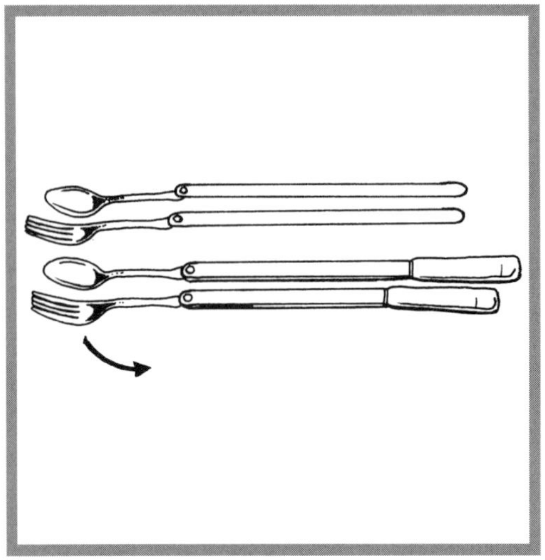

Flatware
Extension handles
Adjustable angles

114

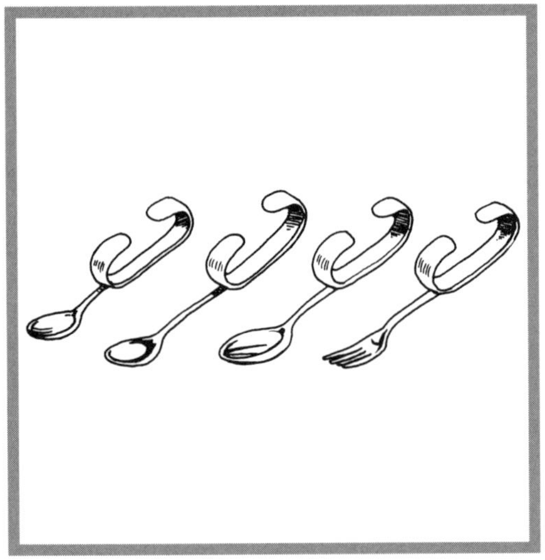

Flatware
On horizontal palm clips
Standard heads
Adjustable coated clips

115

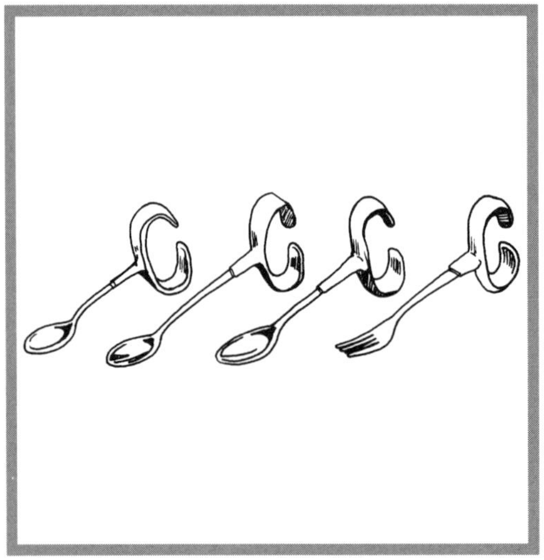

Flatware
On vertical palm clips
Standard heads
Adjustable coated clips

116

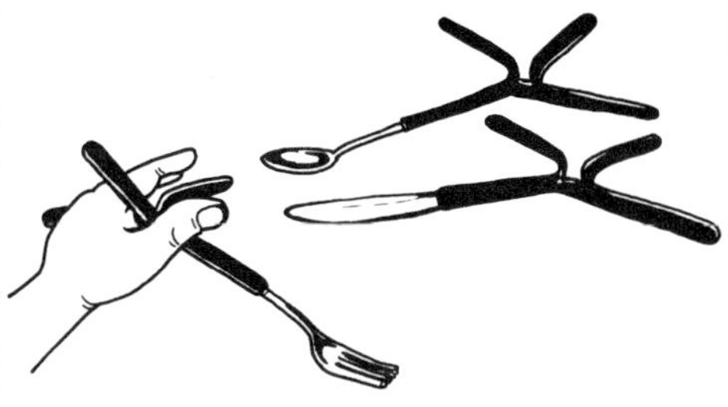

Flatware
With thumb/forefinger grips
Adjustable grips
Plastic coated grips

117

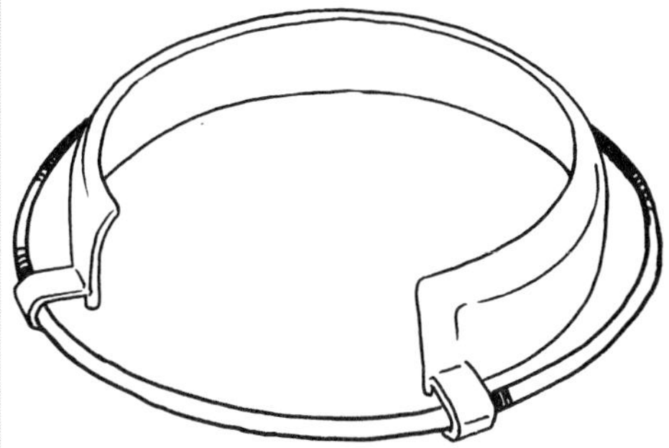

Food guard for plate
Clips inside plate
6 to 8 inch plate

118

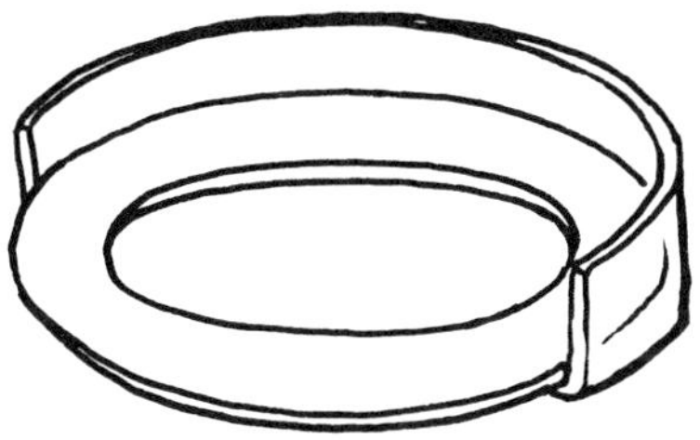

Food guard for plate
Snaps around rim
6 to 8 inch plate
Clear plastic

119

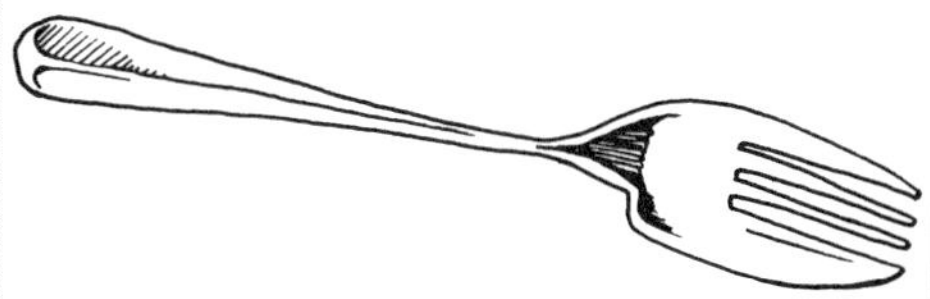

Fork
Side cutter
For Left hand use
Semi-sharp edge right tine

120

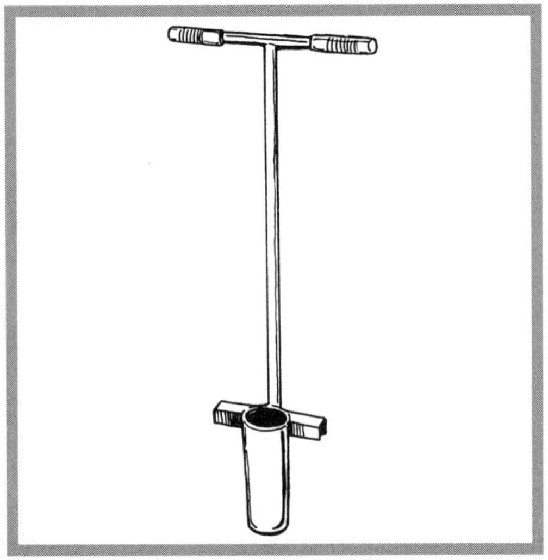

121

Garden bulb planter
T-handle
34 inches long
With foot treads

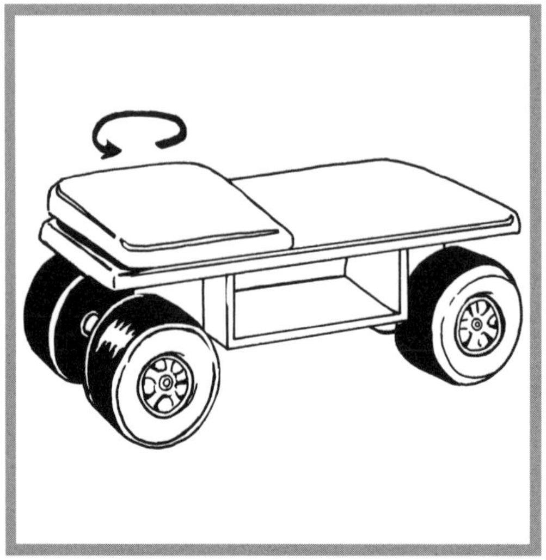

122

Garden workseat
Wide tires
Seat 10 inches high
With storage trays

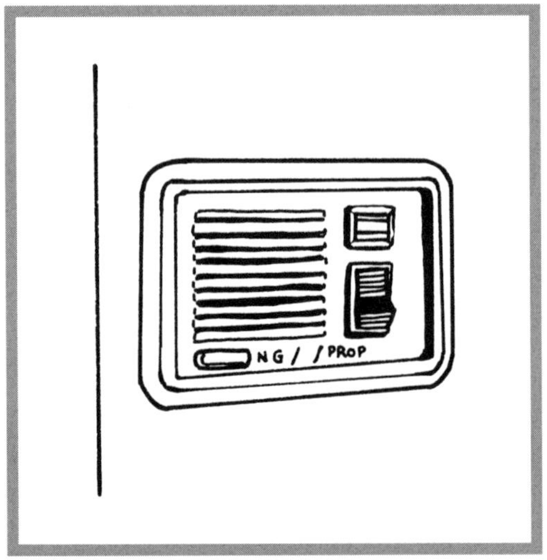

123

Gas detector alarm
Natural gas and
propane
85 decibel sound
AC powered

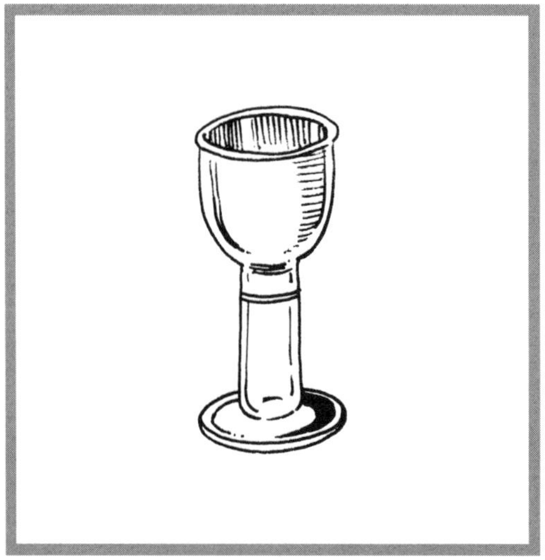

124

Goblet
Tall wide stem grip
Break resistant

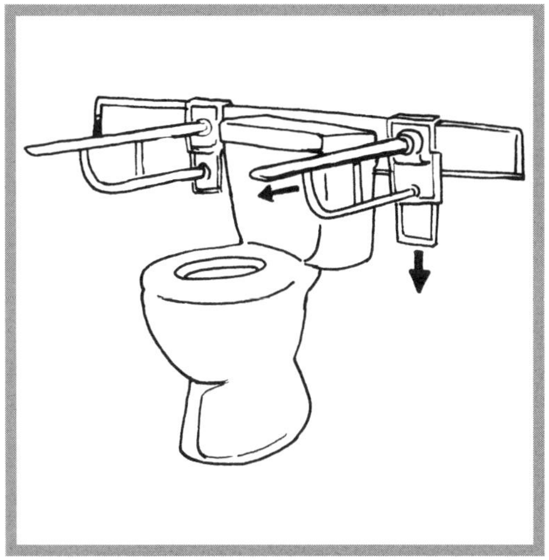

Grab bar
Hinged wall mounted
Horizontal loop bar
Adjustable horizontal/vertical

125

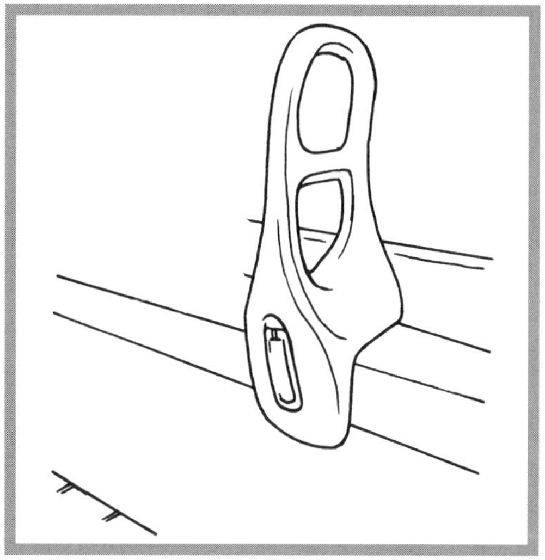

Grab bar
Tub edge cam clamp
Bi-level
Flowing molded shape

126

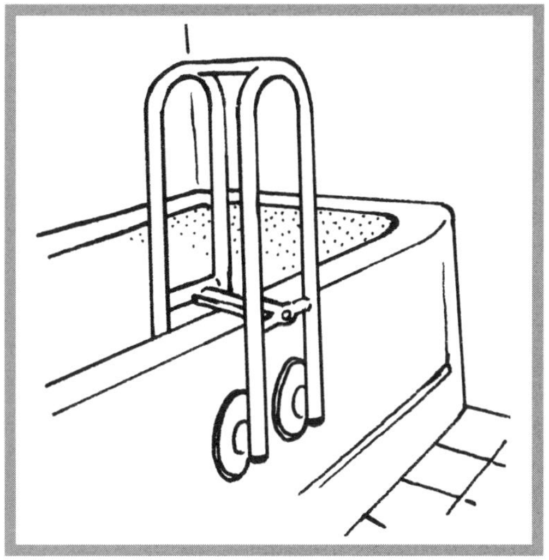

Grab bar
Tub edge screw clamp
Bi-level loop with crossbar

127

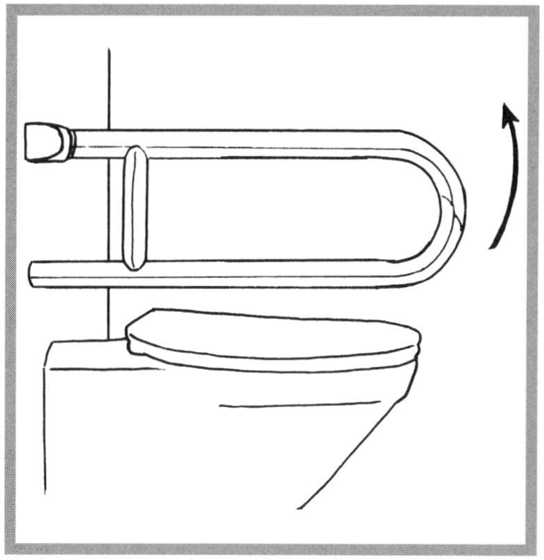

Grab bar
Wall
Single loop grip
Folds upward against wall

128

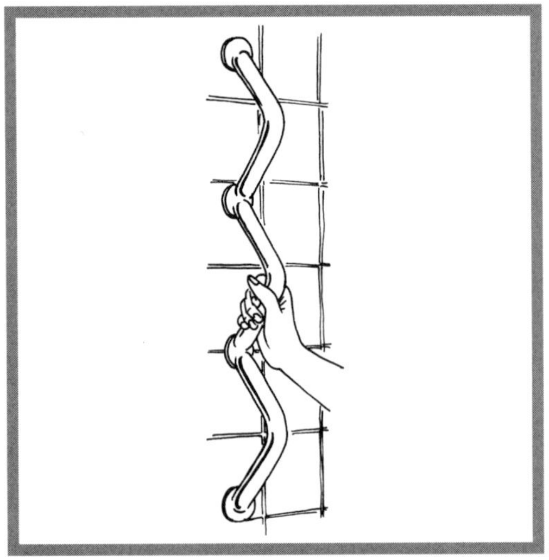

Grab bar
Wall
Tri loop grip

129

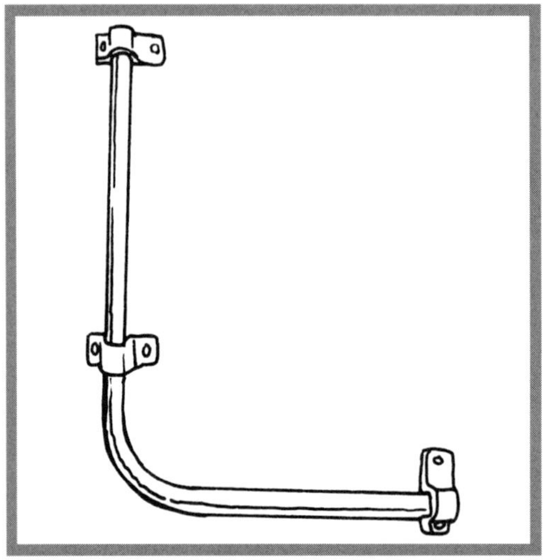

Grab bar
Wall
Two arms 90 degree angle right

130

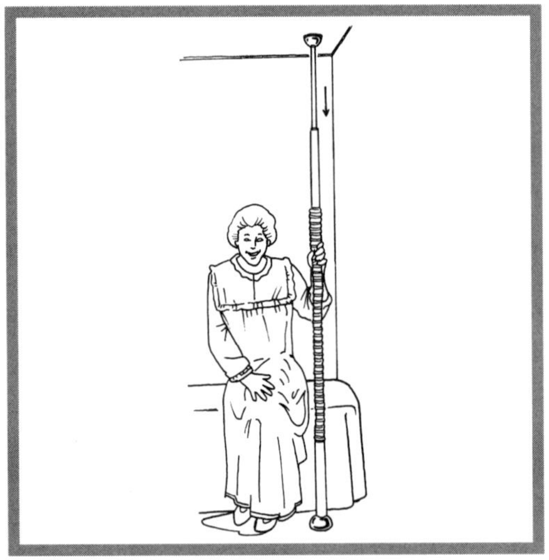

Grab pole
Vertical
Tension mount floor to ceiling

131

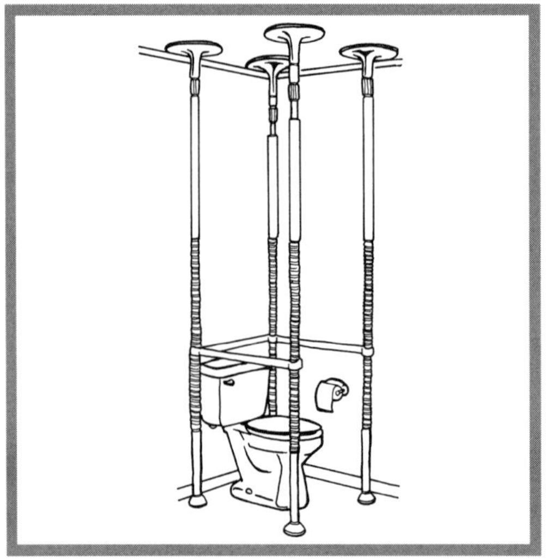

Grab pole system
Vertical poles
Tension mount floor to ceiling
A set with connectors

132

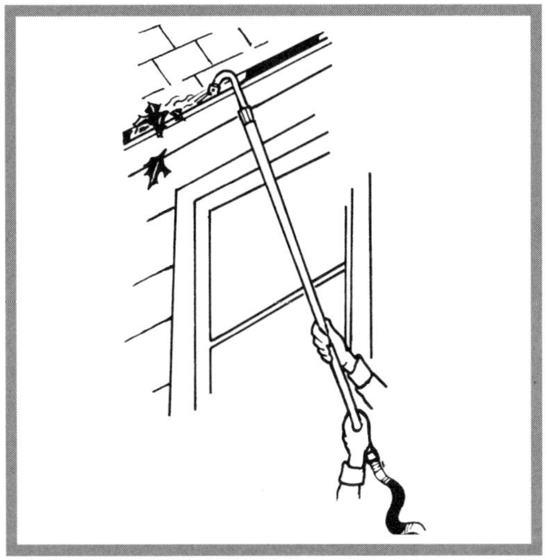

Gutter cleaner
Garden hose powered
Telescoping handle

133

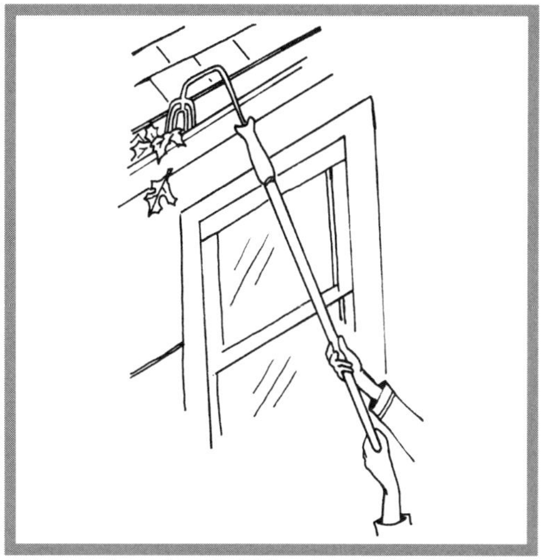

Gutter rake
Curved fork
Extendible handle

134

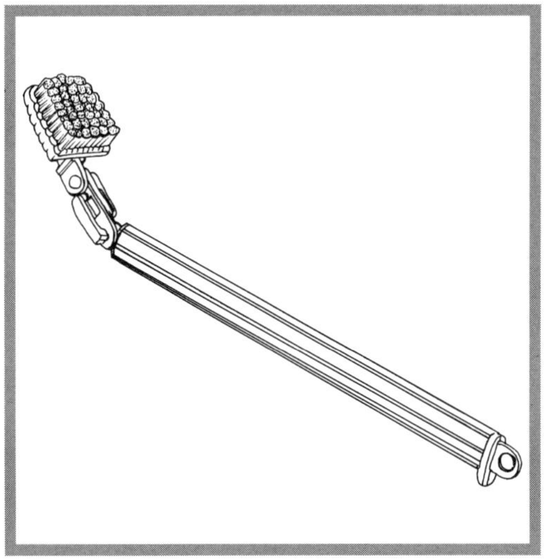

Hair brush
16 inch built-up handle
Adjustable angle

135

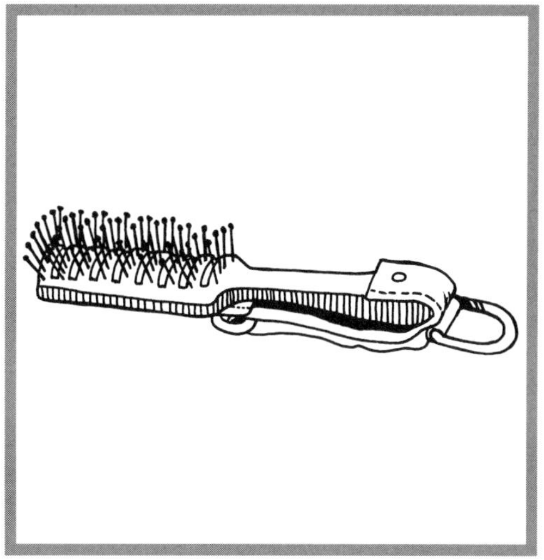

Hair brush
Velcro hand strap
D-ring closure
Stiff bristles

136

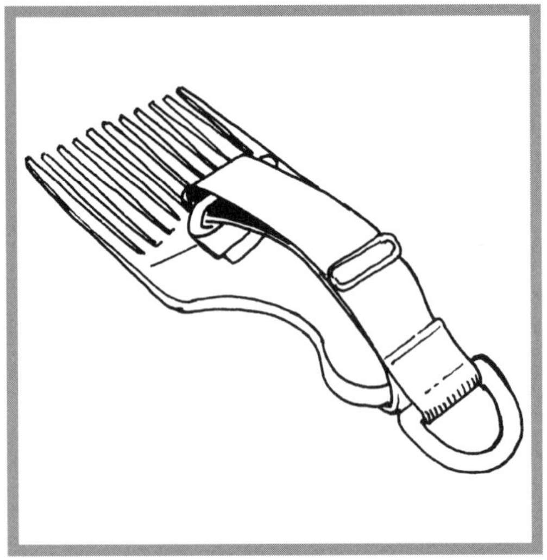

Hair lift comb
With cuff for hand
Velcro D-ring closure

137

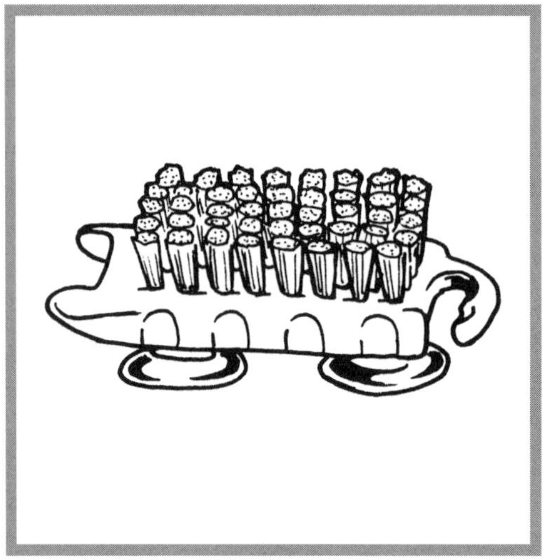

Hand brush
Suction cup base
Base with finger grooves
Hook for hanging

138

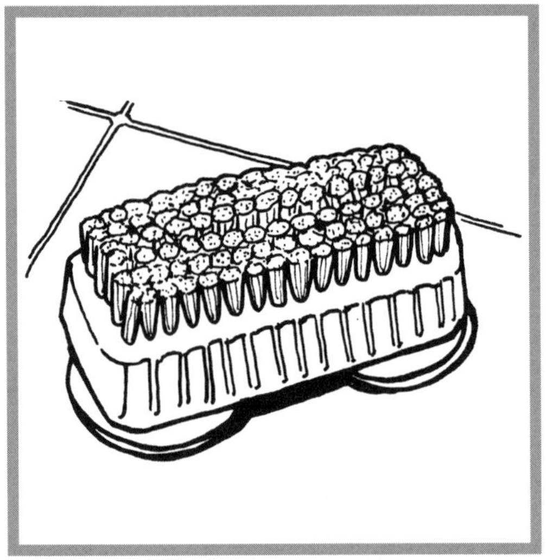

Hand brush
Suction cup base
Short bristles

139

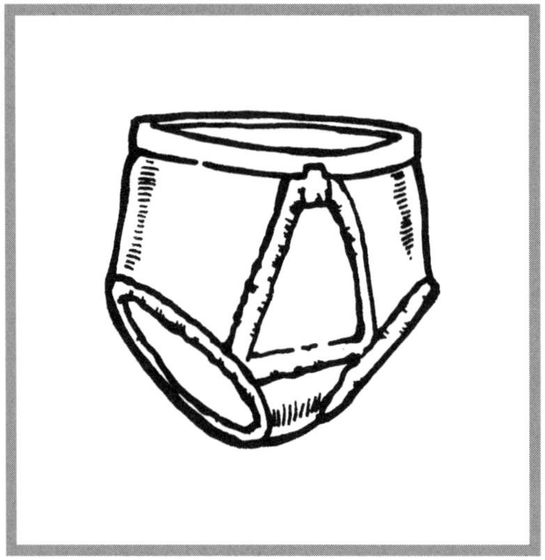

Incontinence brief men's
Full brief with fly
Light absorbent not waterproof
Machine washable

140

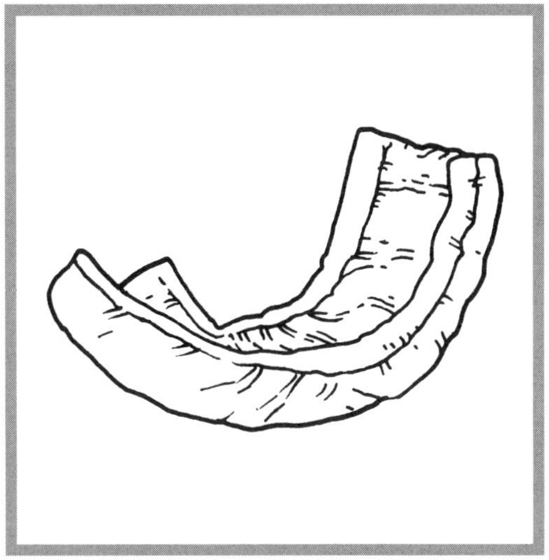

Incontinence pad disposable
Use in incontinence pants
Heavy absorbent
Fits in liner pouch

141

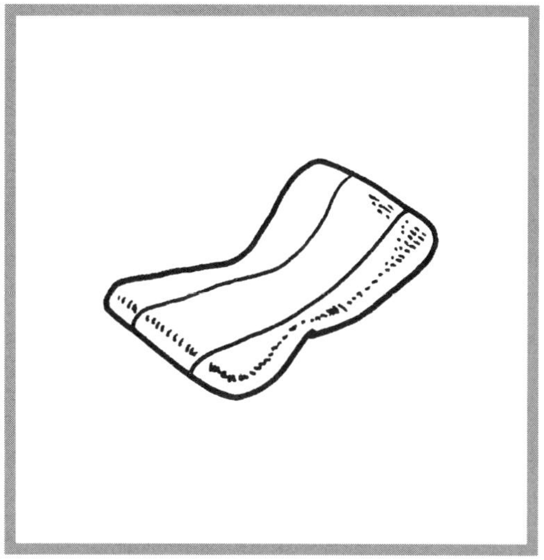

Incontinence pad disposable
Use in incontinence pants
Light absorbent

142

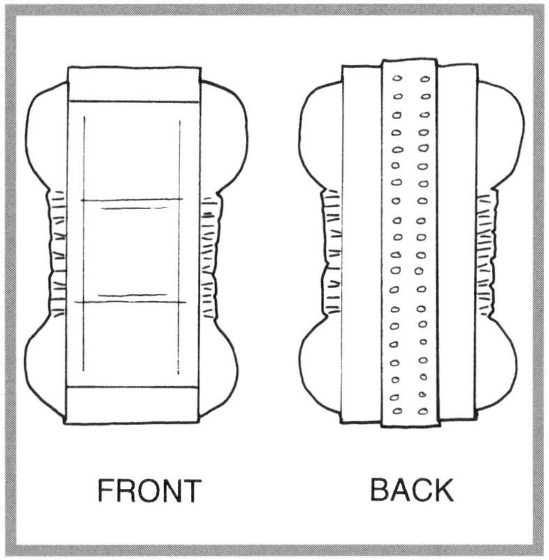

Incontinence pad disposable
Use in regular underwear
Light absorbent
Adheres to underwear

143

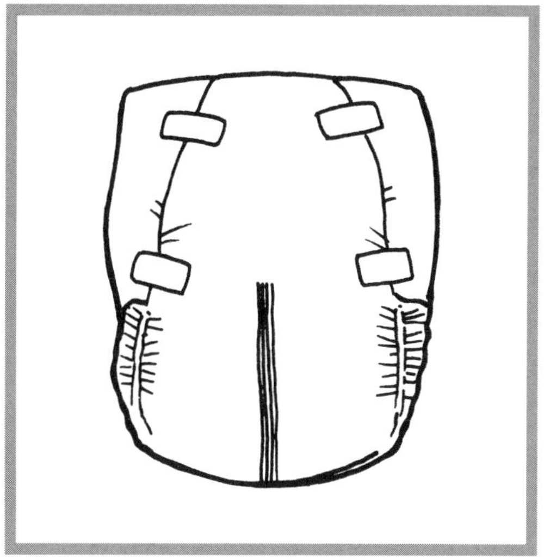

Incontinence shield disposable
Adhesive tab side closure
Heavy absorbent waterproof
Full side coverage

144

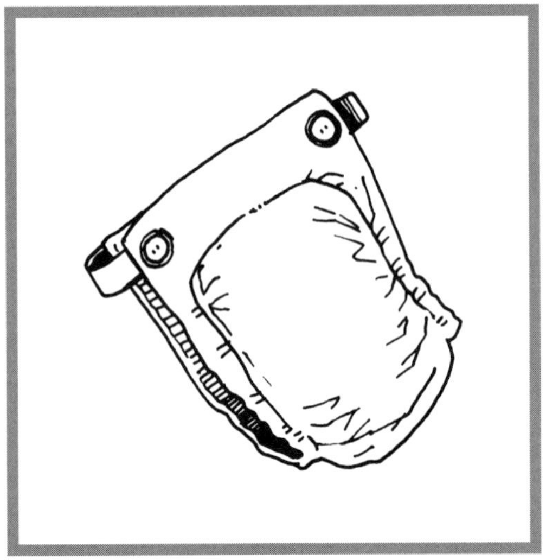

145

Incontinence shield disposable
With waist band no sides
Heavy absorbent waterproof
Elastic edges at legs

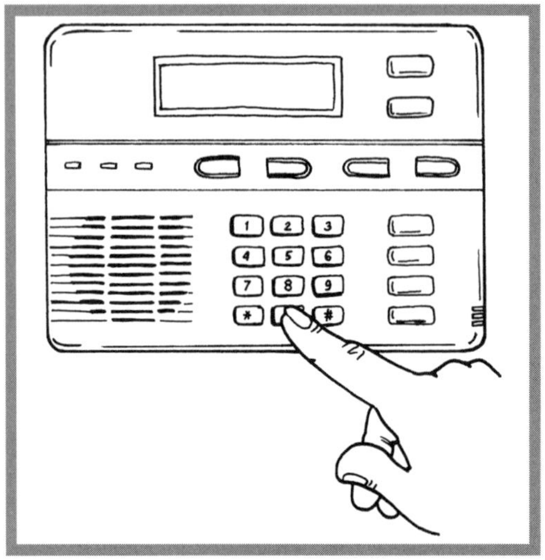

146

Intercom
FM radio wireless 3 channel
Set of sender and receiver
AC powered

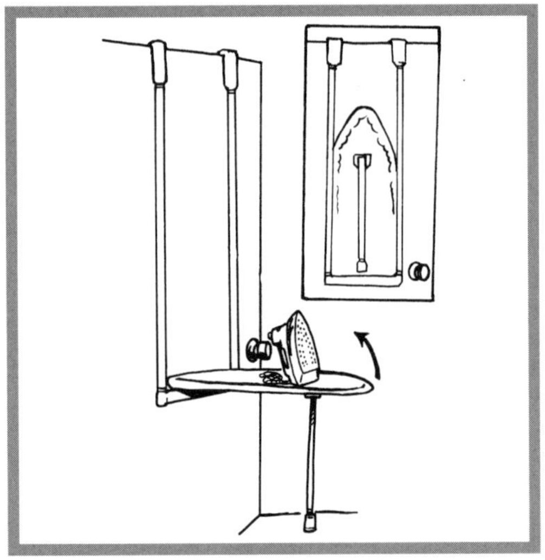

147

Ironing board
Over-door mount
Folds up to door
32 x 12 inch board

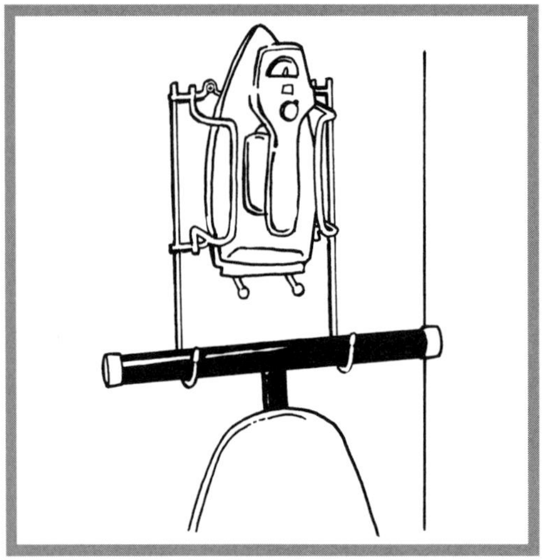

148

Ironing board organizer
Wall mounted
Basket & hook
Holds board & iron

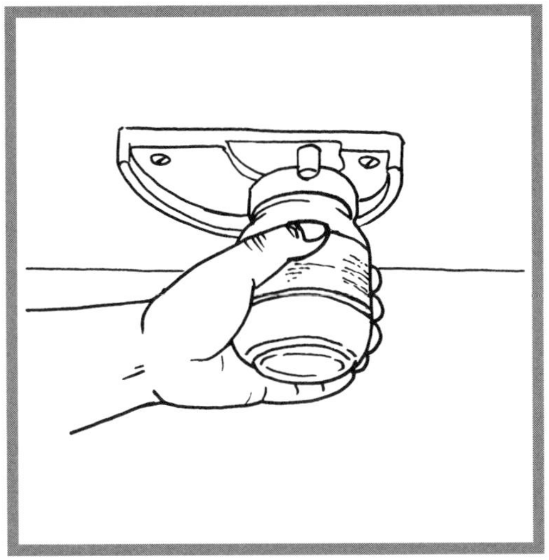

149

Jar opener
One-hand operation
Mounted cam gripper
Under cabinet mount

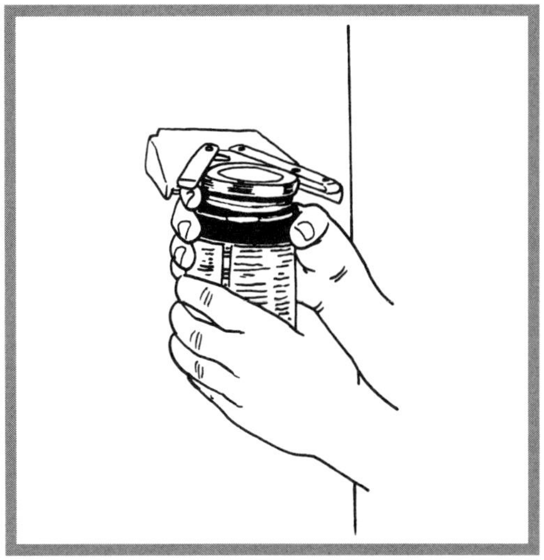

150

Jar opener
One-hand operation
Mounted wedge gripper
Rigid wall mount

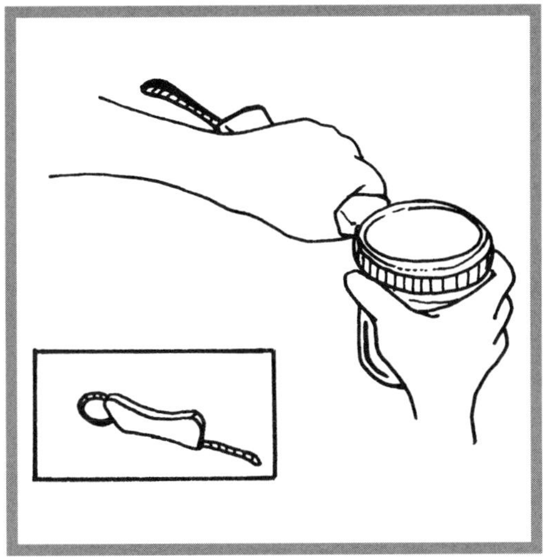

151

Jar opener
Two hands needed to operate
Band wrench

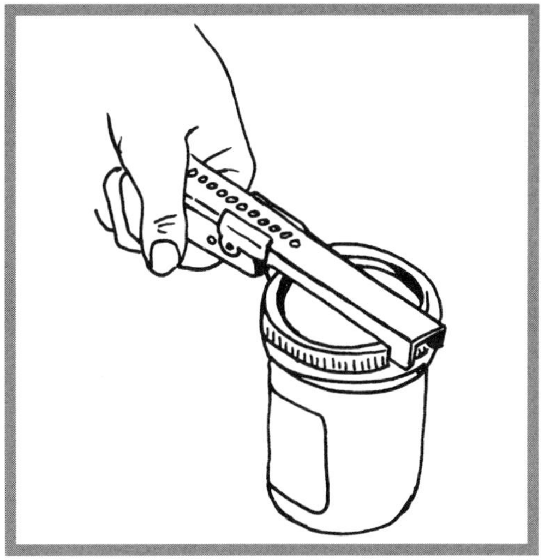

152

Jar opener
Two hands needed to operate
Lever wrench

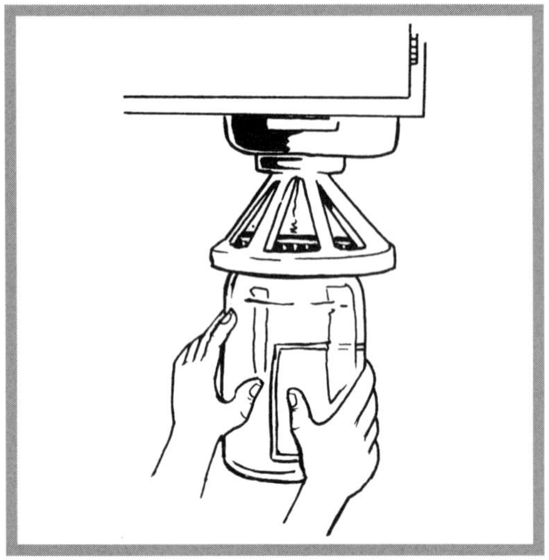

Jar opener motorized
One-hand operation
Cone gripper
Under cabinet mount

153

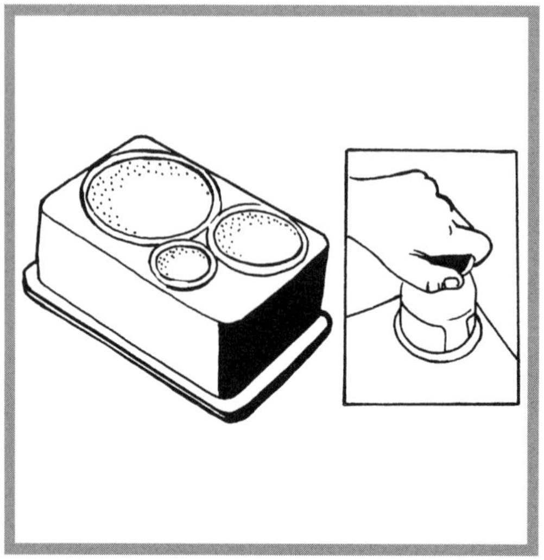

Jar/bottle holder
One-hand operation
Rubber base cone grippers
1 to 4 inch jars

154

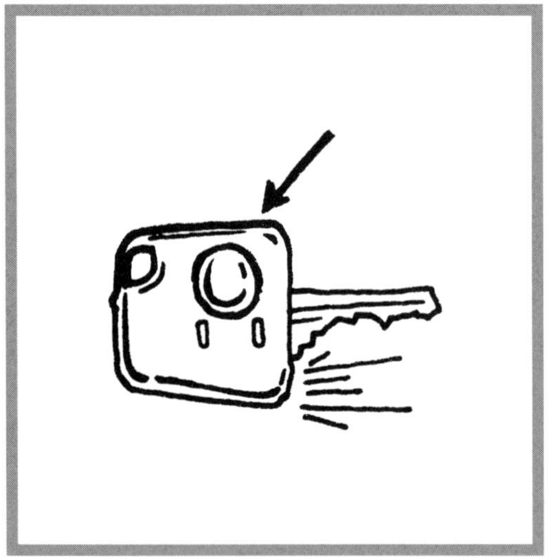

Key cover with light
Thumb button switch
Color coded-4 colors
Battery powered

155

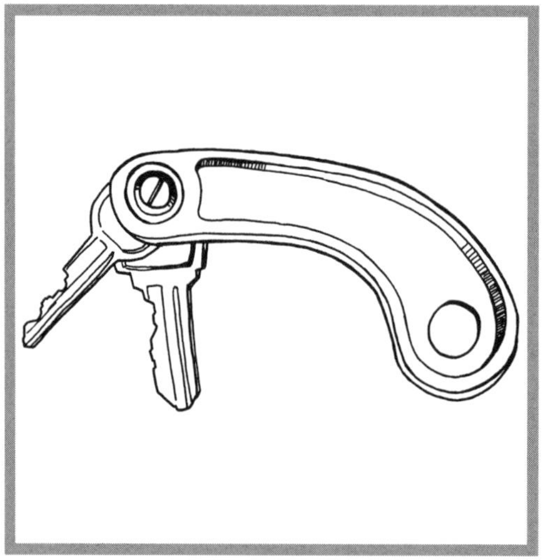

Key holder/handle
Curved handle
2 keys

156

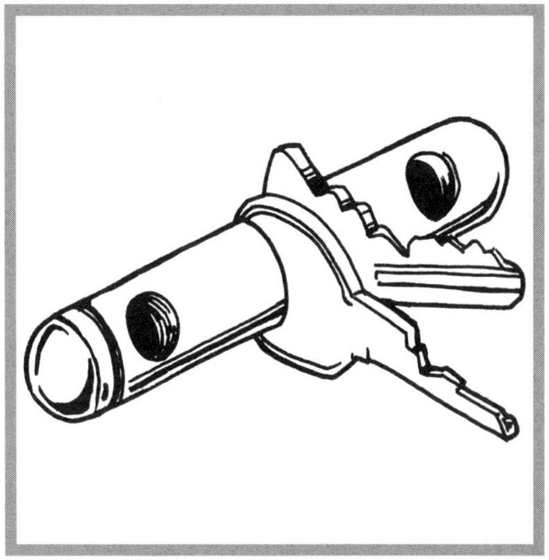

157

Key holder/handle
T-handle

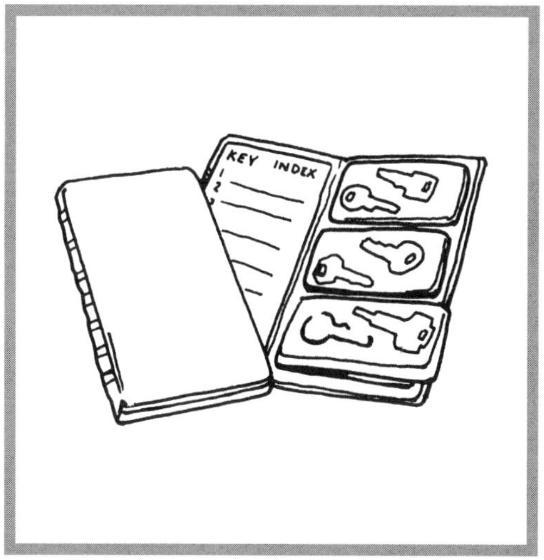

158

Key organizer
Book style
With write-on index
Holds several keys

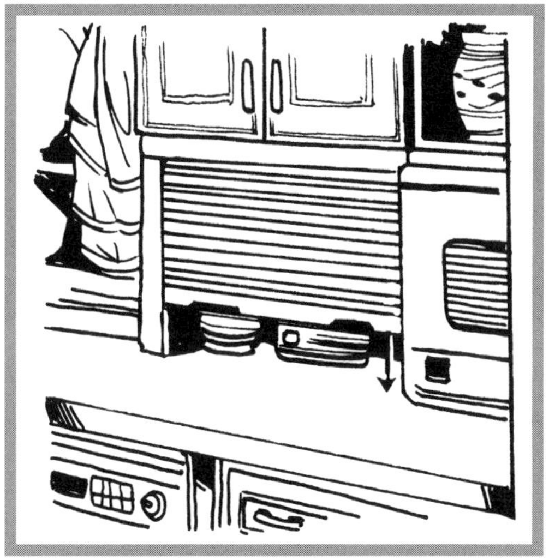

159

Kitchen cabinet door
Tambour
Roll-up

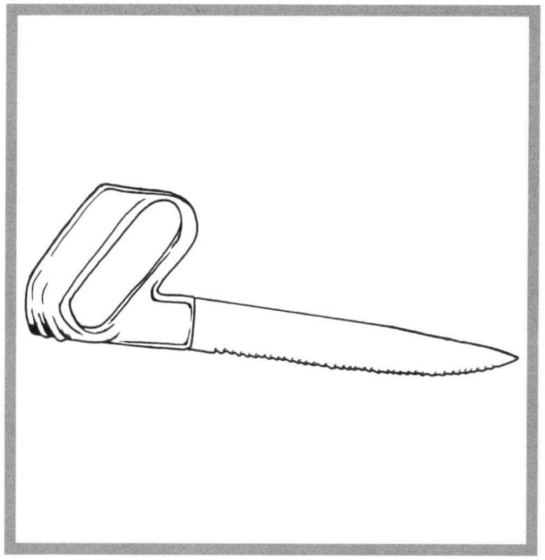

160

Kitchen knife
120 degree handle
Serrated blade

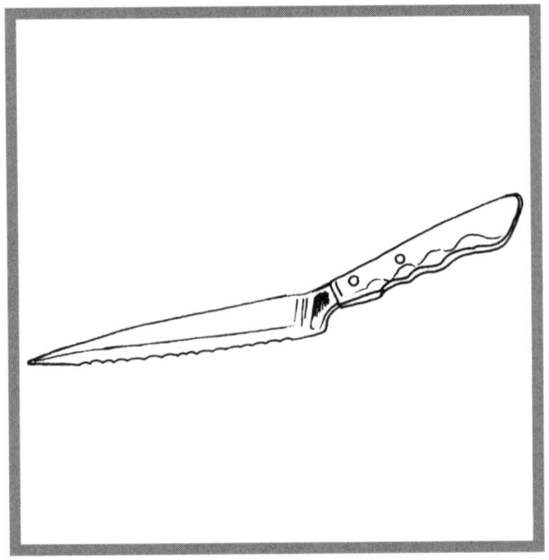

Kitchen knife
30 degree handle
Serrated blade

161

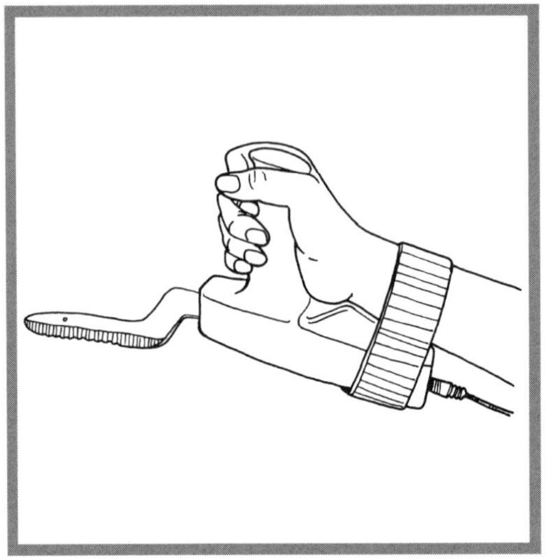

Kitchen knife
90 degree handle
Electric
With wrist support band

162

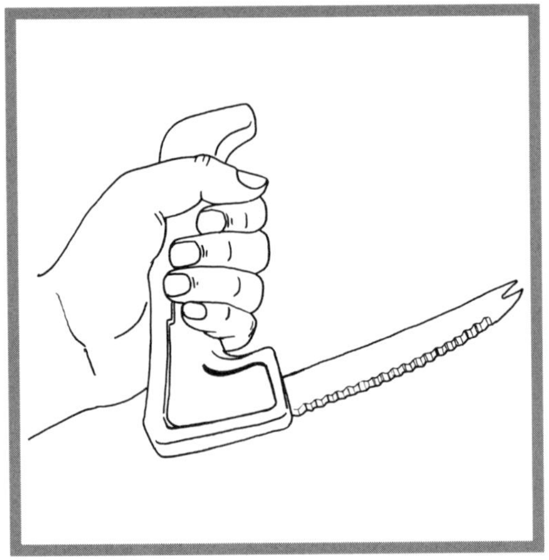

Kitchen knife
90-degree handle
Serrated blade

163

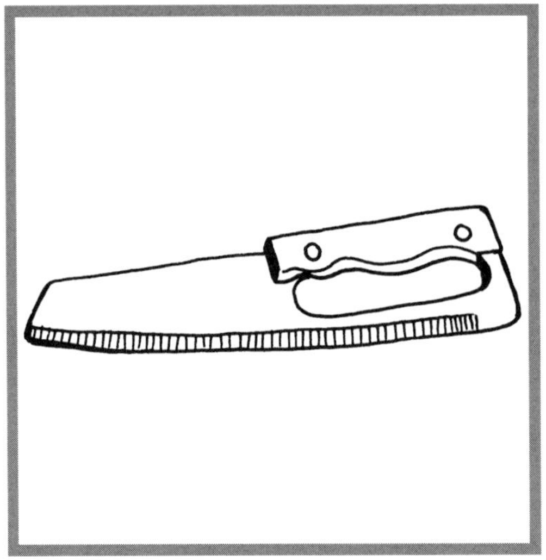

Kitchen knife
Cutout handle
Long blade

164

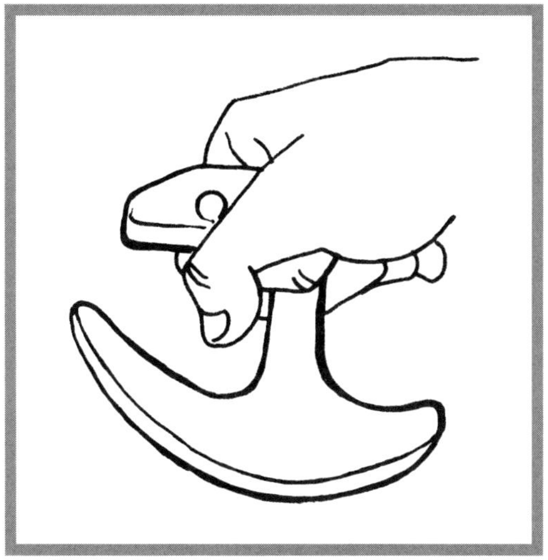

Kitchen knife
Top palmar handle
Crescent blade
Blade parallel to handle

165

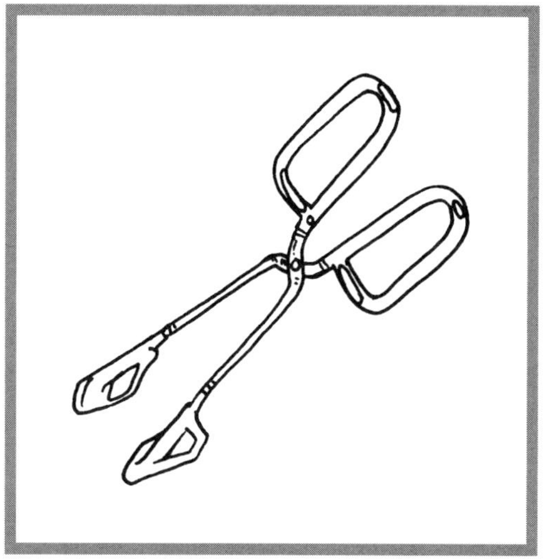

Kitchen tongs
Loop ends
Soft plastic coating

166

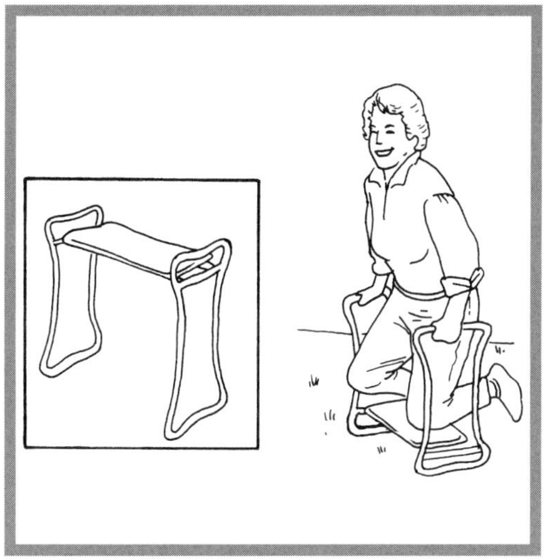

Kneeler and bench
Cushioned
Handles become legs

167

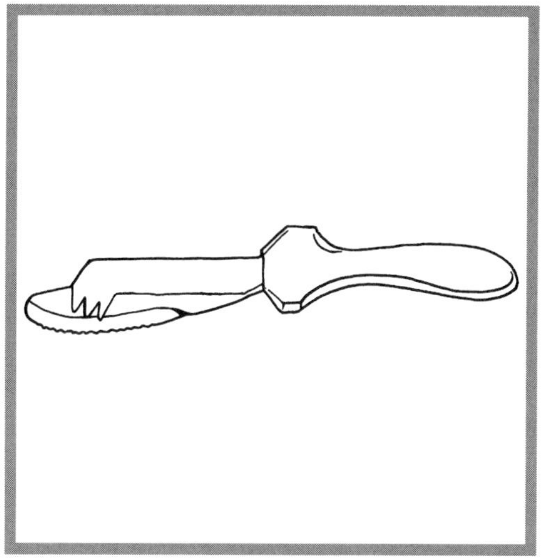

Knife/fork combo
Handle with guard
Rocker blade knife on spring
Right angle fork tines

168

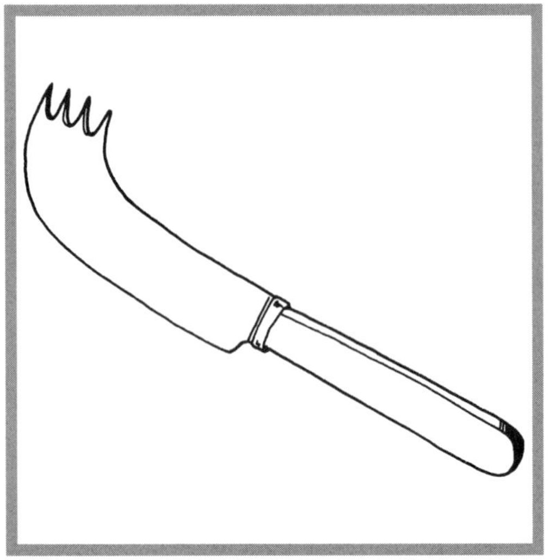

169

Knife/fork combo
Straight handle
Right angle tines

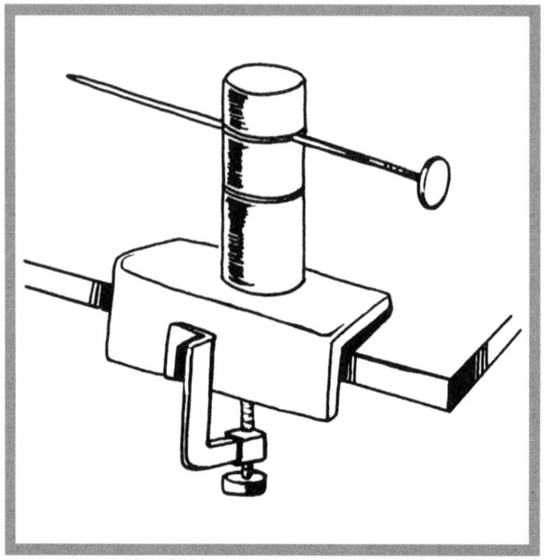

170

Knitting aid
Needle holder
Clamps to table edge
Needles 0 through 14 gauge

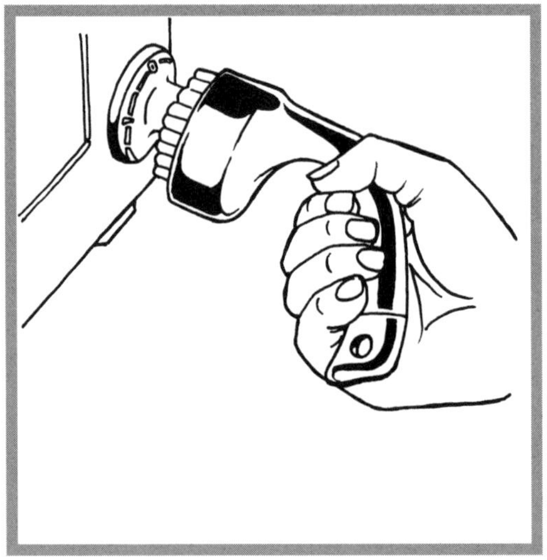

171

Knob turner
Spring loaded pins
Any non-round knob
L-handle

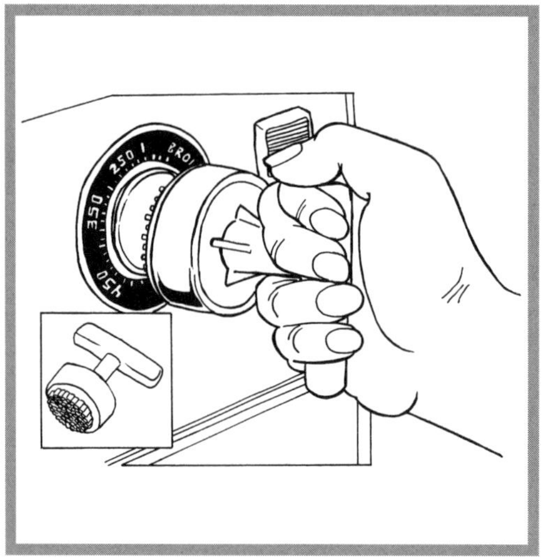

172

Knob turner
Spring loaded pins
Any non-round knob
T-handle

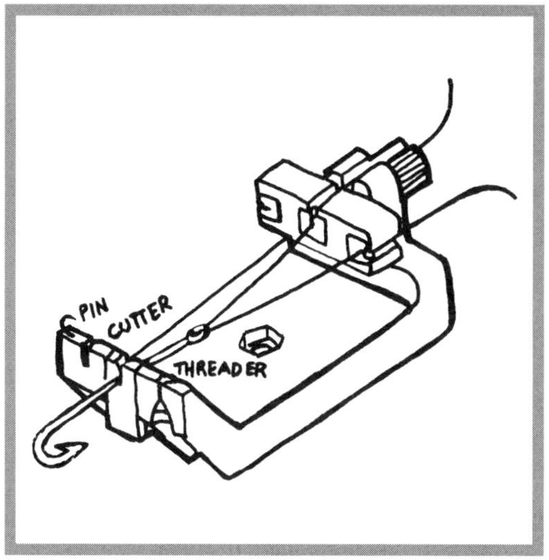

Knot tying/threader
One-hand operated
For fishing lures

173

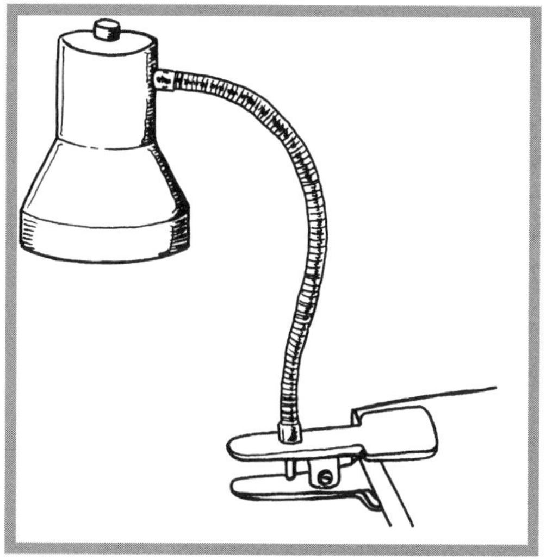

Lamp
Edge clamp
Gooseneck
100 watt

174

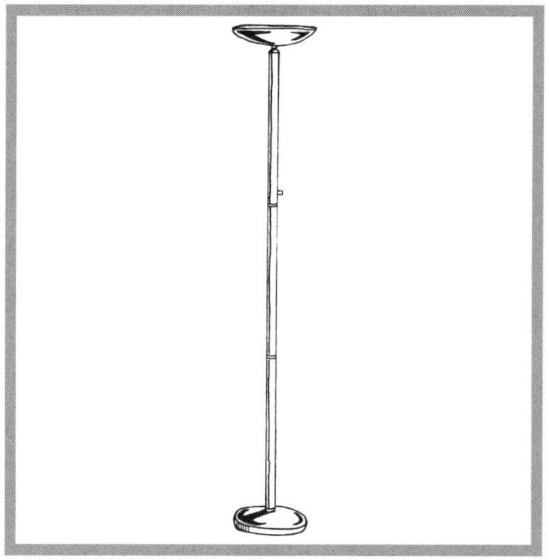

Lamp
Floor torchiere
indirect light
66 inches high

175

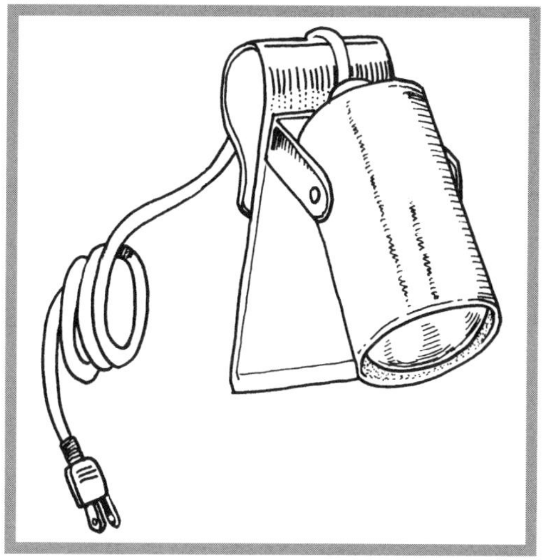

Lamp
Squeeze clamp with
swivel
Reflector bulb

176

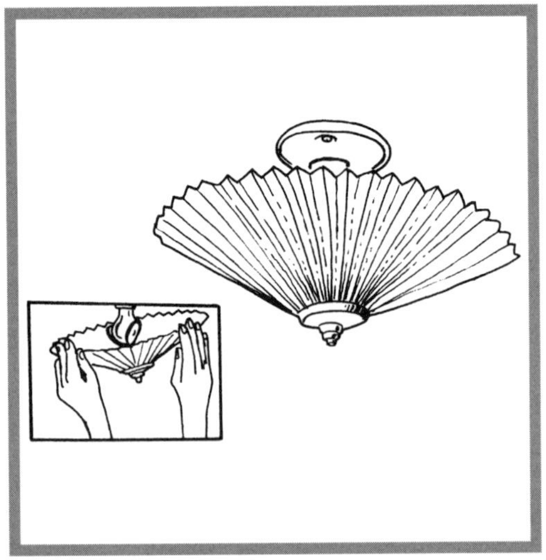

Lamp shade
Fan pleat
Clips onto bare bulb

177

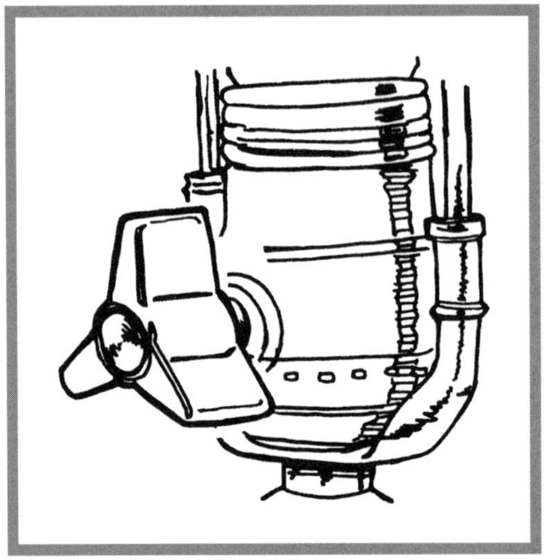

Lamp switch enlarger
3 spoke knob
Standard rotary
Threaded shaft

178

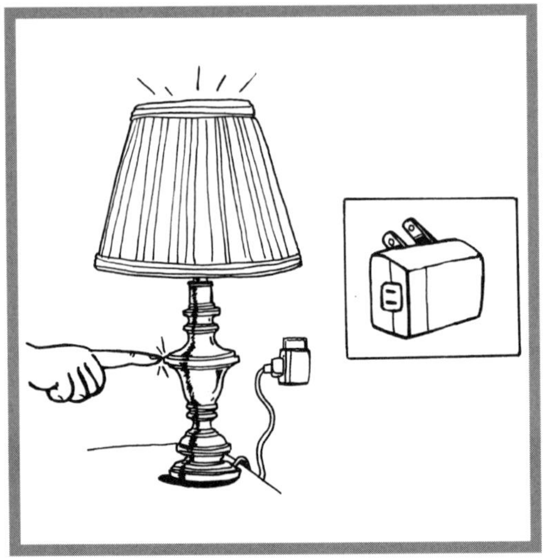

Lamp touch control
Outlet module
3 light levels

179

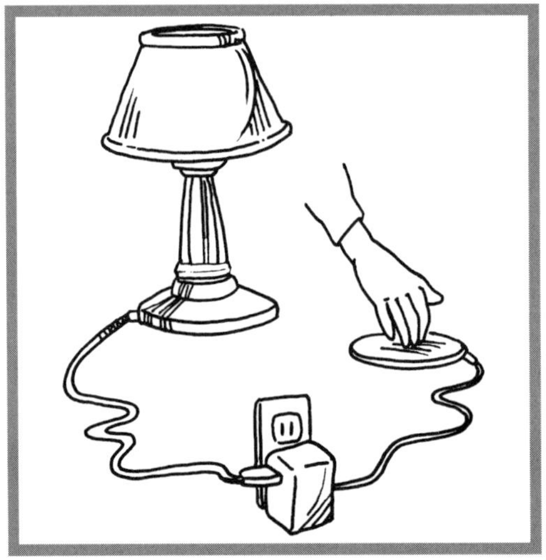

Lamp touch control
Outlet module
3 light levels
Plugs into outlet

180

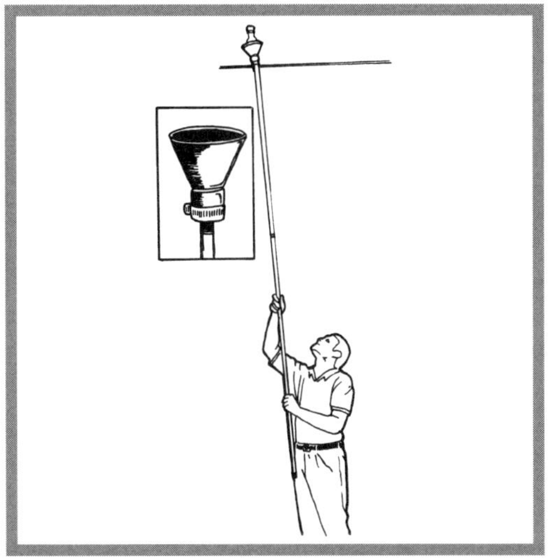

Light bulb changer
For standard bulbs
Accepts extender
Suction cup end

181

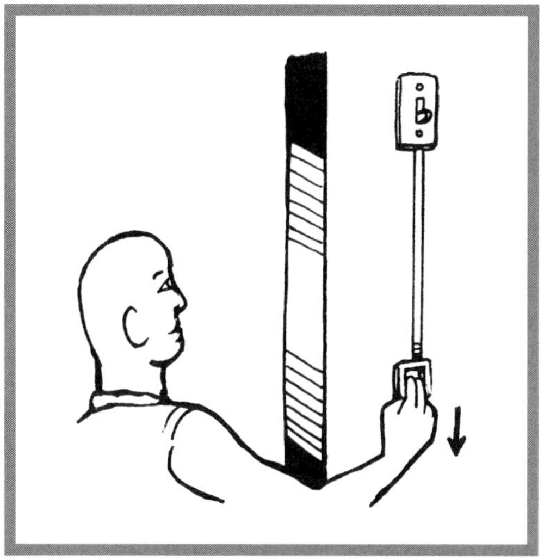

Light switch dropper
Rod and handle
14 inch long

182

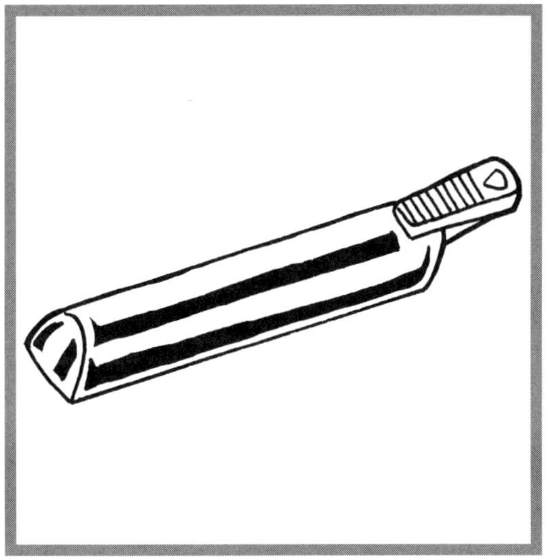

Magnifier
Bar reading
Power in 1.25X - 2.5X range
Magnifies vertically only

183

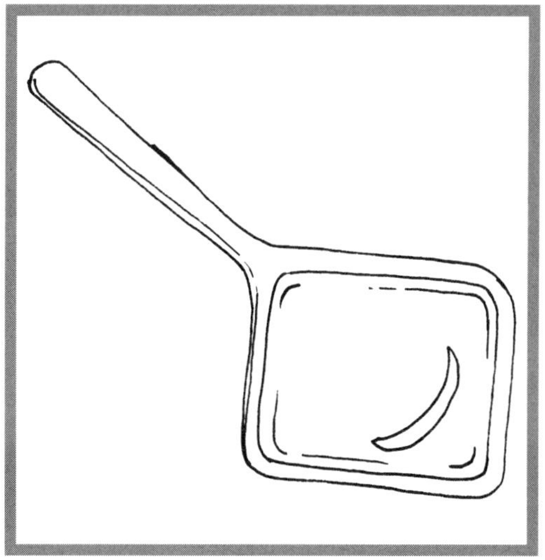

Magnifier
Hand rectangular reading
For object distance 10 inches

184

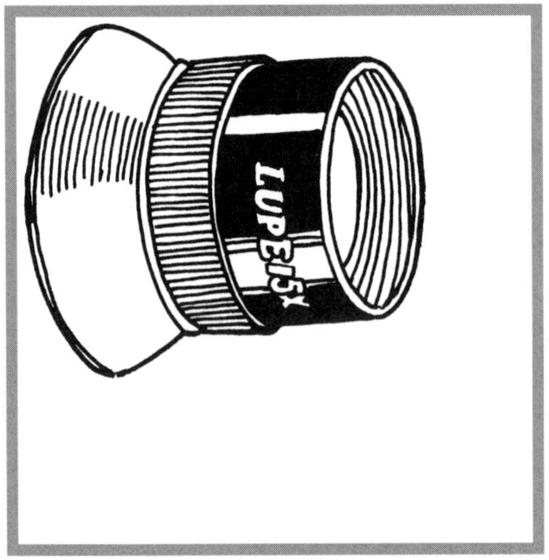

Magnifier
Loupe for very fine detail
Power in 12.1X - 20X range
Monocle

185

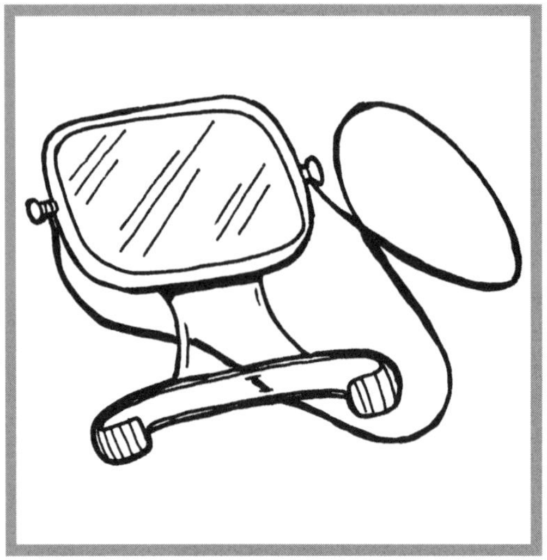

Magnifier
Neck suspended reading
Power in 1.25X - 2.5X range

186

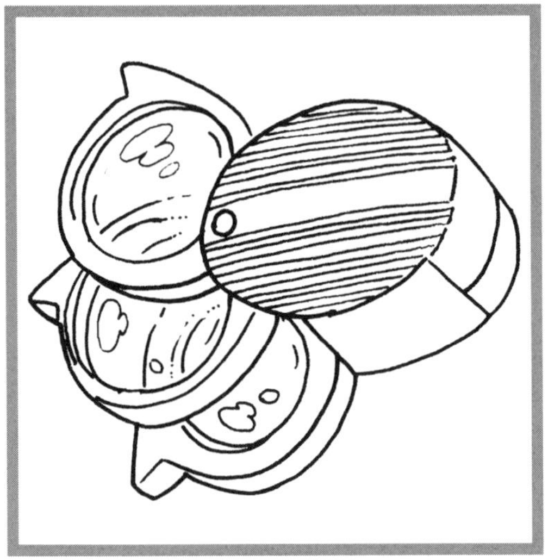

Magnifier
Pocket detail with case
Powers 4X & 6X & 10X & 20X

187

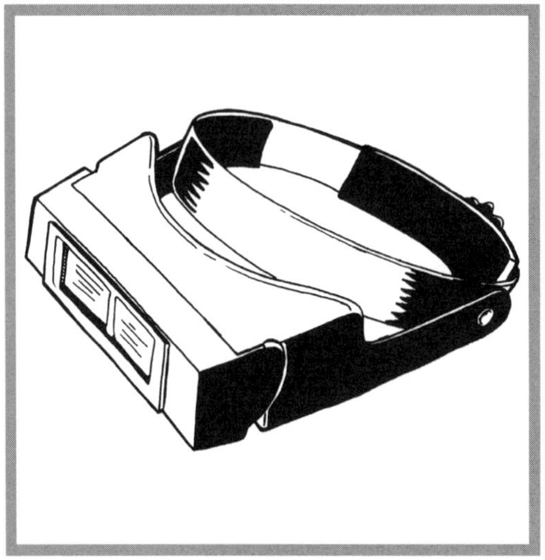

Magnifier
Spectacle type
Power in 1.25X - 2.5X range
Adjustable head band

188

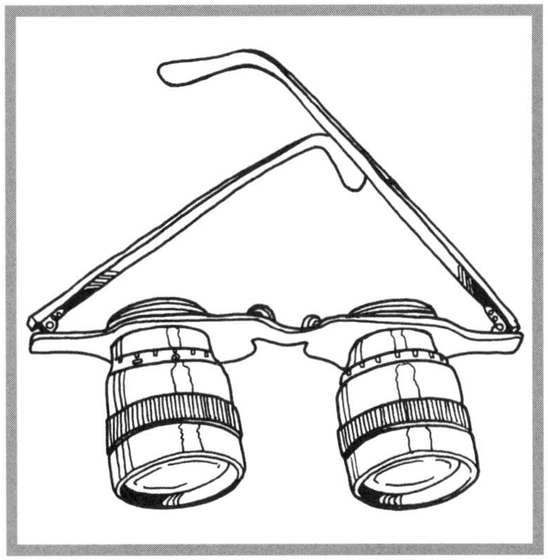

Magnifier
Spectacle type
Power in 2.6X - 4X range
Wear like glasses

189

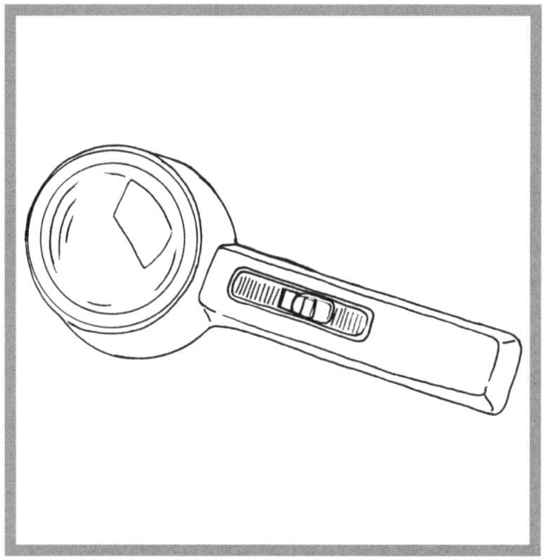

Magnifier with light
Hand held detail
Power in 4.1X - 6X range

190

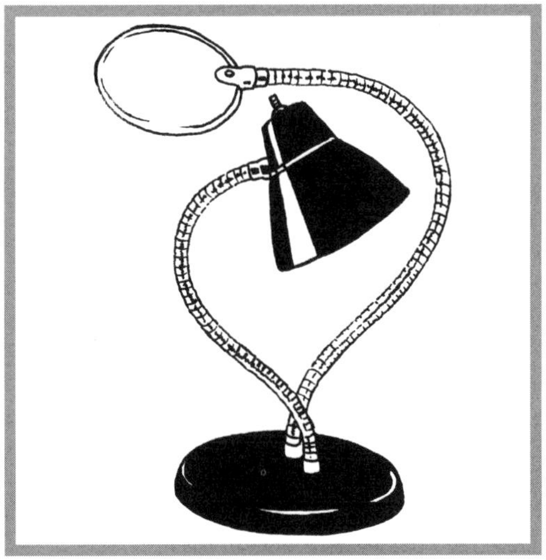

Magnifier with light
Stand with 2 goosenecks
Power in 2.6X - 4X range
60 watt incandescent bulb

191

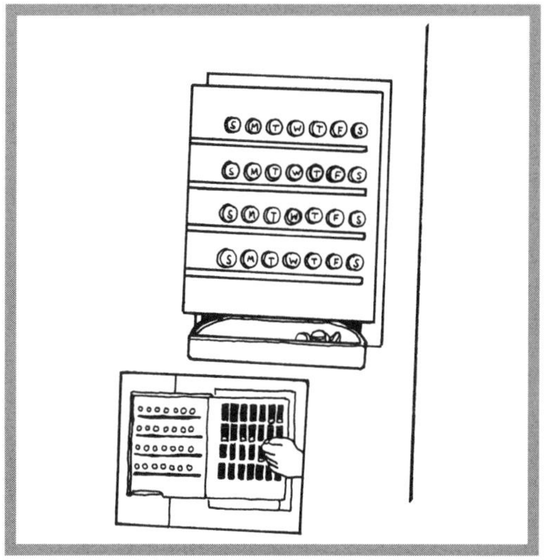

Medication manager
28 bins
Push button release
Wall mount

192

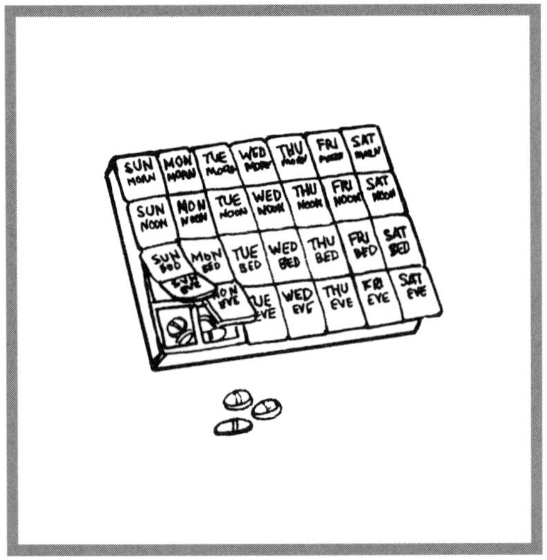

Medication manager
Manual compartments
7 day 4 times/day

193

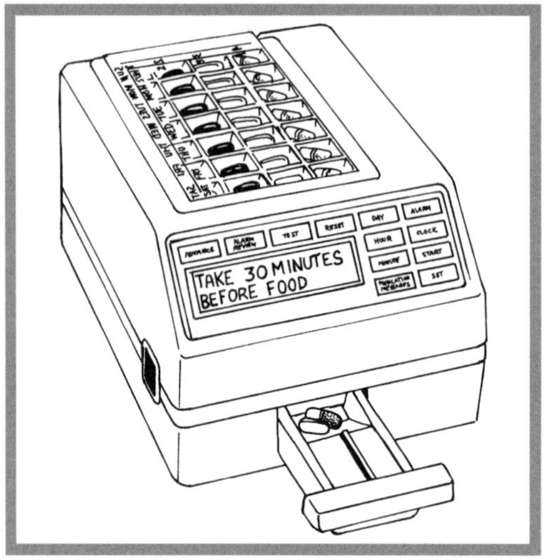

Medication manager
Programmable
7 day 4 times/day
LCD reminder display

194

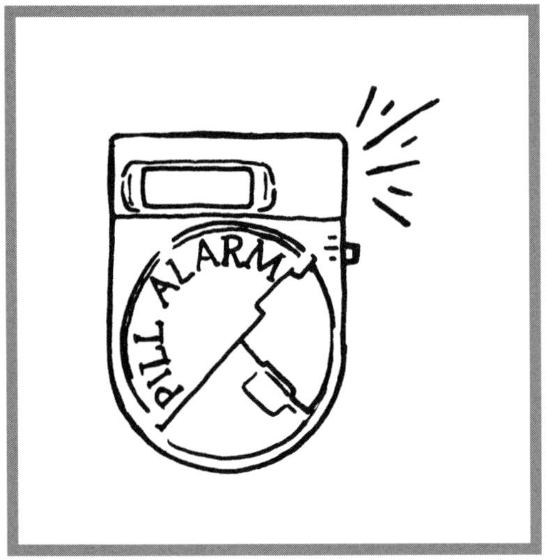

Medication manager
Programmable signal
Beeps and resets

195

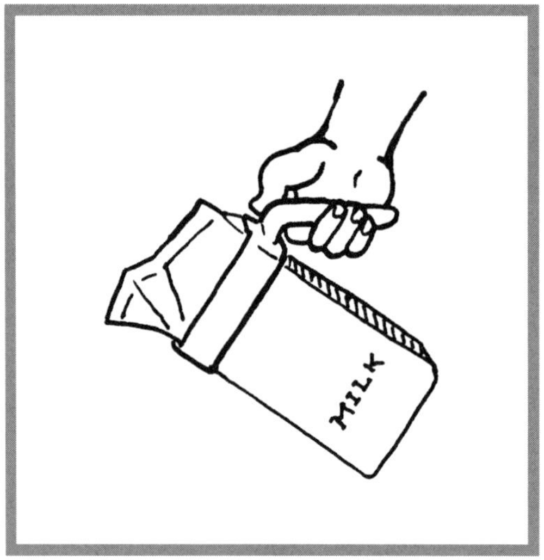

Milk carton handle
For half gallon
Slips over carton

196

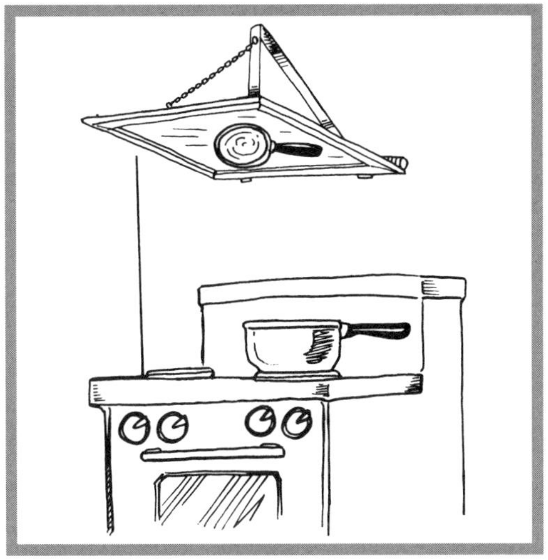

197

Mirror
Over-stove
Wall mount
Adjustable angle

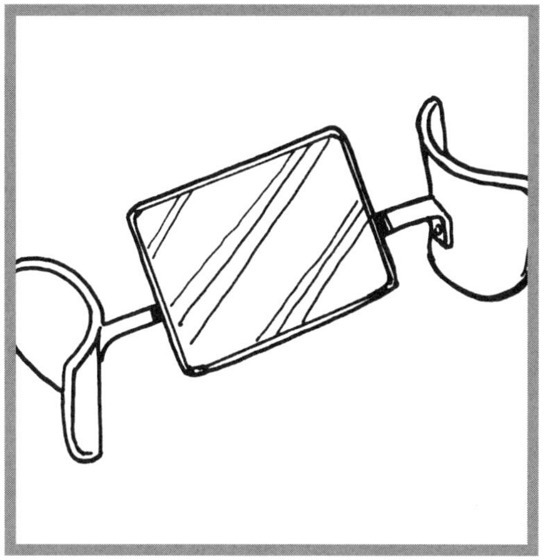

198

Mirror self inspection
On knee spreaders
6 x 4 inch pivoting
9 inch abduction

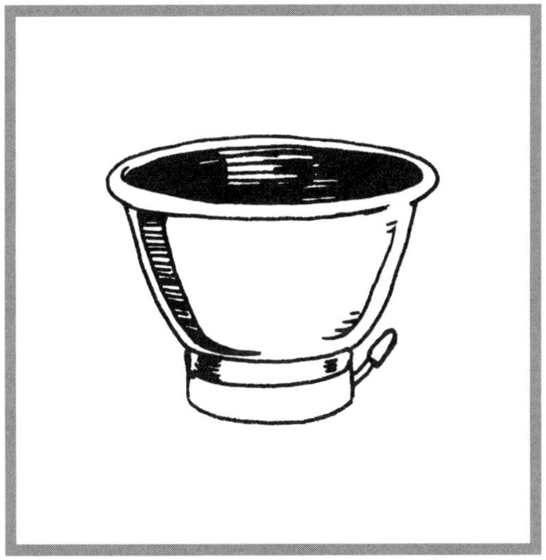

199

Mixing bowl
One-hand operated
suction base
7.5 inch diameter

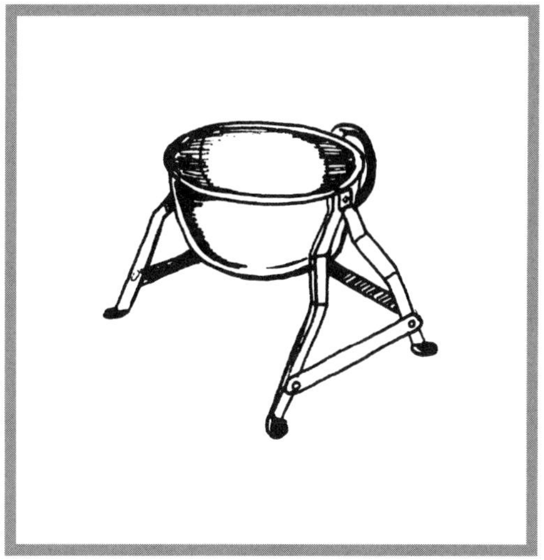

200

Mixing bowl & holder
One hand operated tilt
frame
3 quart
All steel with rubber
feet

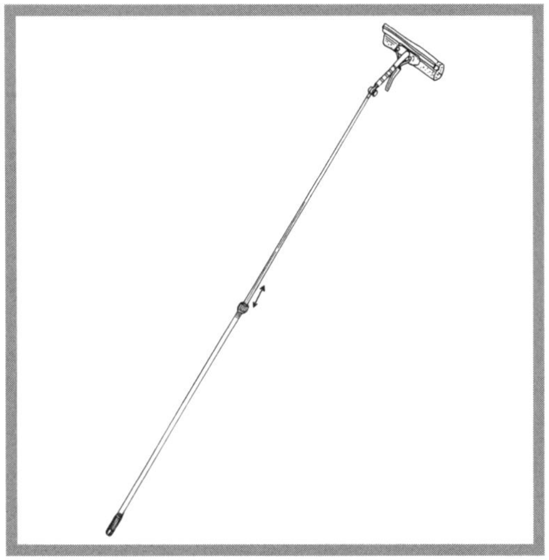

Mop on extension handle
Sponge head with rollers
Handle adjusts to 7 feet
Hinged head

201

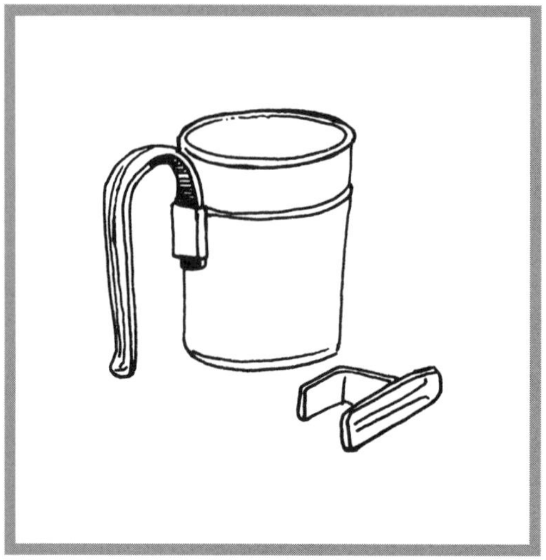

Mug
Short and long loop handles
Interchangeable handles

202

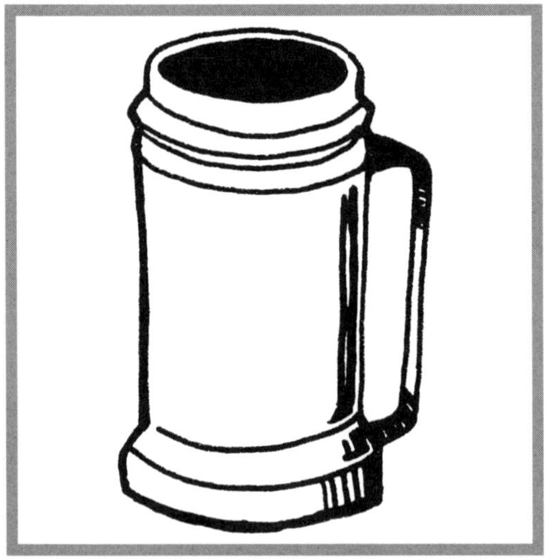

Mug
Single large handle
No lid
Insulated

203

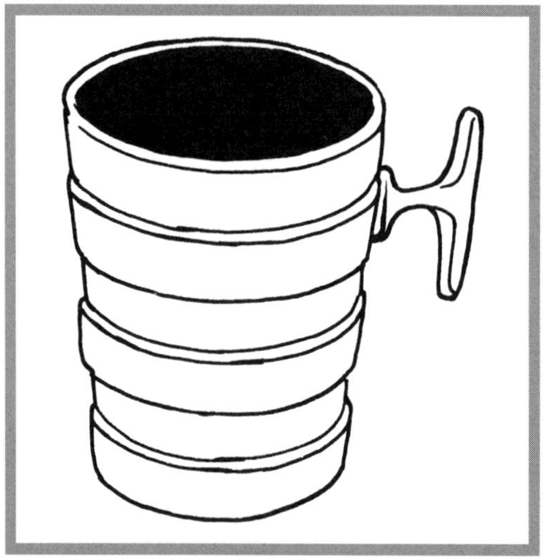

Mug
T-handle
No lid

204

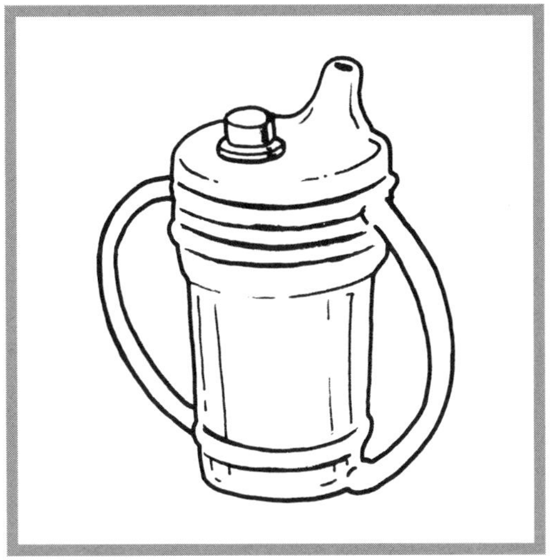

205

Mug
Two large handles
Lid with spout

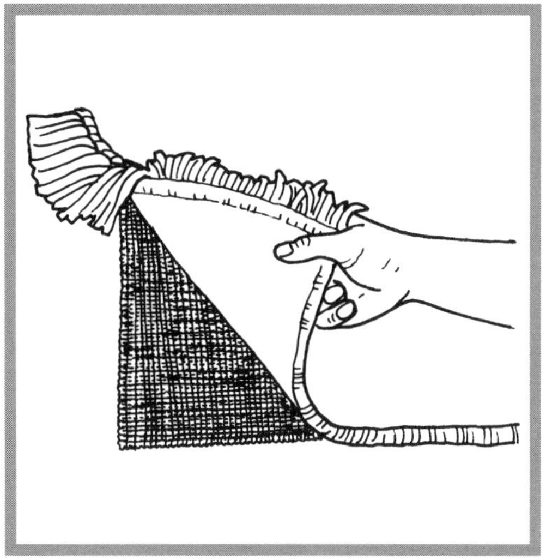

206

Non-skid matting
For rug to floor
9 x 12 feet

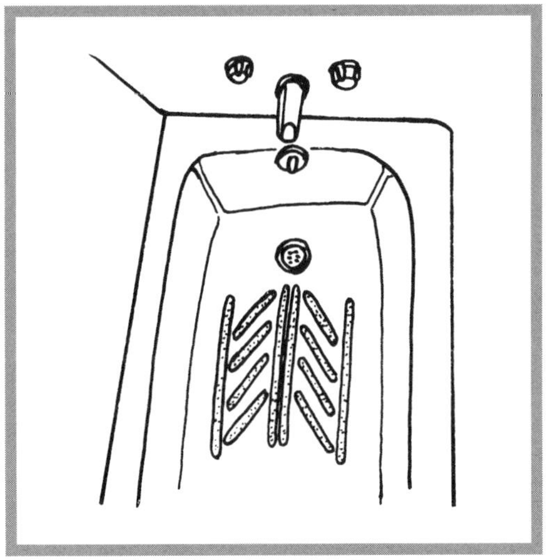

207

Non-skid strips
Adhesive back
For bathtubs

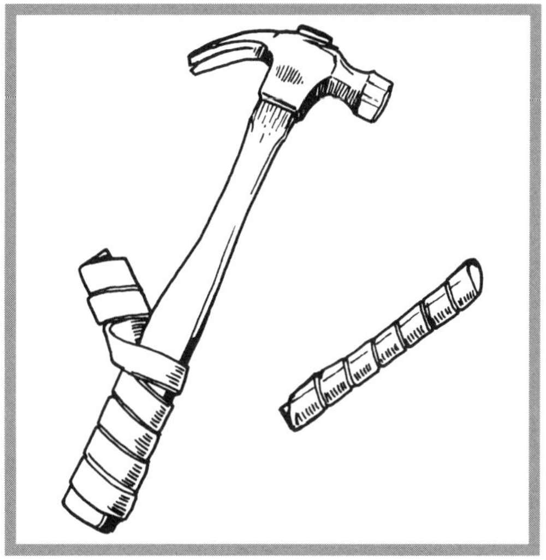

208

Non-slip strips
Adhesive back
For handles
High-tack soft plastic

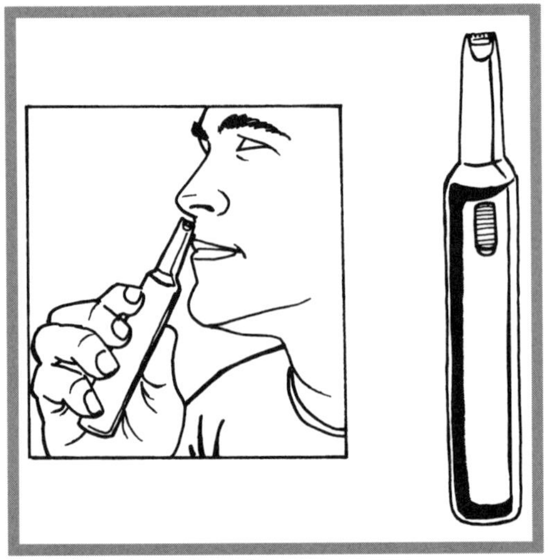

Nose/ear hair trimmer
Tubular blade
Cordless non-recharge

209

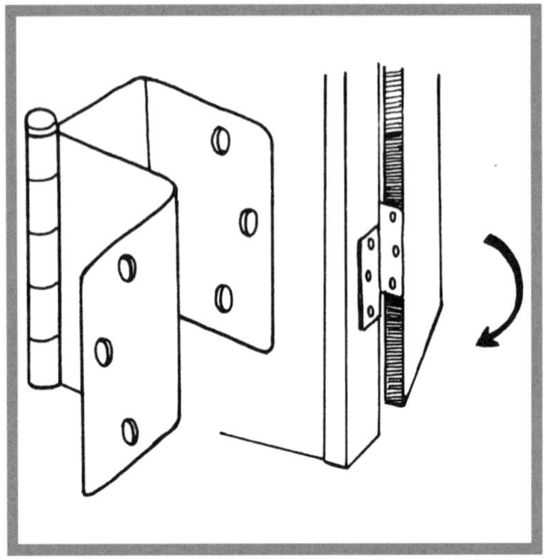

Offset door hinge
Adds 2 inches to width
Use existing holes

210

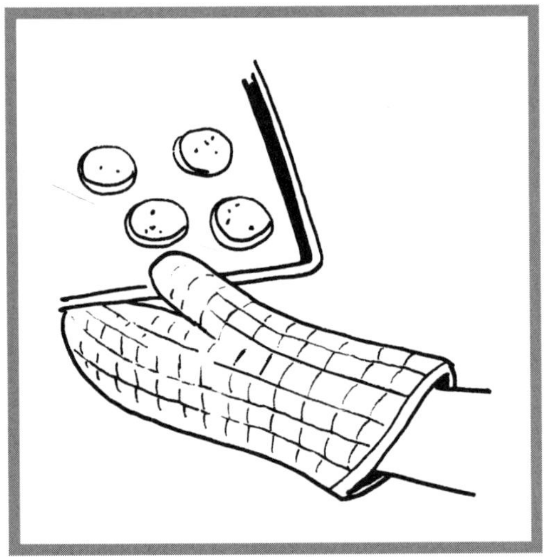

Oven mitt
16 inches long
Flame resistant

211

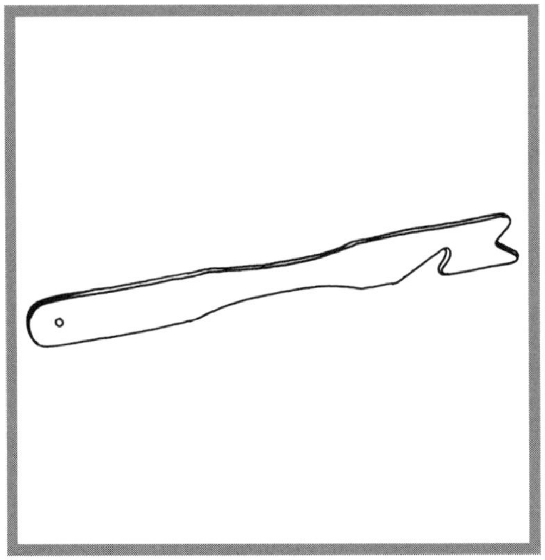

Oven rack stick
Notched for oven
12 inches
To push and pull

212

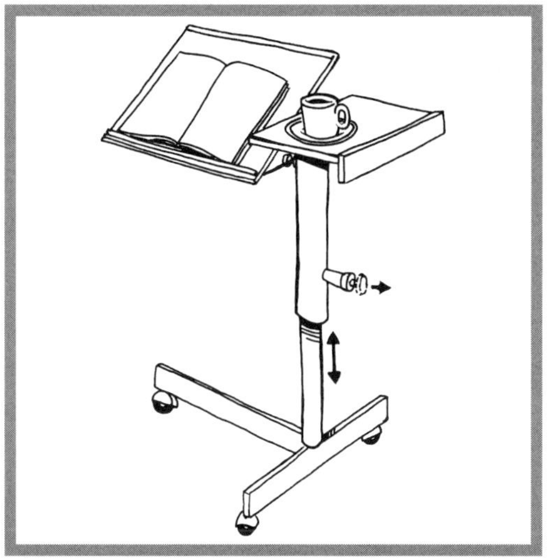

213

Overbed table
Floor base split tilting top
Adjustable height
T-base

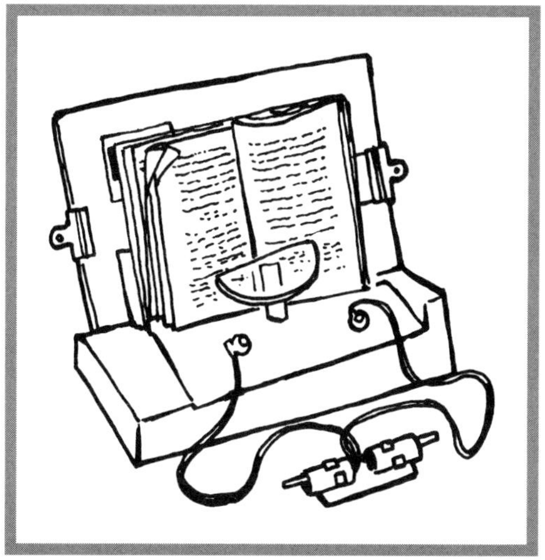

214

Page turner
Book holder
Microswitch actuated

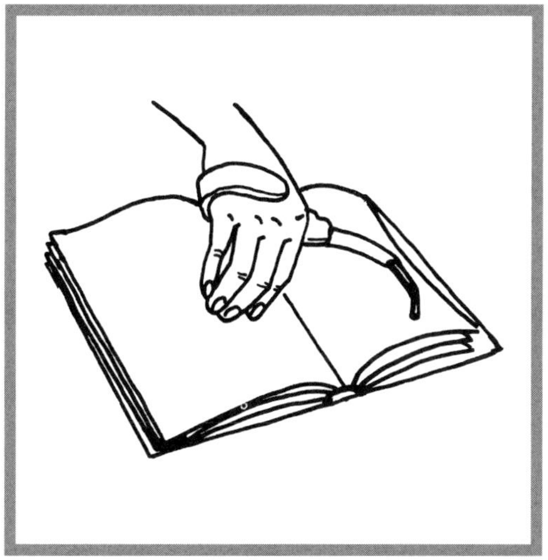

215

Page turning stick
Hand clip mount
Curved rubber tip

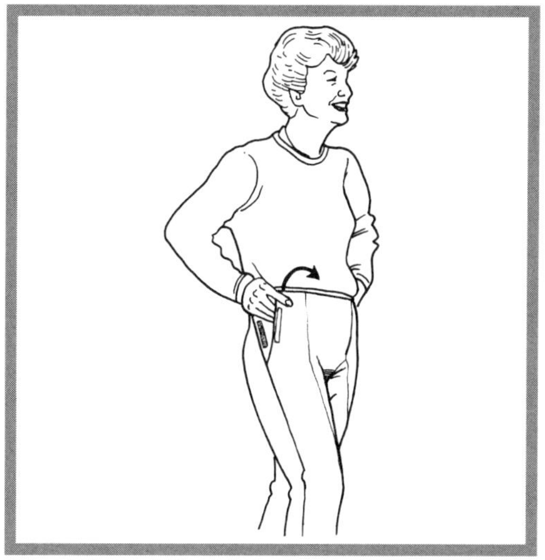

216

Pants
Women's drop front
Velcro closure

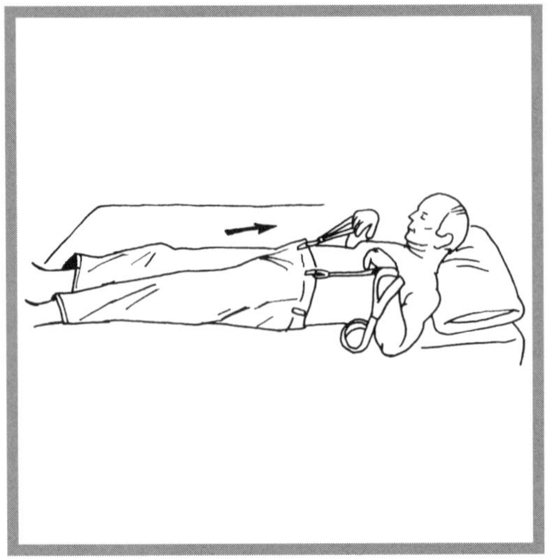

Pants pull
Loop webbing
Hooks into belt loop
Pull and roll body

217

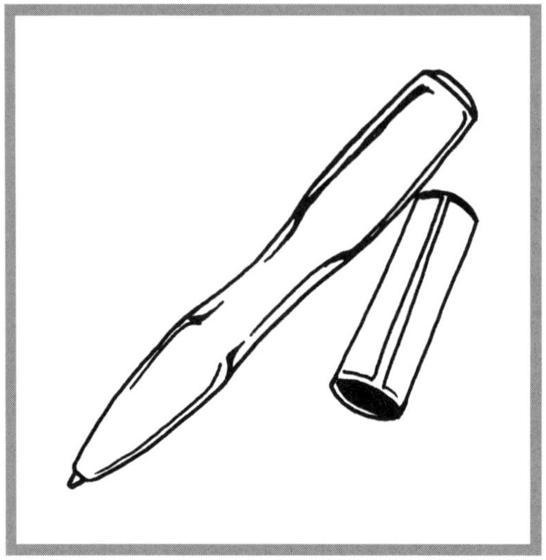

Pen
Contoured & built-up
Fixed weight
Refillable ball point

218

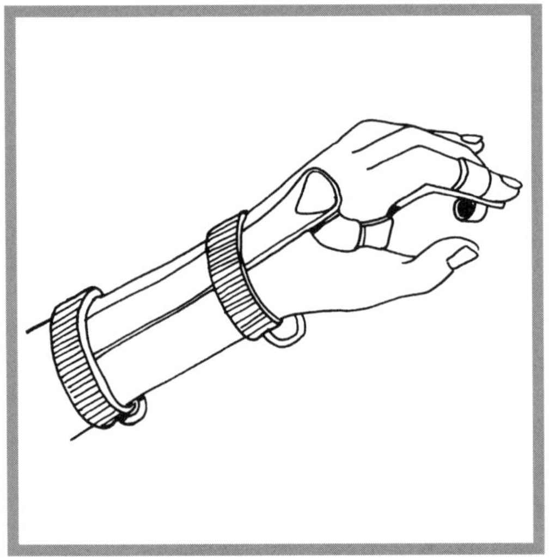

Pen holder
Palm clip/finger/wrist support
For Left hand use

219

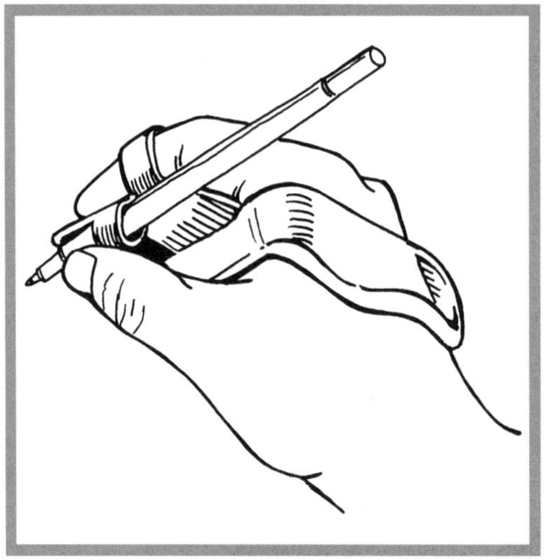

Pen holder
Palmar cuff & finger support
For Right hand use
For large hand

220

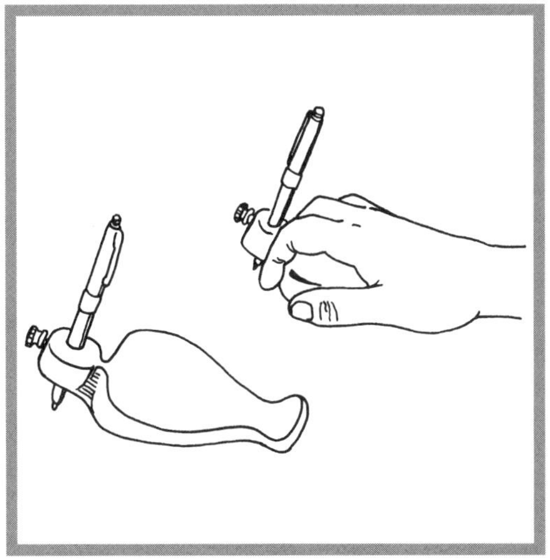

Pen holder sliding
Palmar support
Bird shaped
Holds pen or pencil

221

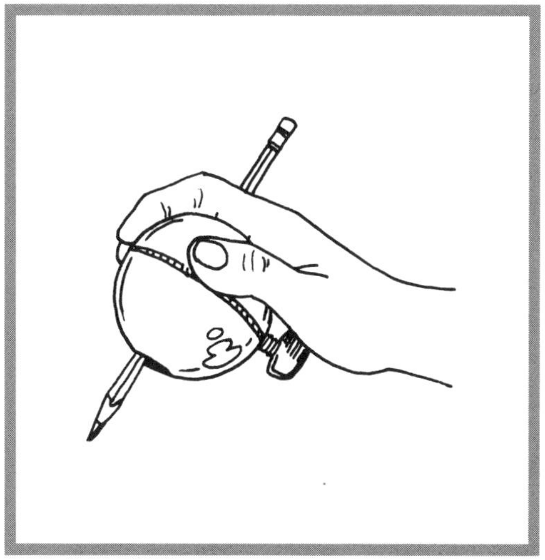

Pen-and-pencil grip
Ball-shaped
For standard pencil
Large enough to fill hand

222

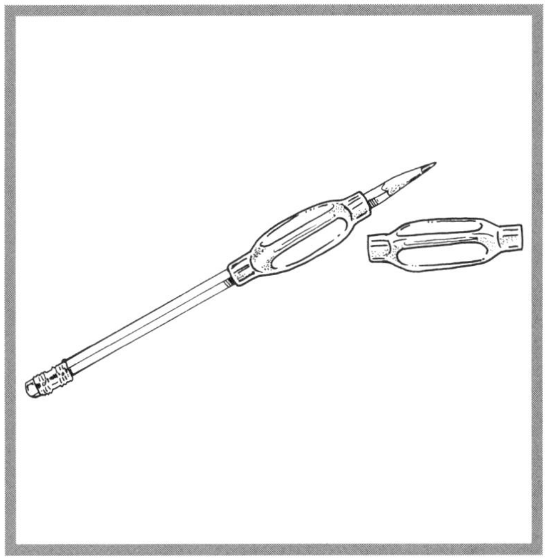

Pen-and-pencil grip
Bulb-shaped
For standard pencil
Non-rolling

223

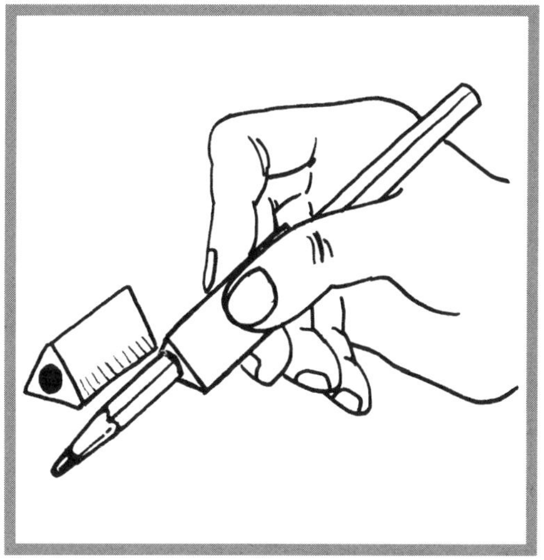

Pen-and-pencil grip
Slip-on gripper
Triangular
Fixed length

224

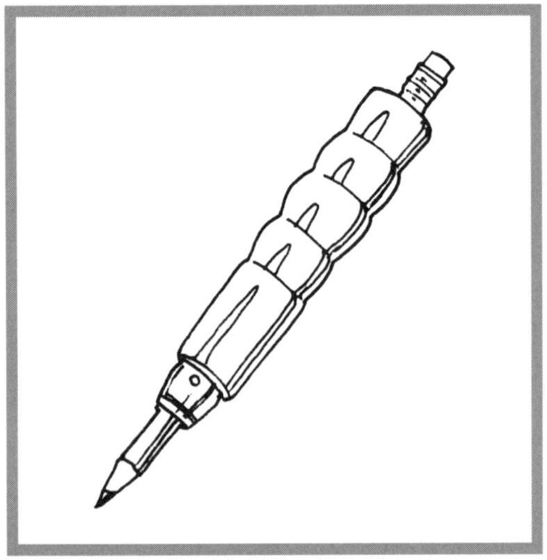

Pen-and-pencil holder
Built up and weighted
Adjustable weights

225

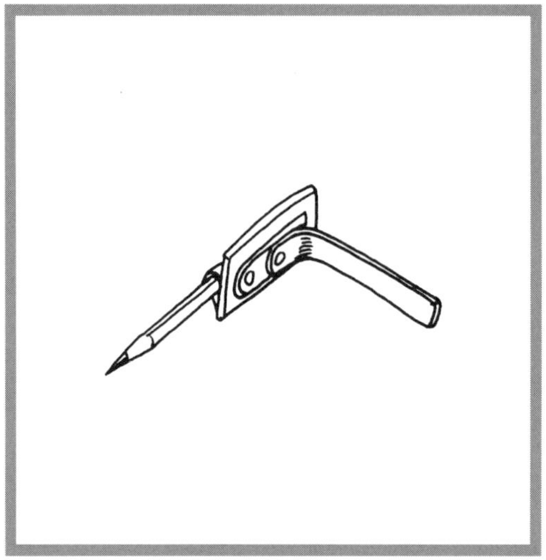

Pen-and-pencil holder
Right angle holder block
Fits universal cuff pocket

226

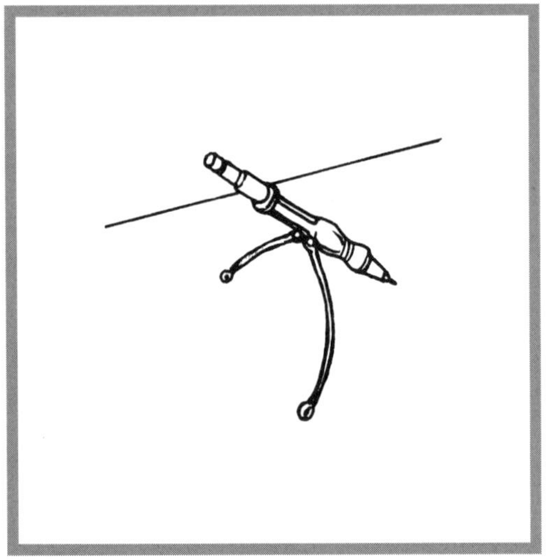

Pencil with holder
Spring wire frame
For use with either hand
Mechanical pencil permanent

227

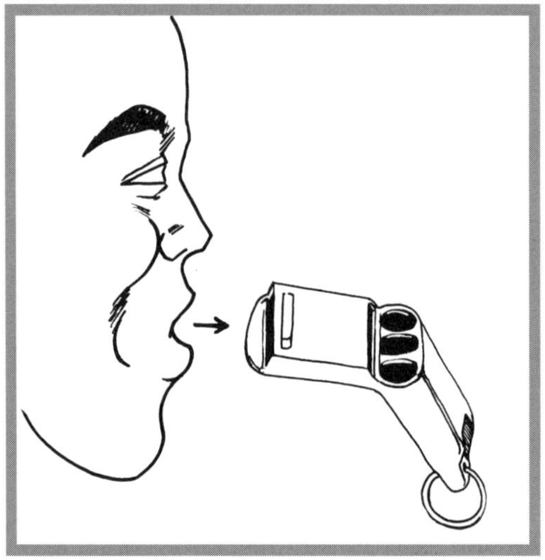

Personal alerting device
Carried on neck cord
Whistle

228

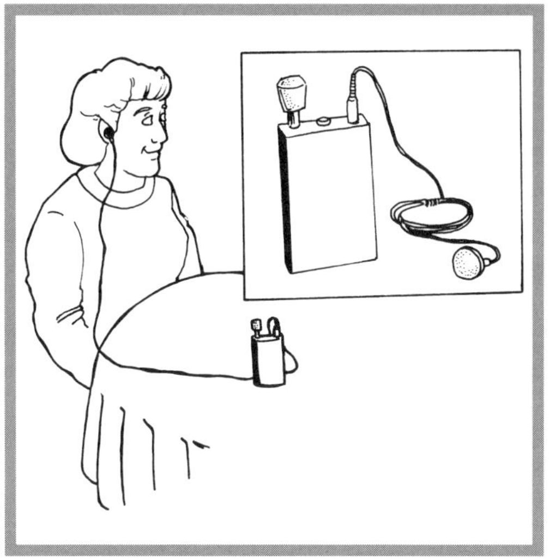

229

Personal sound amplifier
Table or pocket model
Mike-amplifier/cord/earphone
Battery powered

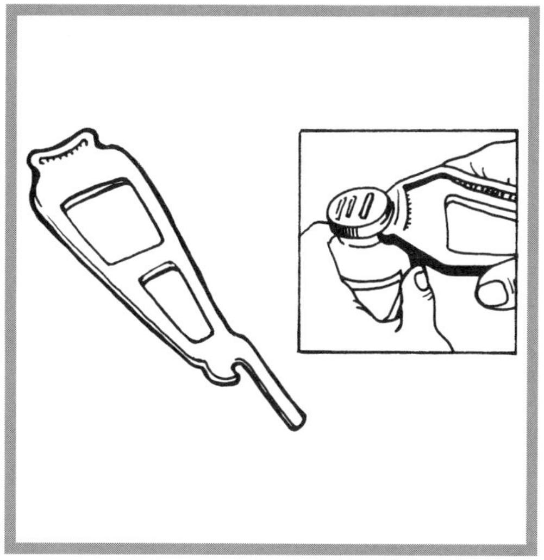

230

Pill bottle opener
Two hands needed to operate
Wedge lever

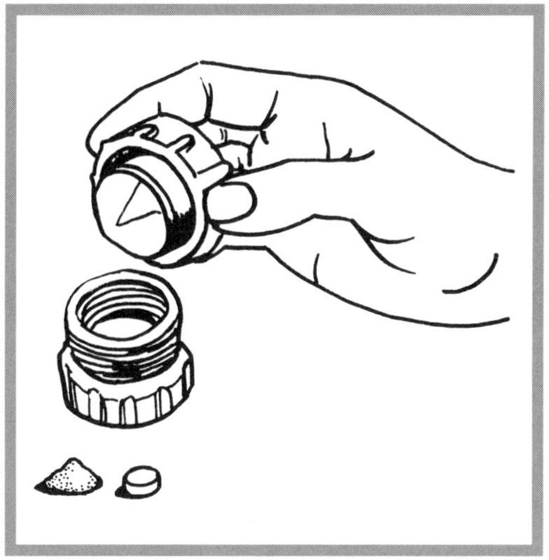

231

Pill crusher
Durable plastic
Twist operated

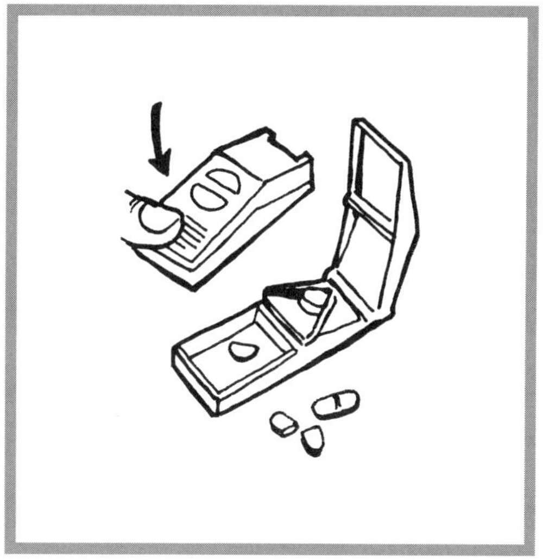

232

Pill splitter
Close lid to split
Does not crush pill

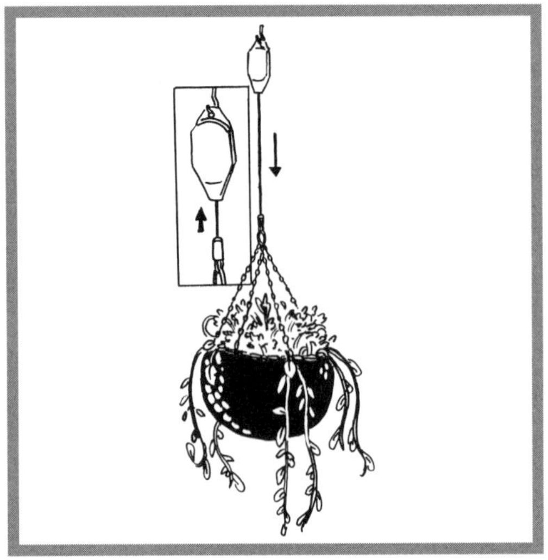

233

Plant hanger
Pulley operated
Holds 25 pounds
Lowers 3 feet

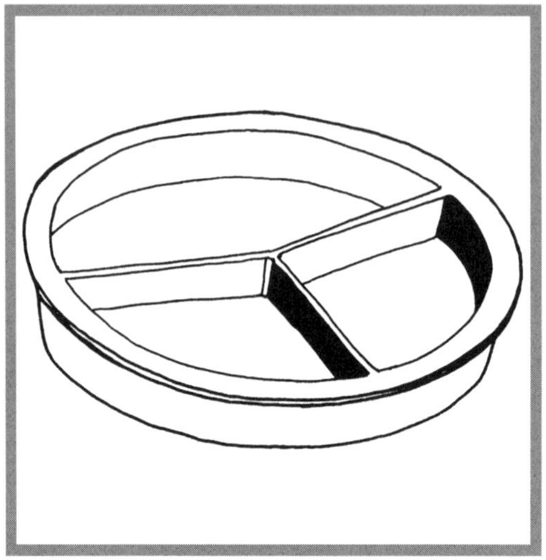

234

Plate
Divided 3 section high sided
10 inch round

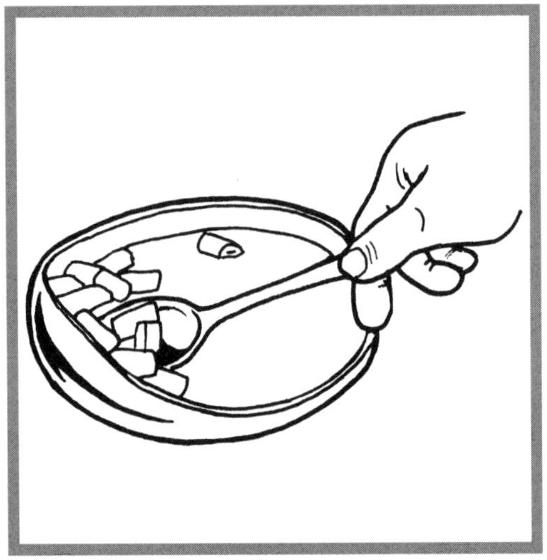

235

Plate
Scoop back or side

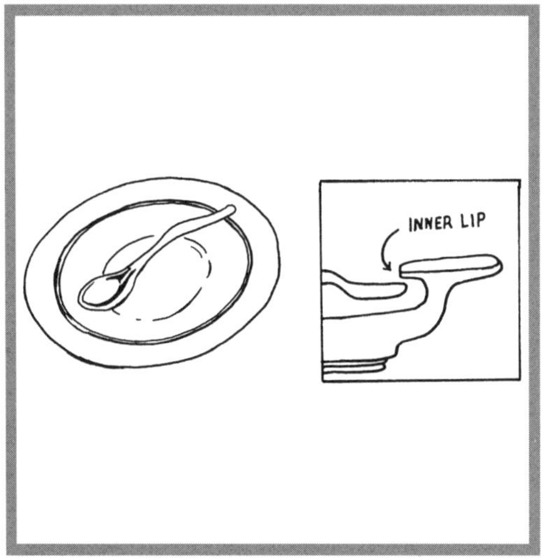

236

Plate
With inner lip

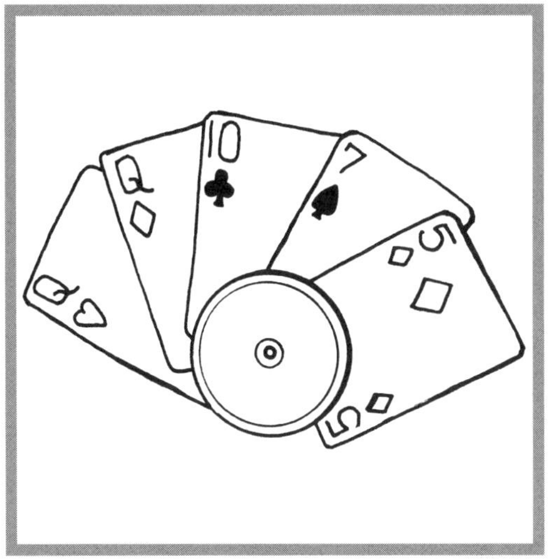

Playing card holder
Hand held spring
loaded disks

237

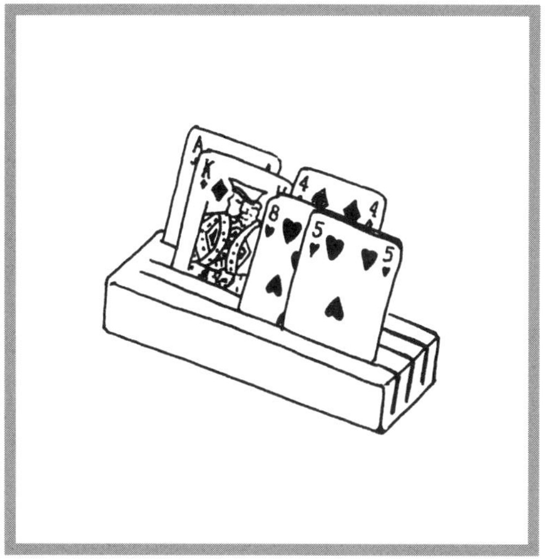

Playing card holder
Slotted block type
4 angled slots

238

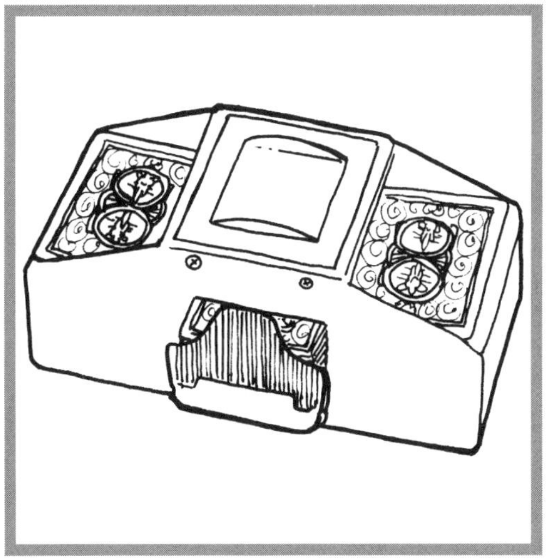

Playing card shuffler
One-deck
Battery powered

239

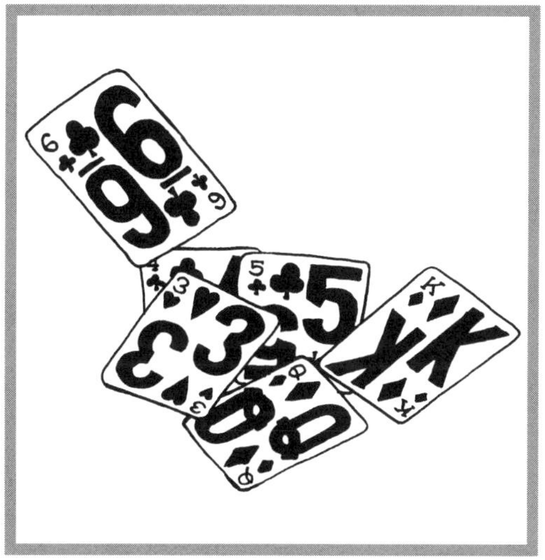

Playing cards
2-inch numbers
Poker sized cards
4 color codes

240

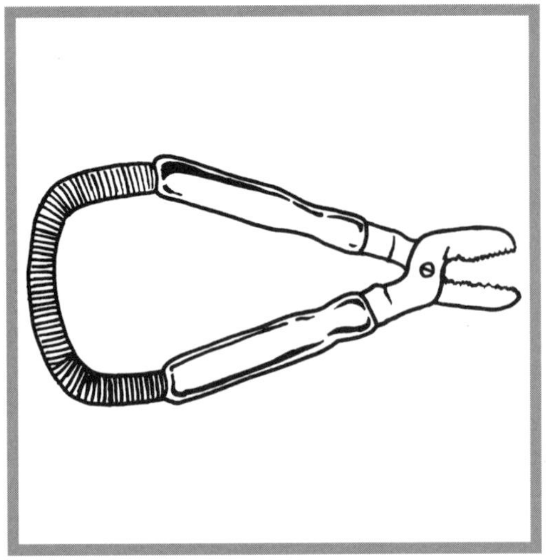

241

Pliers
Loop handle
Self-opening

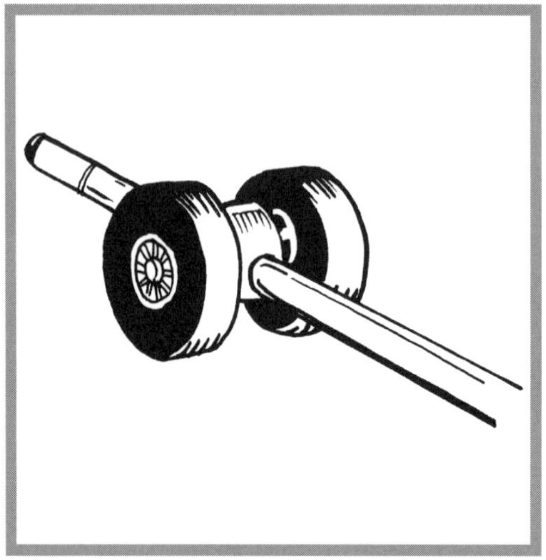

242

Pool cue bridge
Bridge on wheels
With fixed cue

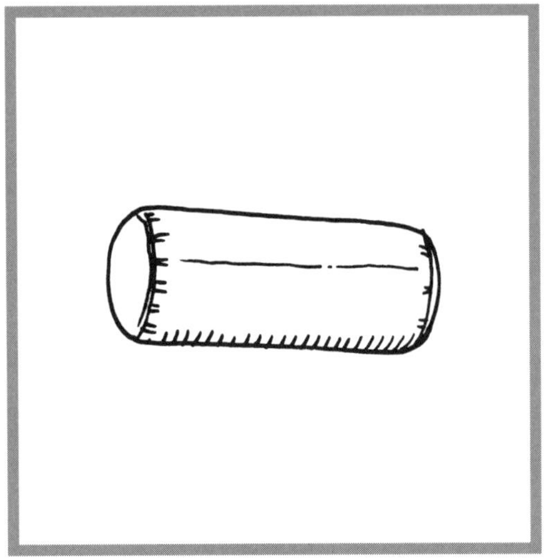

243

Positioning cushion
Bolster type
Firm

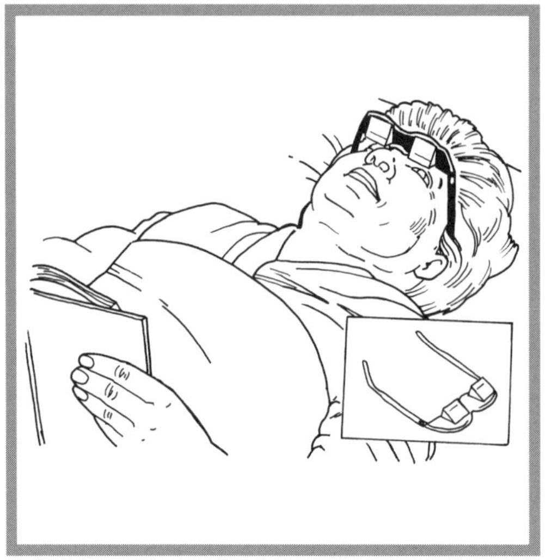

244

Prism glasses
Not over regular glasses
Up to 90 degree view

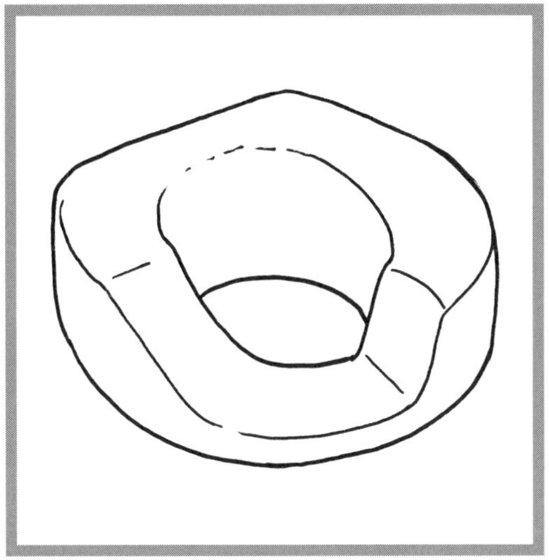

Raised toilet seat
4 inch height
No grips or rails
Right cut-out

245

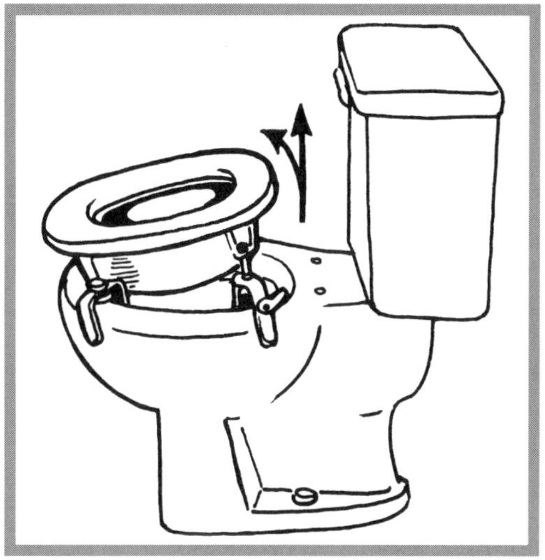

Raised toilet seat
Adjustable height
No grips or rails
Adjustable slope to front

246

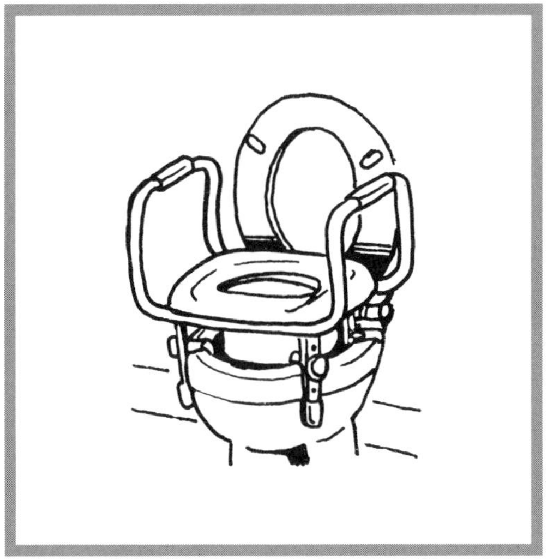

Raised toilet seat
Adjustable height
With hand rails
Doughnut seat

247

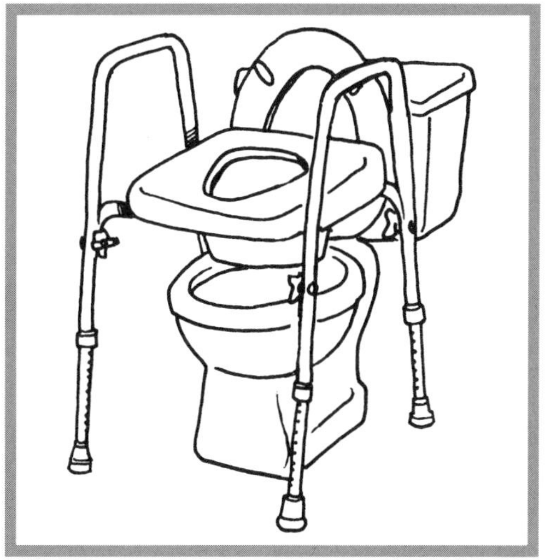

Raised toilet seat
Adjustable height
With hand rails

248

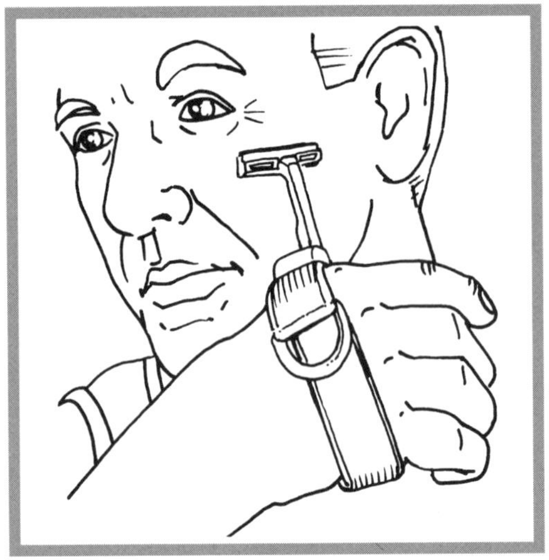

249

Razor holder
For Trac II razor
With palm cuff

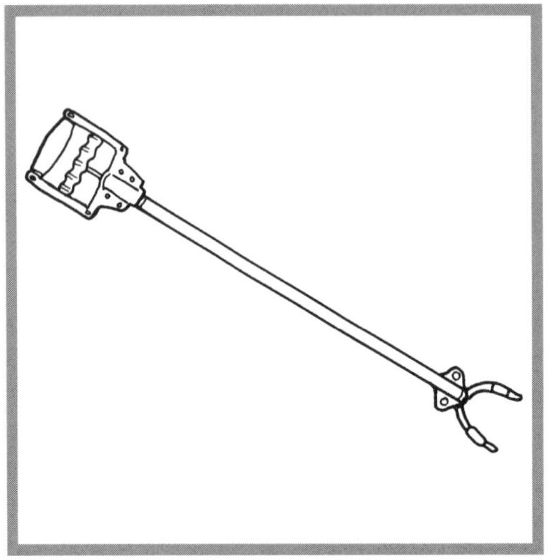

250

Reacher
D-grip
Squeeze operated horizontal jaws

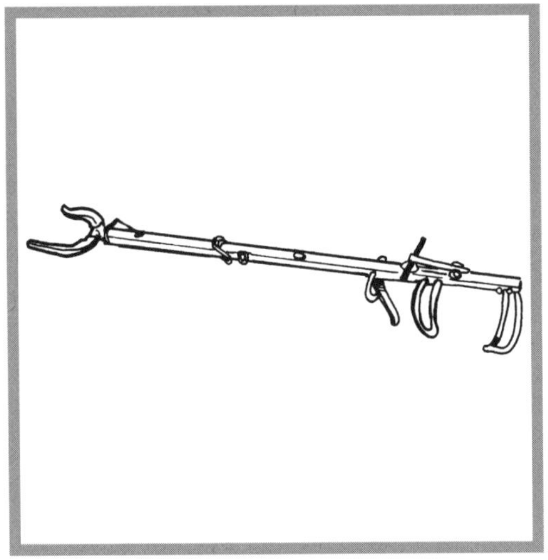

251

Reacher
No grip with wrist support
Wrist extension operated
Horizontal jaws

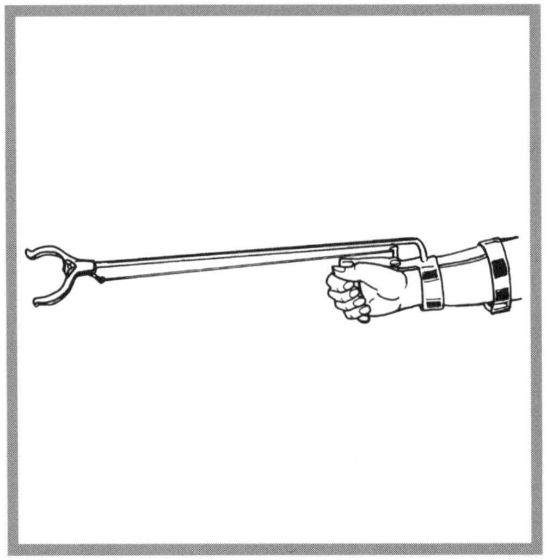

252

Reacher
No grip with wrist support
Wrist flexion operated
Horizontal jaws

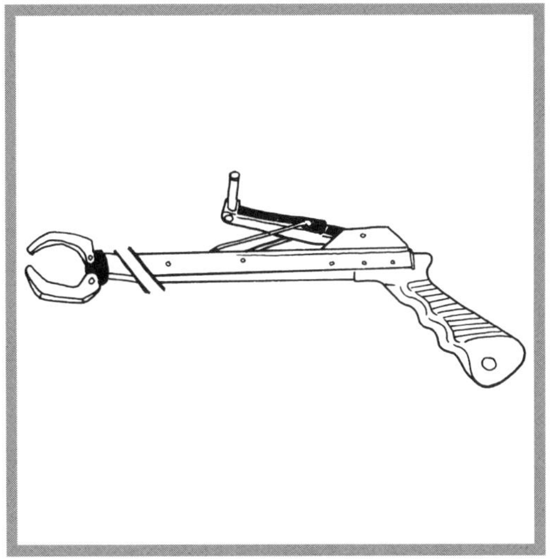

253

Reacher
Pistol grip
Lever operated

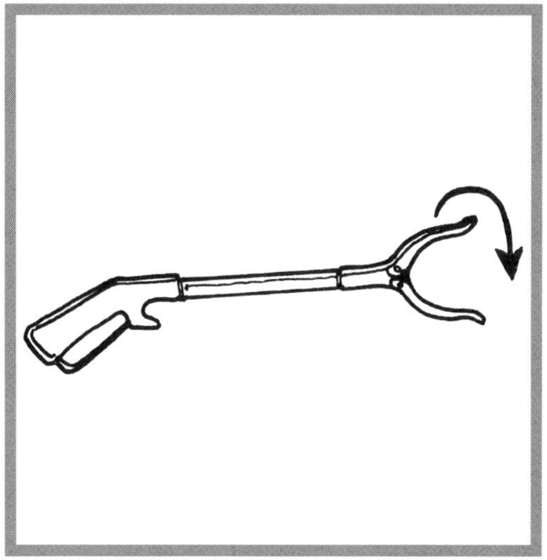

254

Reacher
Pistol grip
Squeeze operated
Rotating jaw - 18 inches long

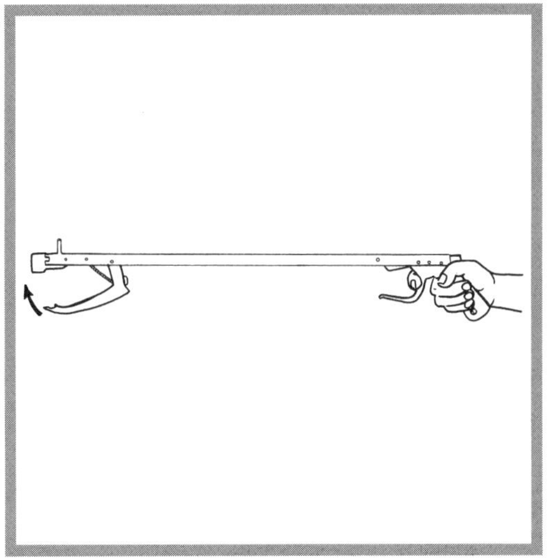

255

Reacher
Pistol grip
Trigger operated
Vertical jaw

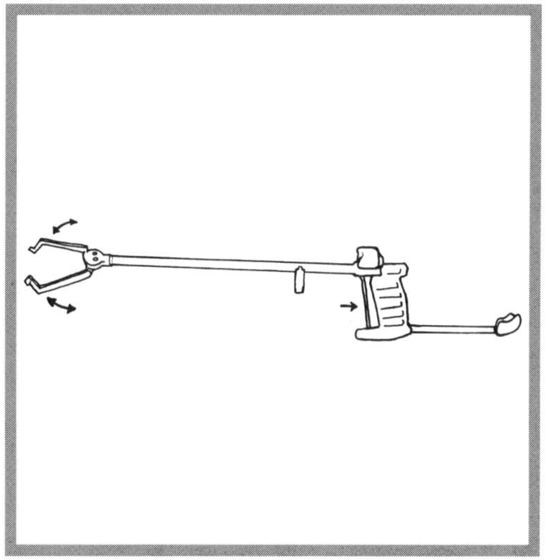

256

Reacher
Pistol grip with wrist support
Squeeze operated
Horizontal jaws

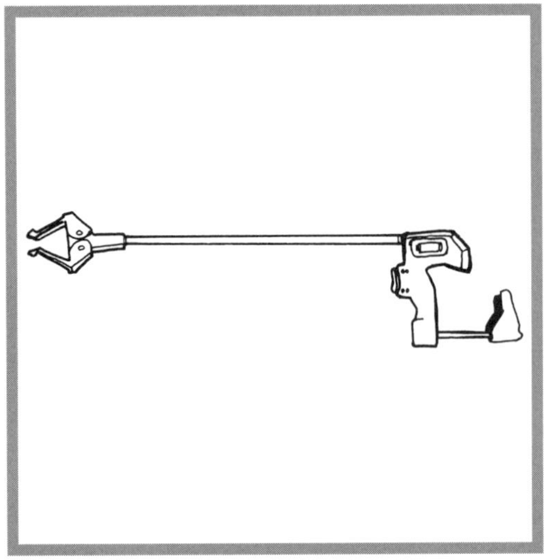

Reacher
Pistol grip with wrist support
Trigger operated
Horizontal jaws

257

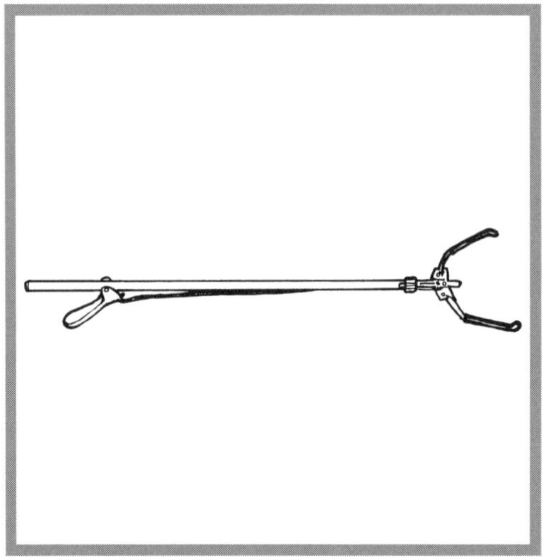

Reacher
Straight handle
Squeeze operated
Horizontal jaws

258

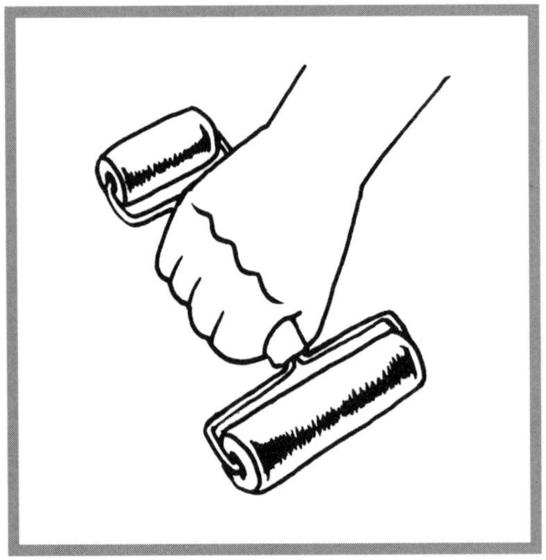

Rolling pin
One-hand operated
2 rollers
Single handle

259

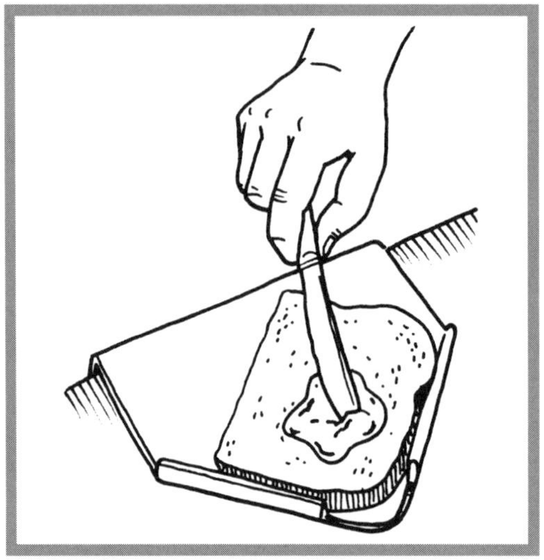

Sandwich board
One-handed
With corner guards

260

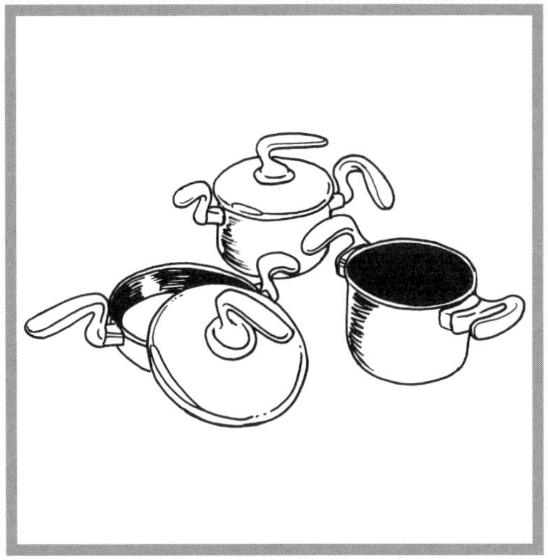

Saucepan
Curled handle grips
Allows two-hand lift

261

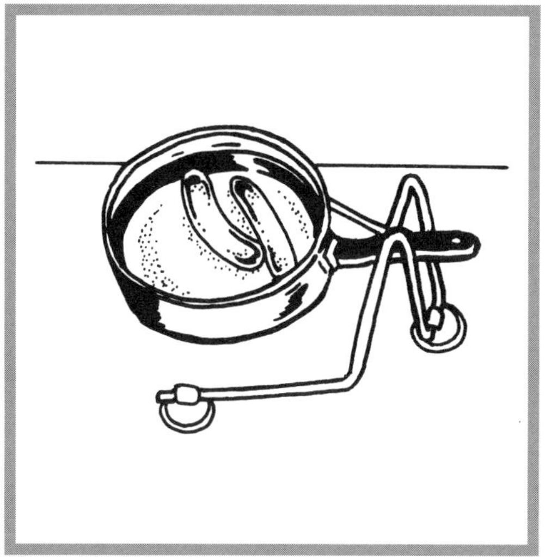

Saucepan stabilizer
Stovetop
Suction feet
For handles 5 inches high

262

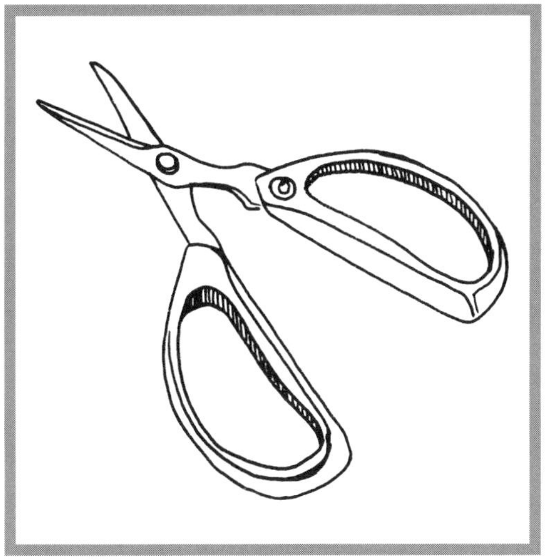

Scissors
Not self-opening
Large loop handles

263

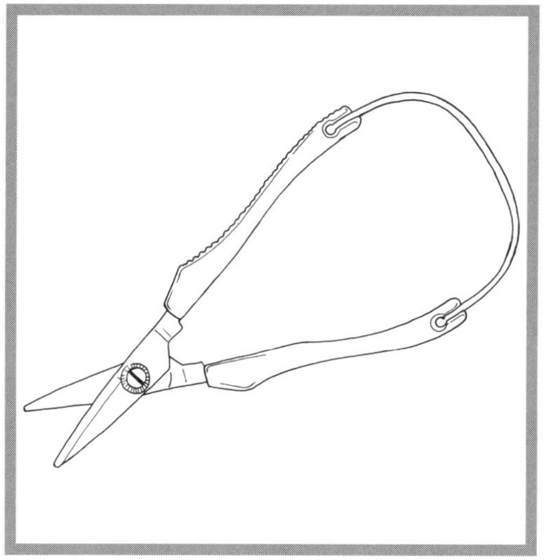

Scissors
Self-opening
End loop

264

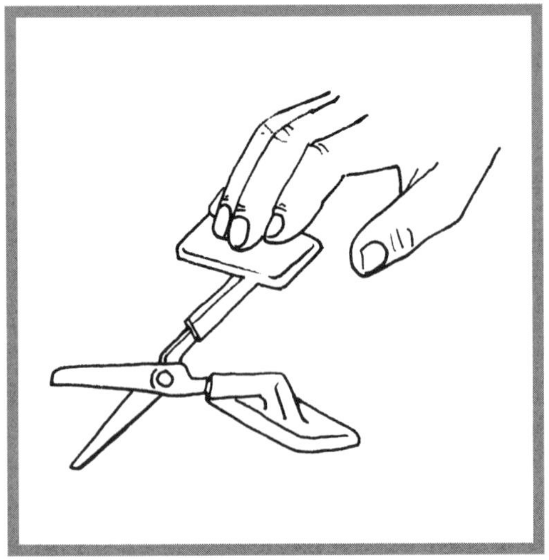

265

Scissors
Self-opening
Spring opening
Press down to cut

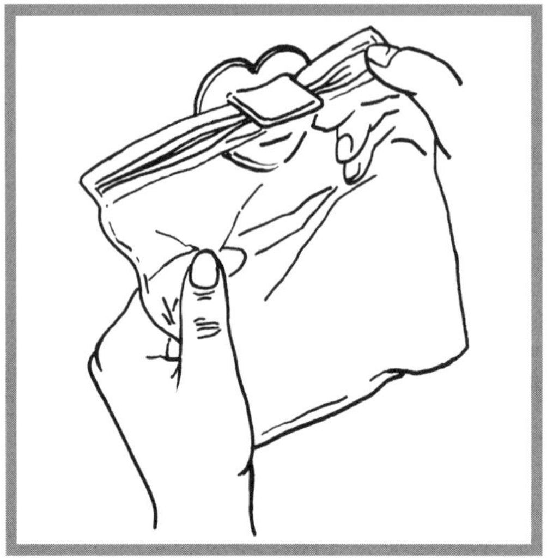

266

Sealer for plastic bags
For zip-type bags
Wall mounted
Pull-through operation

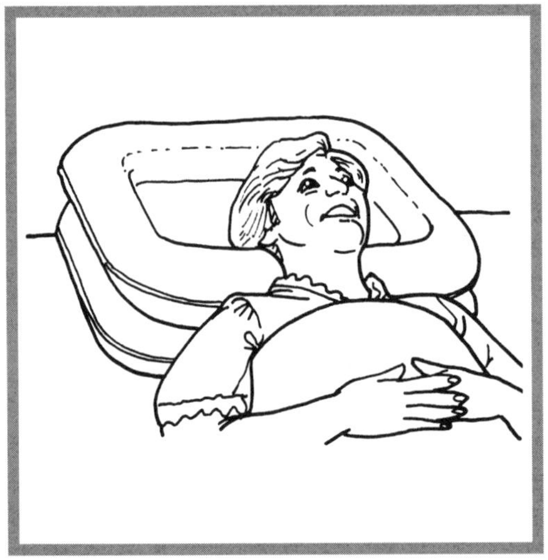

267

Shampoo basin
Inflatable
With drain
28 X 24 X 6 inches

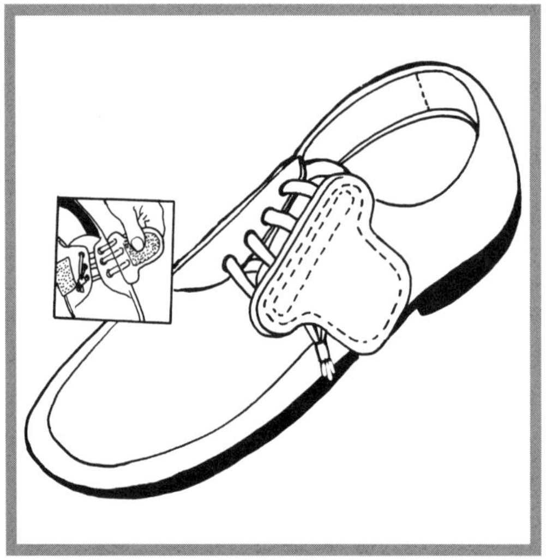

268

Shoe lace fastener
One-hand operated
Four eyelet
Velcro closure

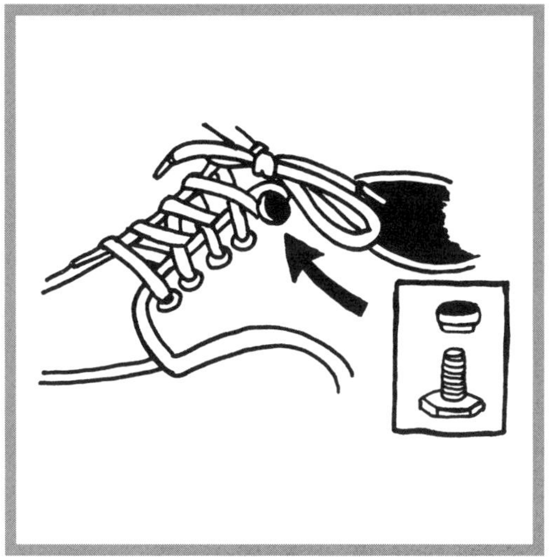

269

Shoe lace fastener
Screw button top lacing hole
Lace left tied
Slack wrapped on button

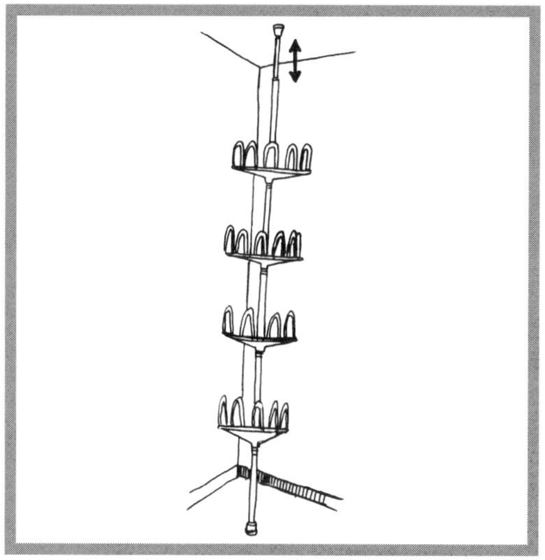

270

Shoe organizer
Tension pole mount
Manual rotating

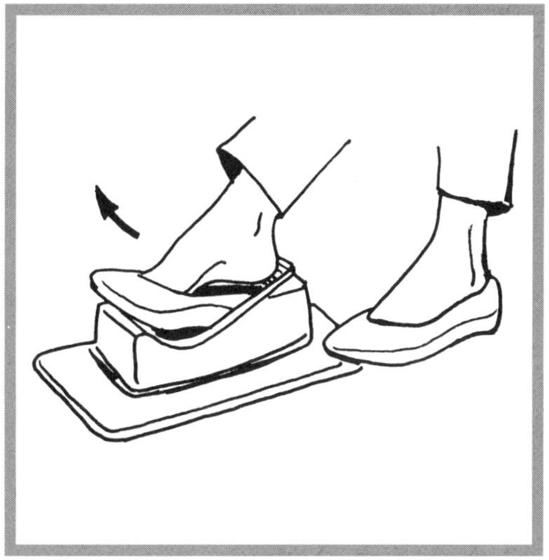

271

Shoe remover
Hands free
Boot-jack type

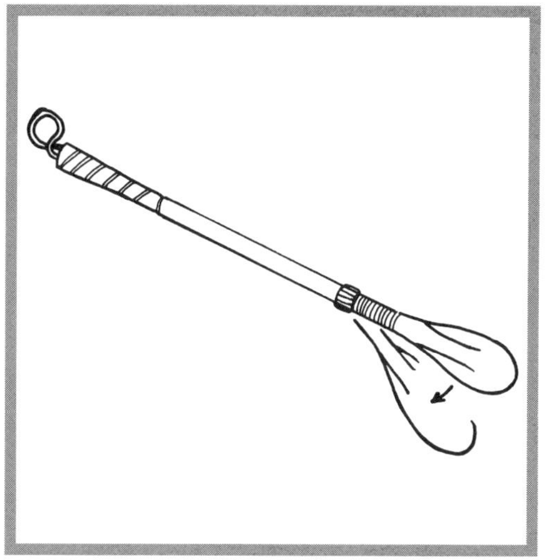

272

Shoehorn
Long handle, 24 inch
Flex spring above blade
Metal blade

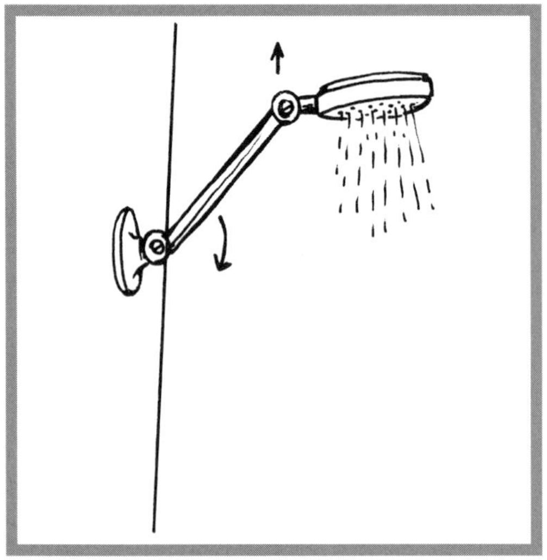

273

Shower arm and head
Adjustable
Attaches to shower arm
Adjustable 9 in pipe

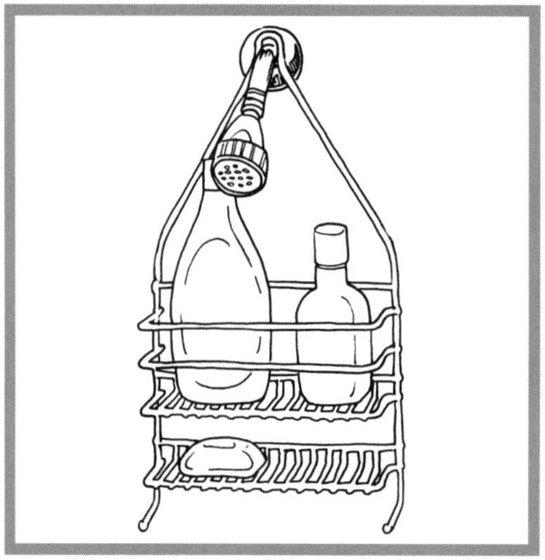

274

Shower caddy
Two shelf
Hangs on shower head

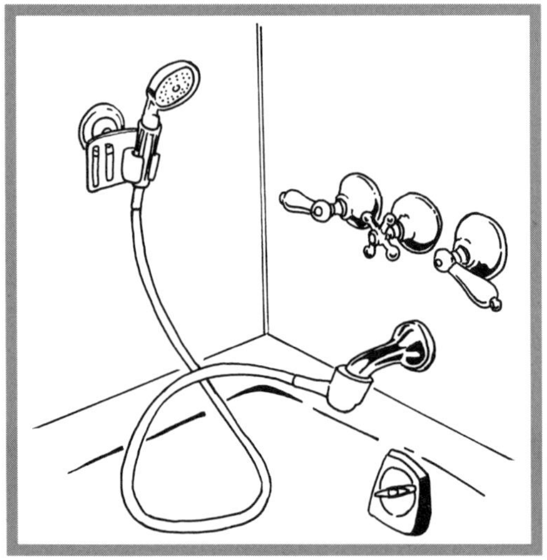

275

Shower hose and head
Hand held
Attaches to faucet
Suction cup bracket

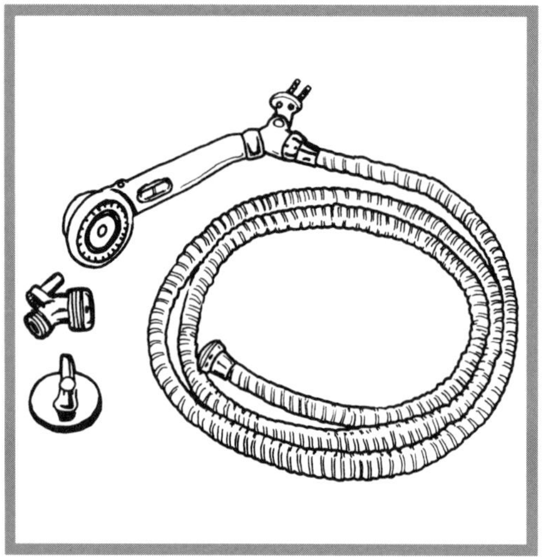

276

Shower hose and head
Hand held
Attaches to shower arm

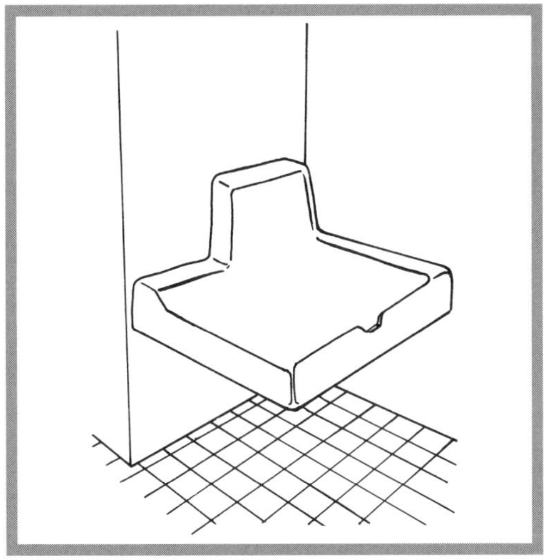

277

Shower seat
Wall mounted
Fixed height

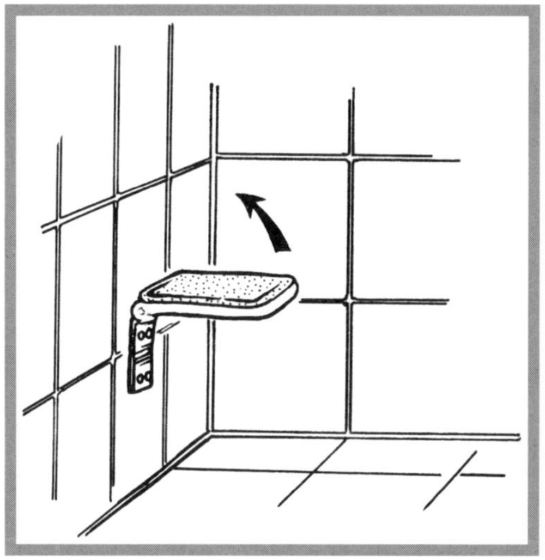

278

Shower seat
Wall mounted
Folding
Padded solid seat

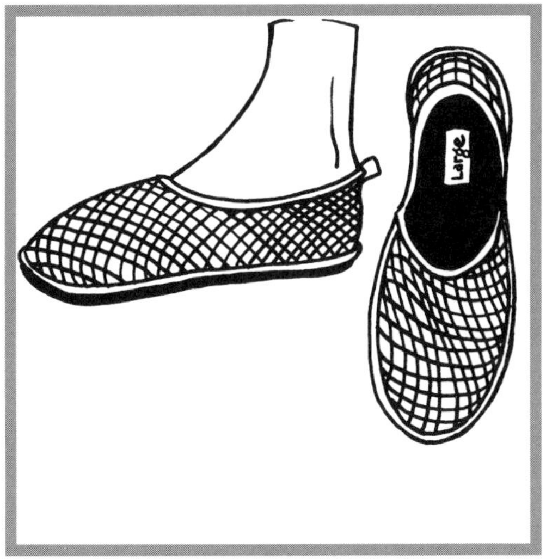

279

Shower slippers
Men's
Large
Nylon mesh uppers

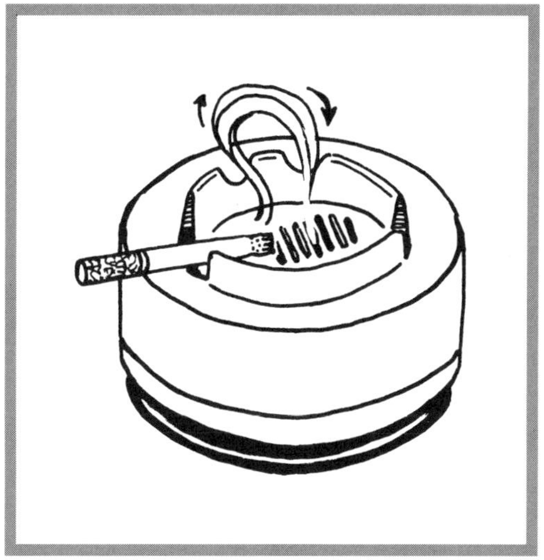

280

Smokeless ashtray
Charcoal filter
Table model
Battery powered

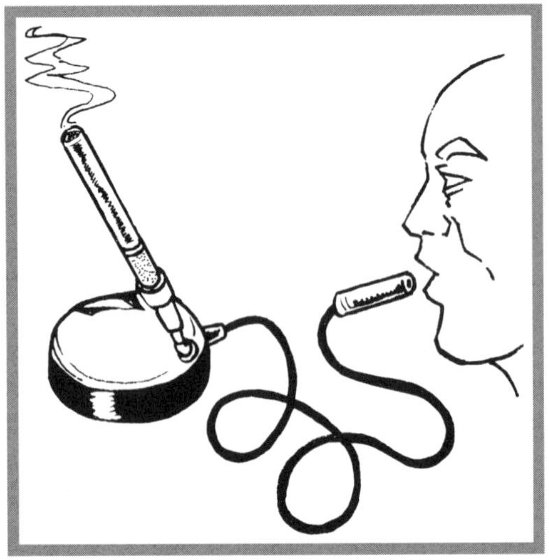

Smoker's aid
Tube & mouthpiece & holder
36 inch tube on tray
Holder for cigarette

281

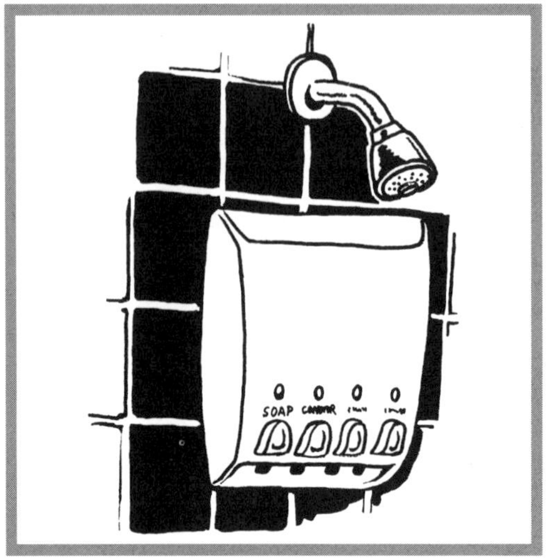

Soap dispenser
One-hand operated/wall mounted
4 section
Dispenses pre-measured amounts

282

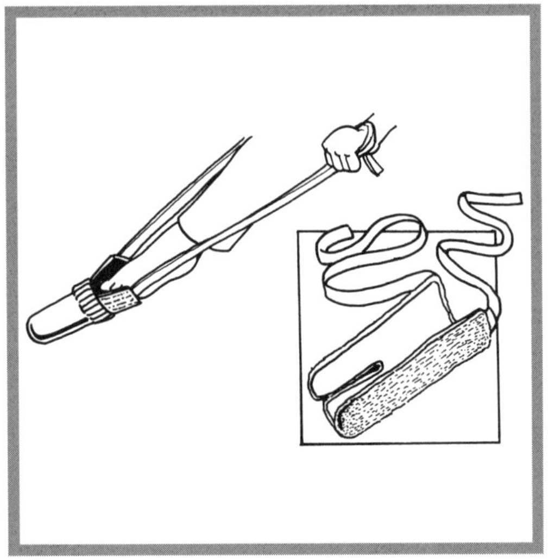

Sock aid
2 hand use
Cord handle
Flexible trough

283

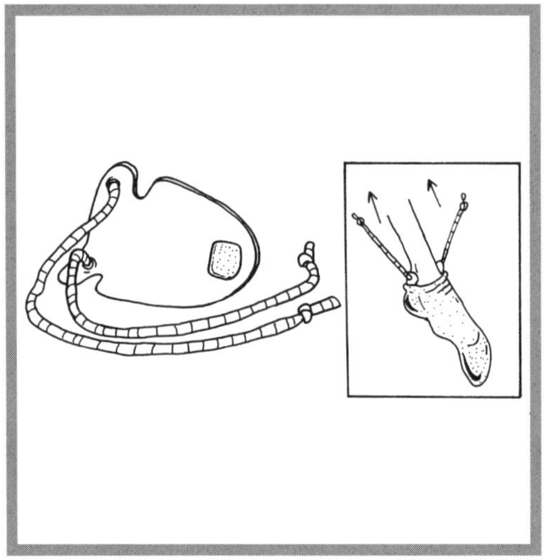

Sock aid
2 hand use
Cord handle
Floppy trough

284

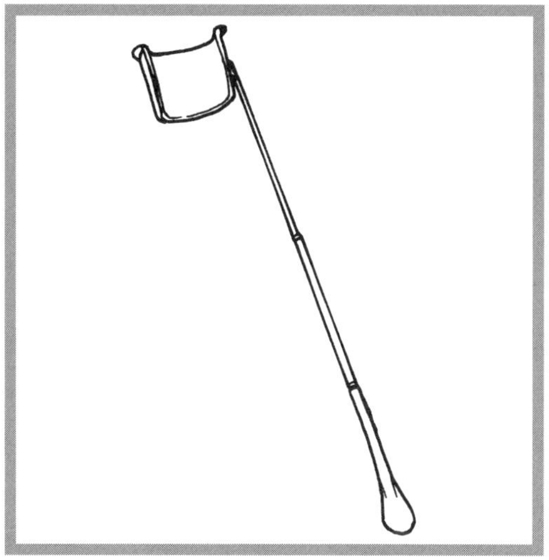

Sock aid with shoehorn
2 hands to load
24 inch shaft
Rigid short trough

285

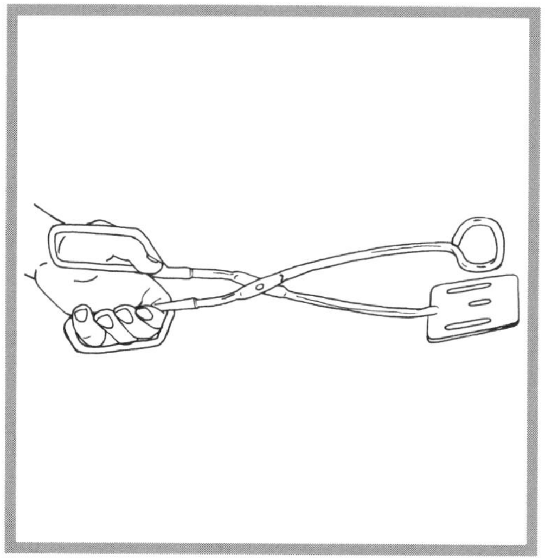

Spatula/tong combination
Extra long handles
Nylon coated handles

286

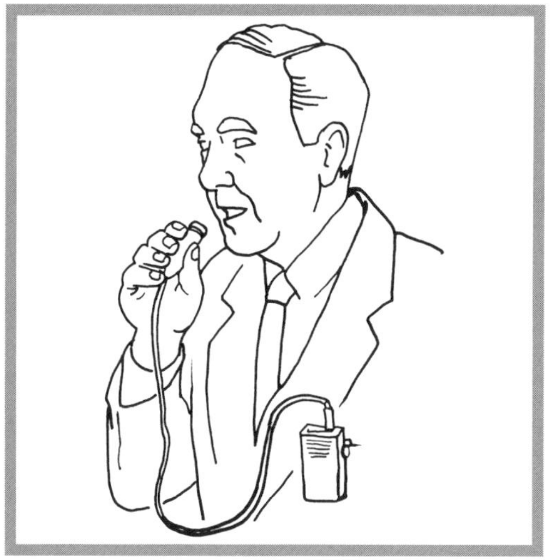

Speech amplifier
Breast pocket model/handheld m
Microphone/amplifier/ speaker
Battery powered

287

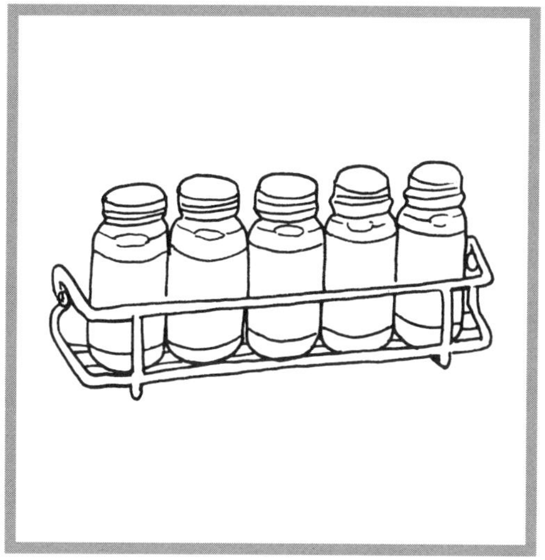

Spice rack
Inside cabinet door
Wire rack
One tier

288

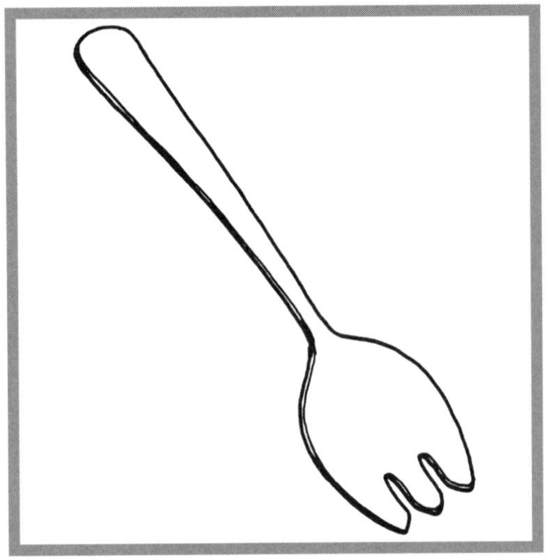

289

Spork
Standard handle

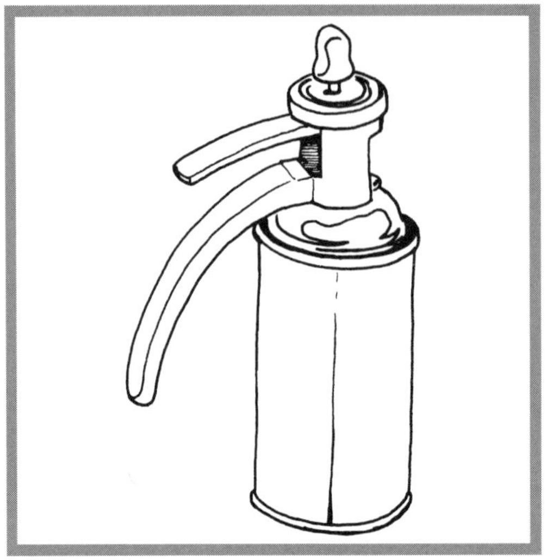

290

Spray can aid
Dispenser handle
Adjustable trigger operated
Large handle

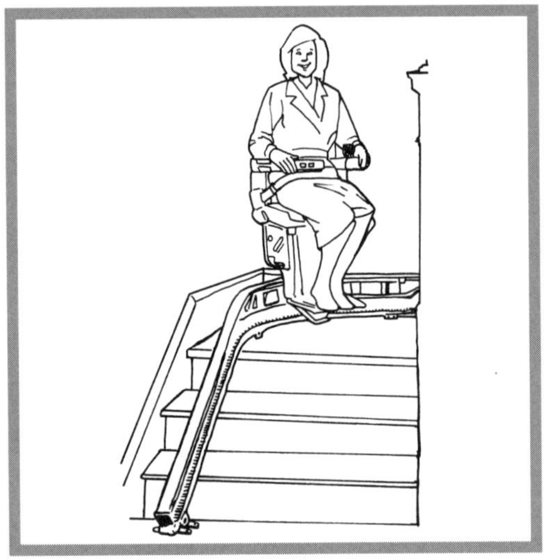

291

Stair lift
Can fit curved staircases
Can have landing
AC powered

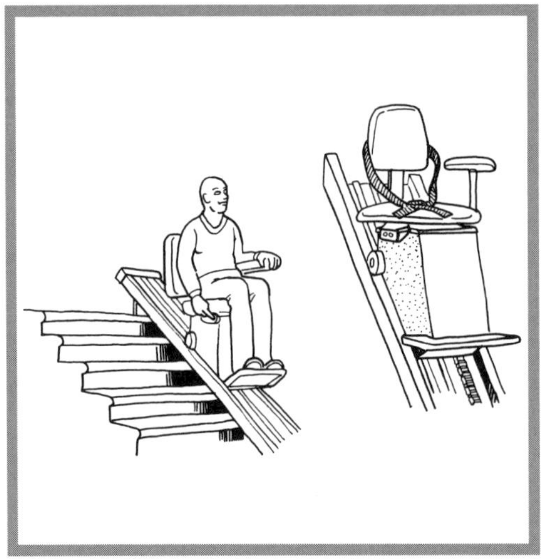

292

Stair lift
Fits straight staircases
Cannot have landing

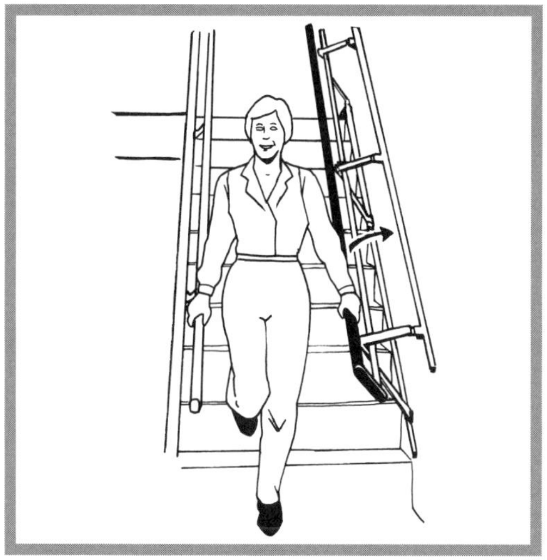

Stair rail extender
Folds out from wall
Narrows the span between rails
Provides second rail

293

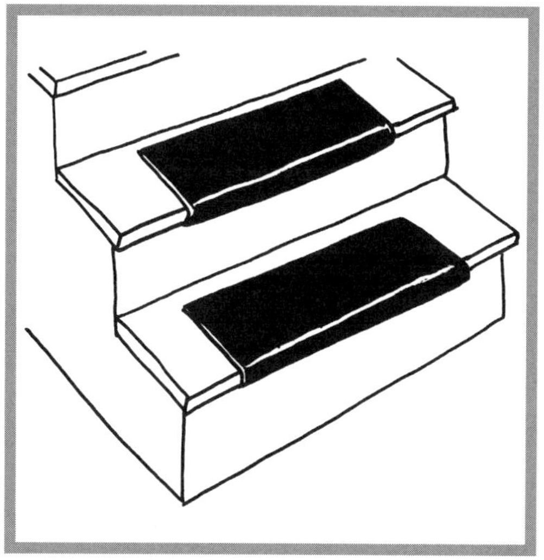

Stair treads
Rubber
10-1/4 x 24 inches

294

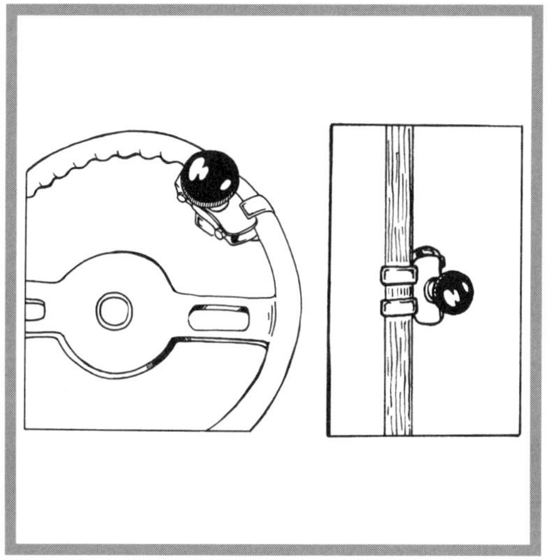

Steering wheel knob
Clamp-on
Spinner knob grip
Can clamp to straight handle

295

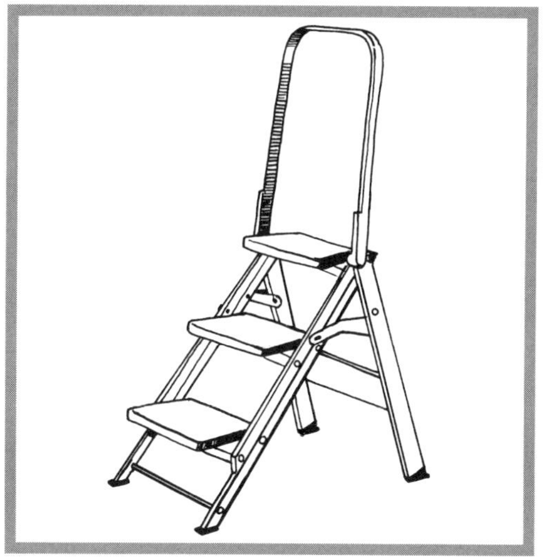

Step ladder
With top hand rail
3 step

296

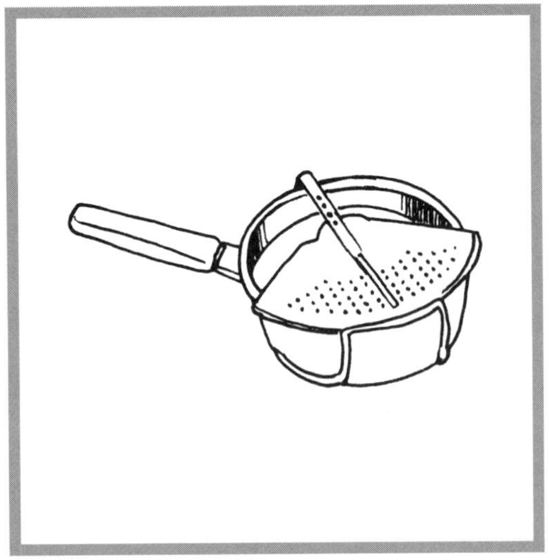

297

Strainer
Attaches to cooking pot
Adjustable to pot size

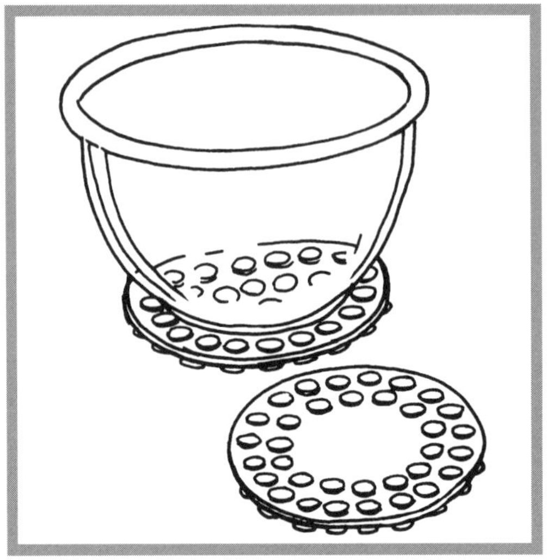

298

Suction disk
Double sided
Multi-cup general
2-1/2 inch

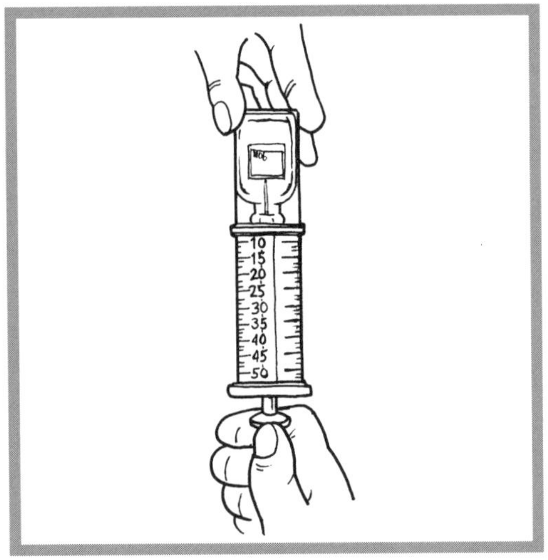

299

Syringe holder
With magnifier
Insulin
One-piece

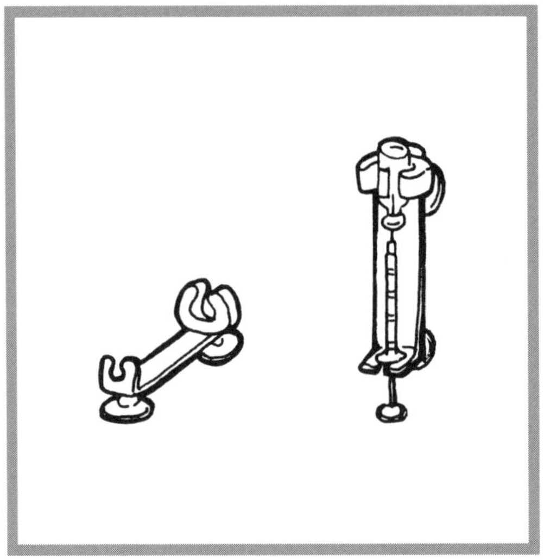

300

Syringe stabilizer
Suction cup base
Holds bottle & guides syringe
Vertical or horizontal mount

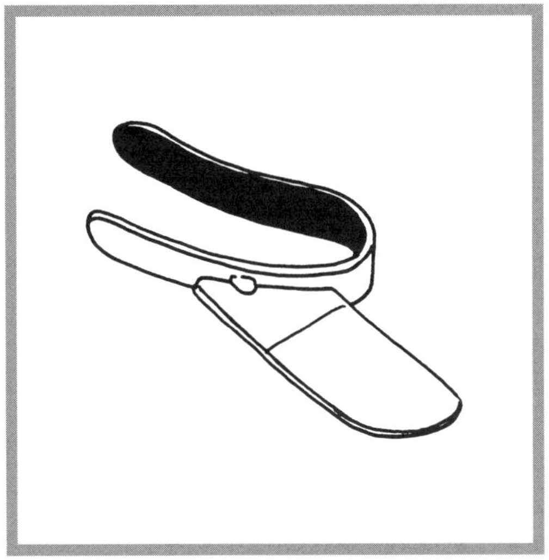

301

Table knife
On palmar clip
Rocker blade

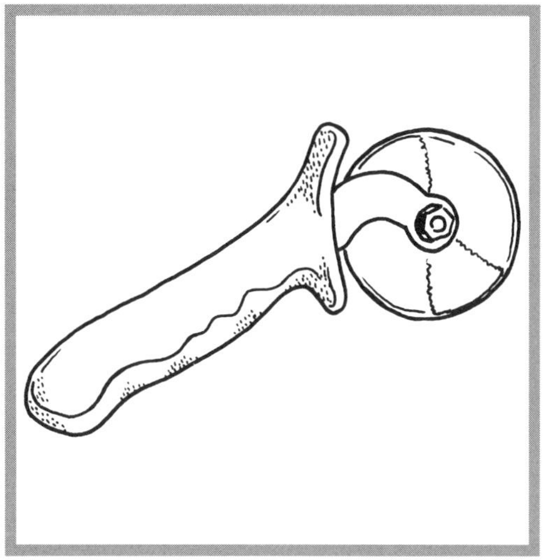

302

Table knife
Straight handle
Rolling blade

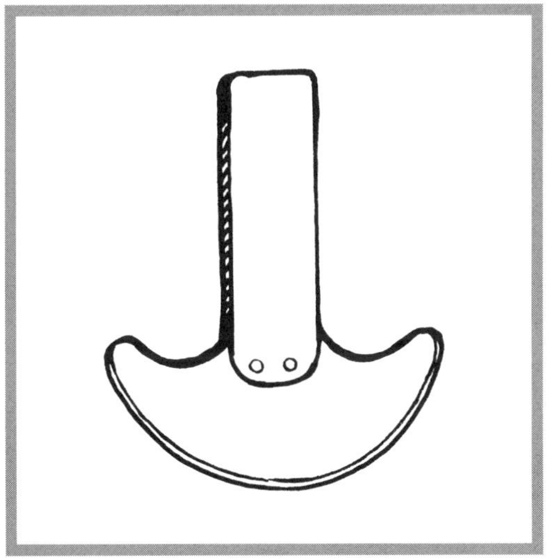

303

Table/kitchen knife
Vertical cylinder handle
Crescent blade
Wooden handle

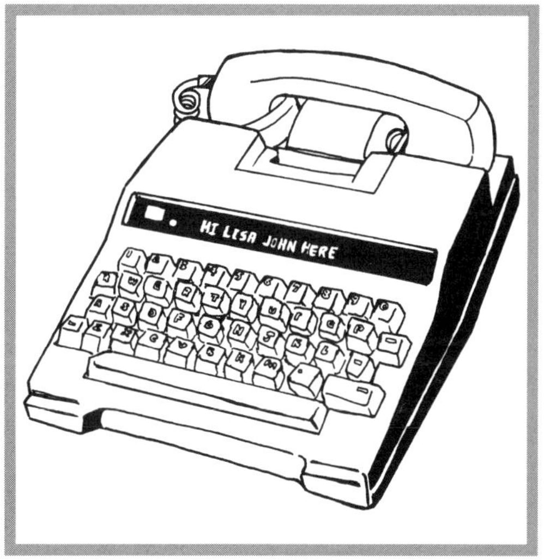

304

TDD
Auto-answer
20 character 1 line display
Signal indicator

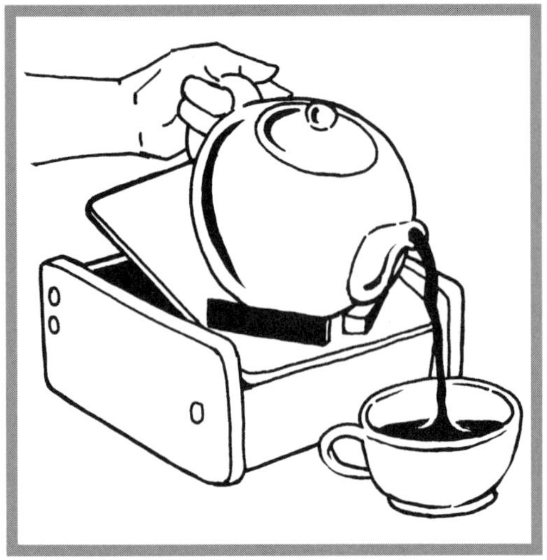

Teapot pourer stand
Holds common teapots
Tilts teapot
Low effort

305

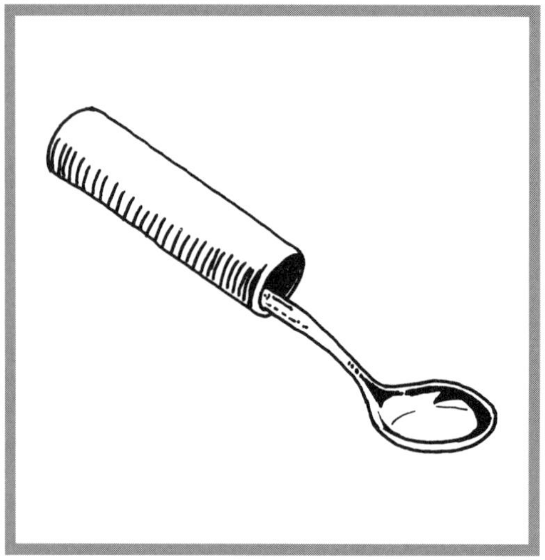

Teaspoon
Built-up tube handle

306

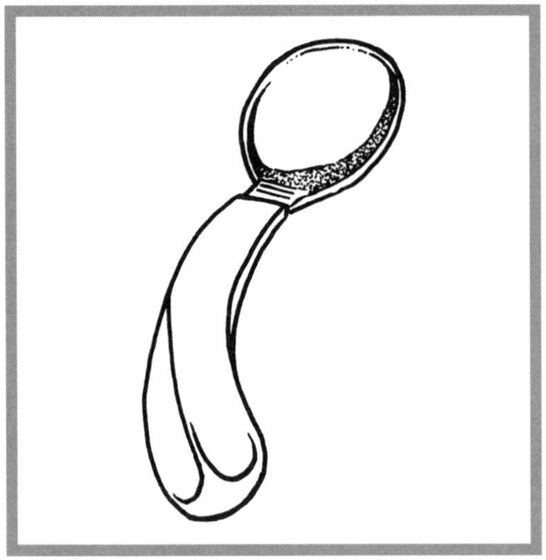

Teaspoon
Curved handle
Shallow bowl
For Left hand

307

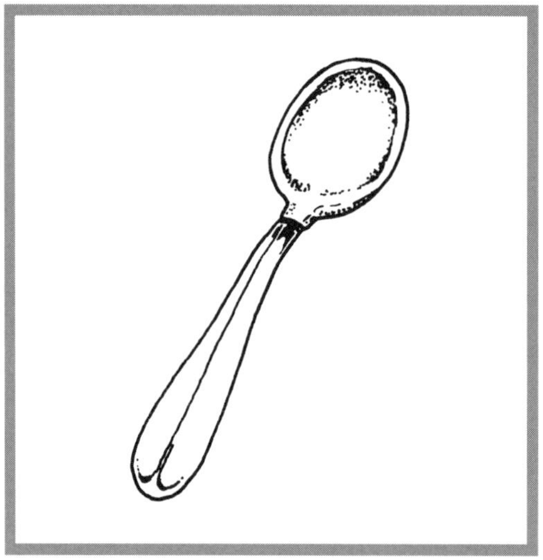

Teaspoon
Standard handle
Soft plastic coated bowl

308

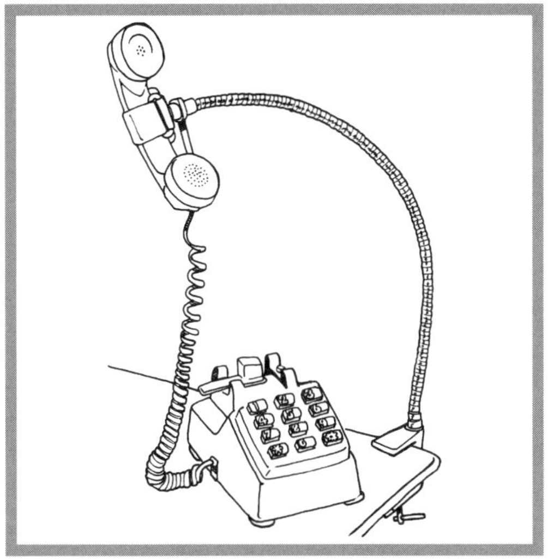

Telephone aid
Gooseneck holder
Table clamp
24 inch/adjustable

309

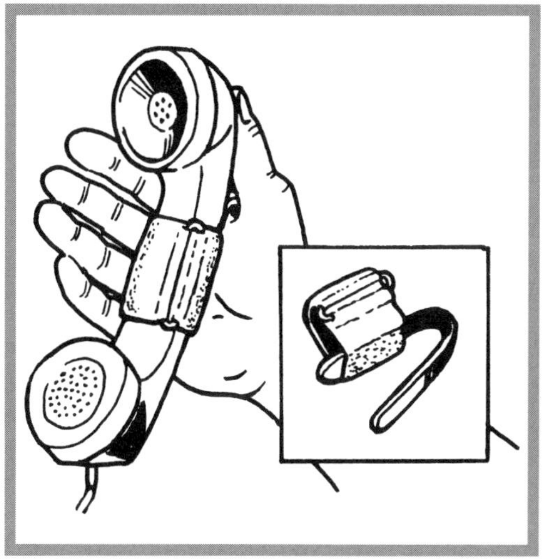

Telephone aid
Palmar clip holder
Fits over palm
Velcro to receiver

310

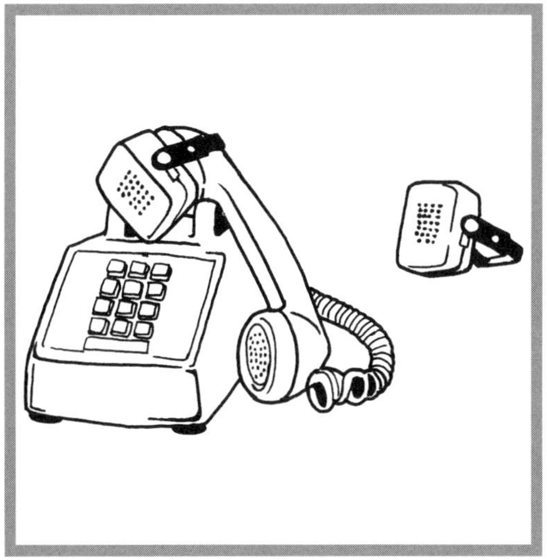

Telephone amplifier
Snap-on module
Slips over receiver

311

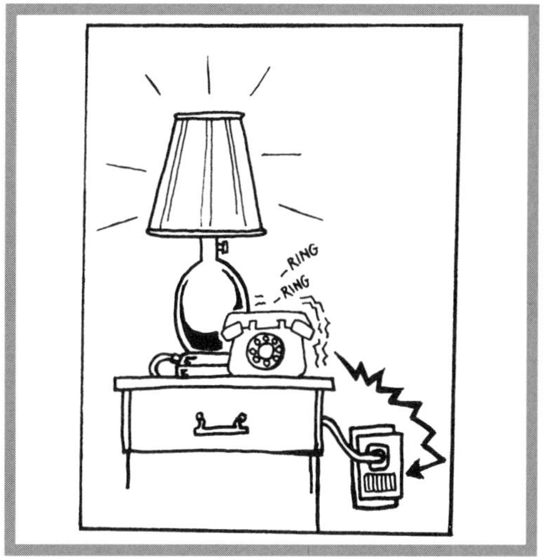

Telephone signaling device
Activates any lamp
Modular jacks

312

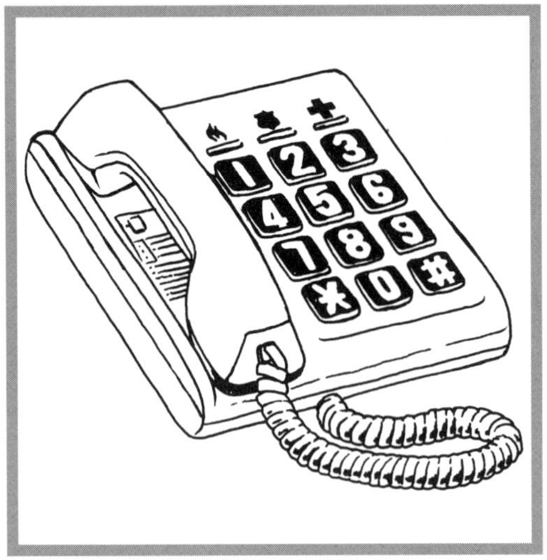

313

Telephone with big buttons
Buttons on phone base

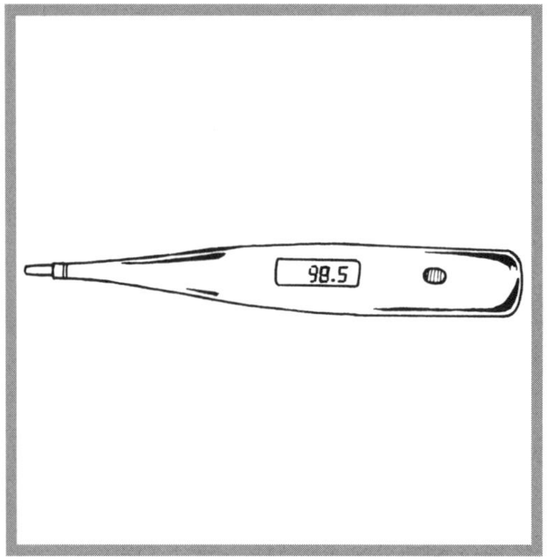

314

Thermometer
Clinical
Small LED readout

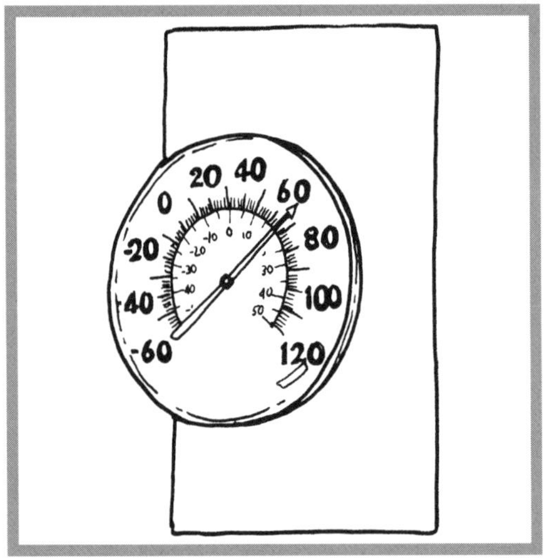

315

Thermometer
Outdoor
Large numbers
18 inch diameter

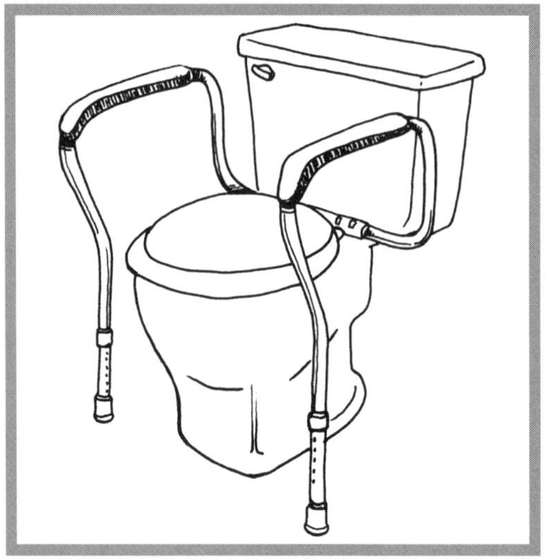

316

Toilet armrest frame
Attaches to toilet
Adjustable height

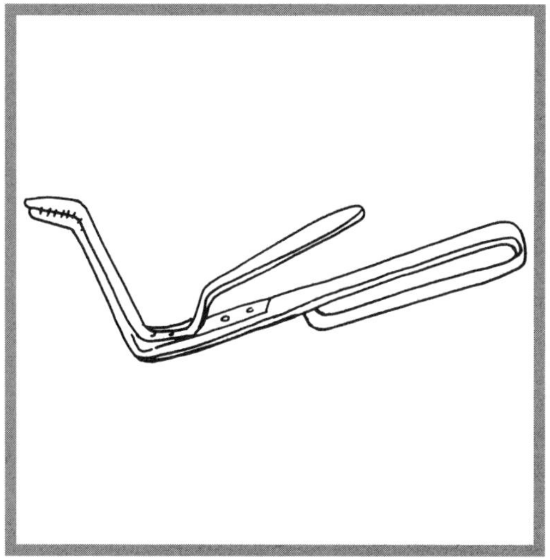

Toilet tissue aid
Angled handle
Spring clip

317

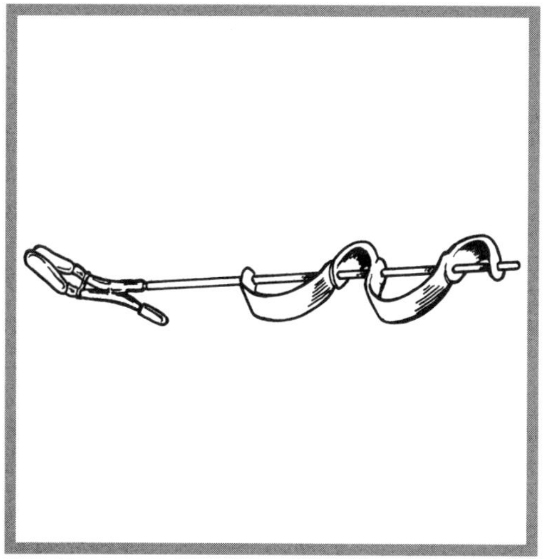

Toilet tissue aid
Hand loops on handle
Spring clips
Plastic clips

318

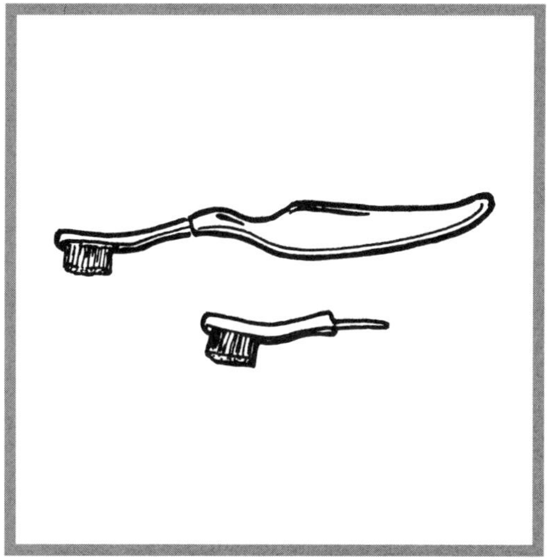

Toothbrush
Built-up handle
Includes 6 heads

319

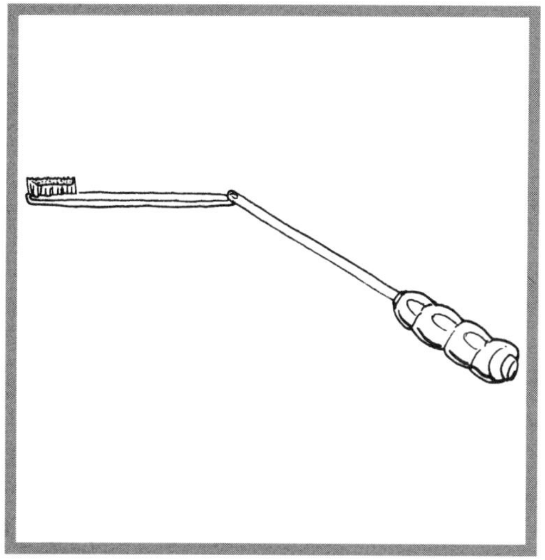

Toothbrush
Long handle
Folding handle
Adjustable angle

320

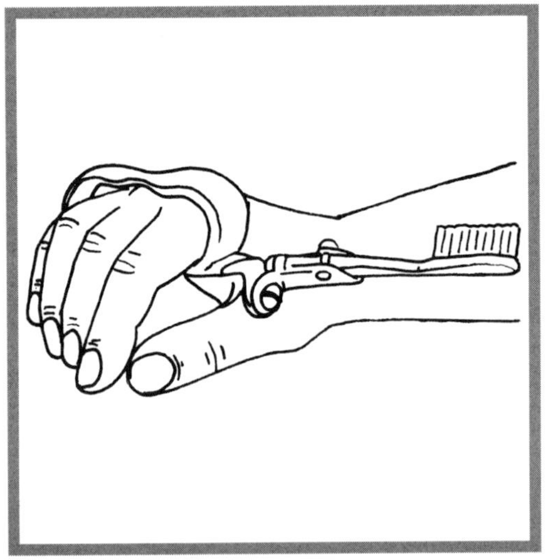

Toothbrush
On horizontal palm cuff
Self-rotating

321

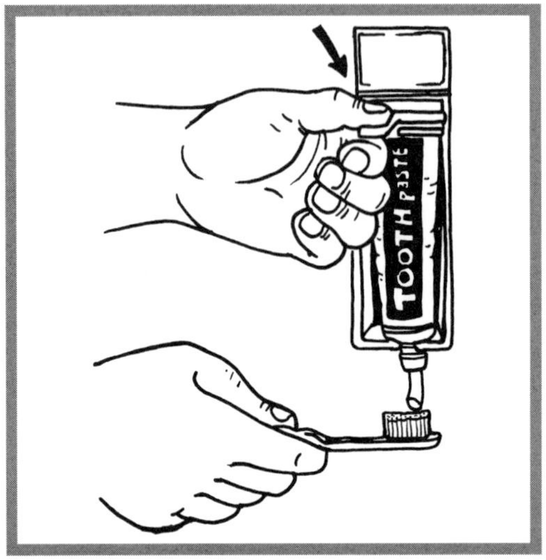

Toothpaste dispenser
One-hand operation
Push-down actuated
Accepts standard tubes

322

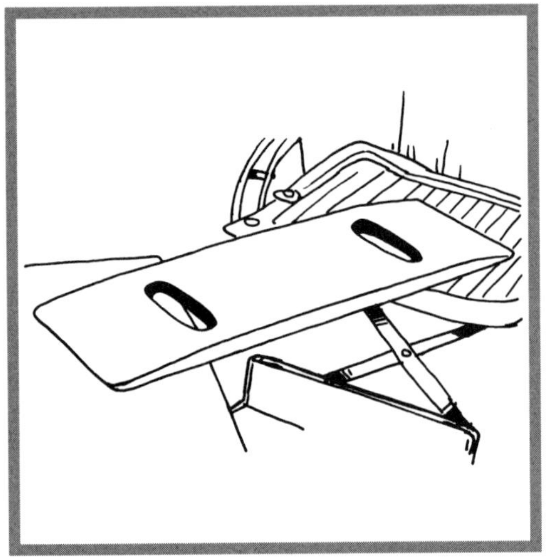

Transfer board
Two hand slots
Tapered ends

323

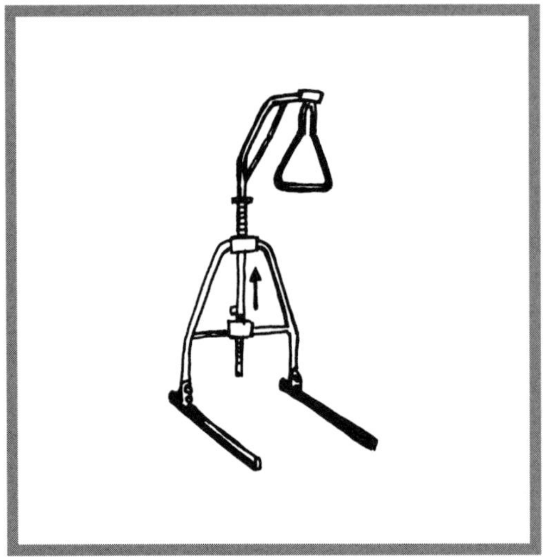

Trapeze bar
Free standing frame
Adjustable height
45 inch opening legs

324

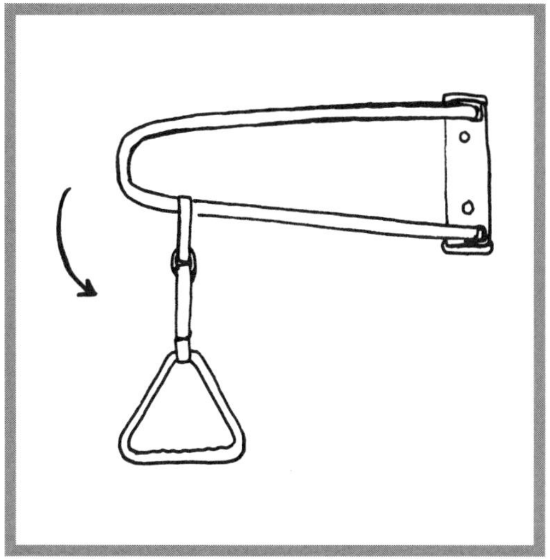

Trapeze bar
On wall mount
Adjusts to 6 angles
Pivots on wall mount

325

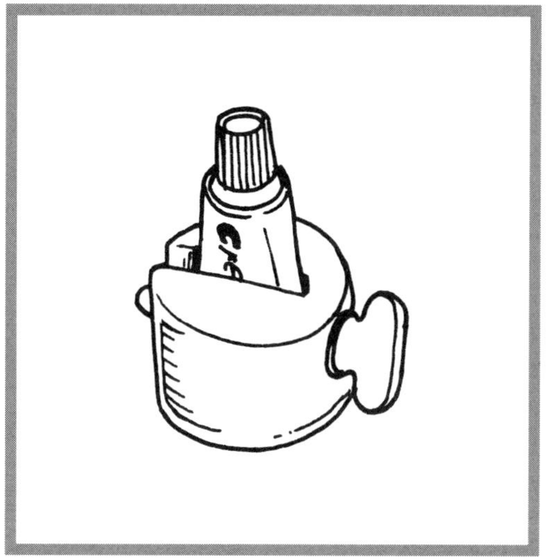

Tube squeezer
Twist-key operated

326

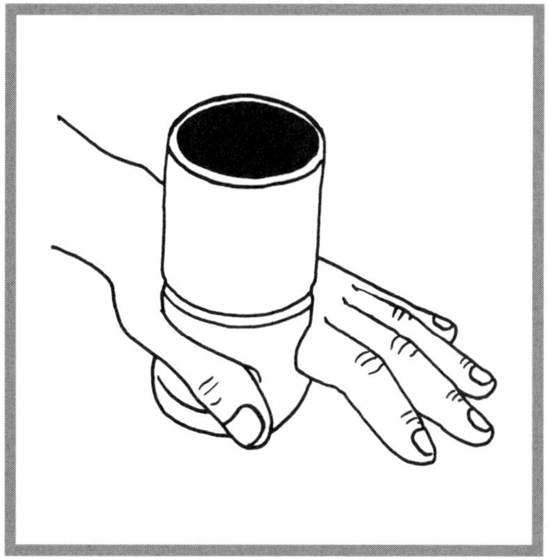

Tumbler
Pedestal grip
No lid

327

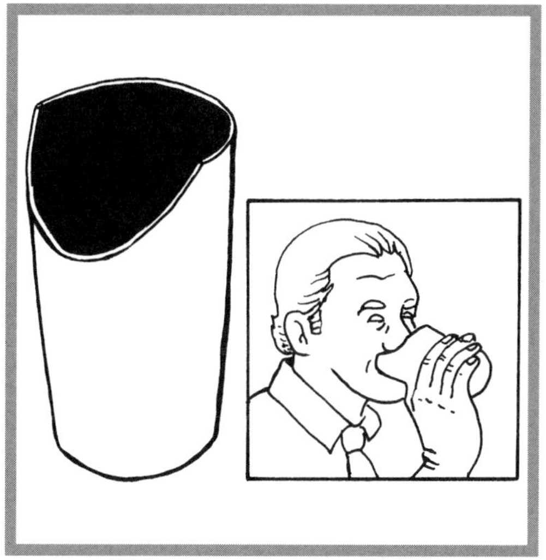

Tumbler with nose cut-out
No handle
No lid

328

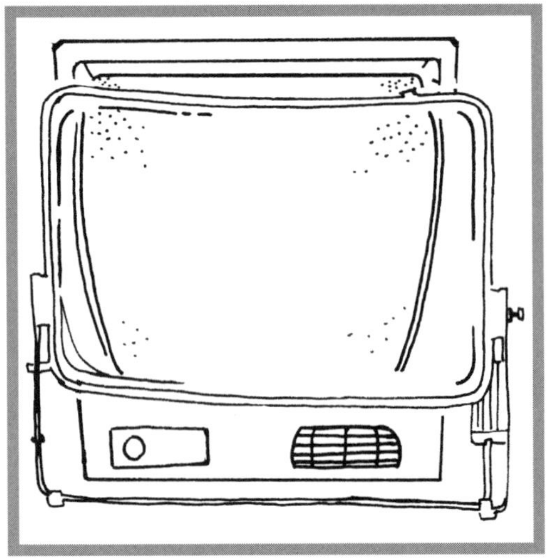

329

TV magnifier
Fits 17-19 inch screens
Enlarges to 25 inch
Adjustable free standing frame

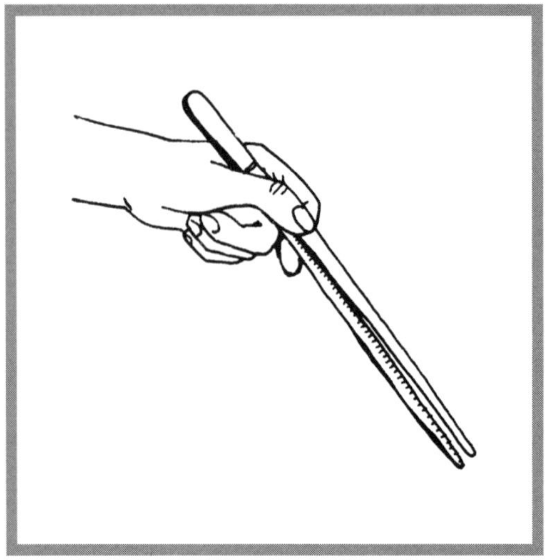

330

Tweezers
10-inch

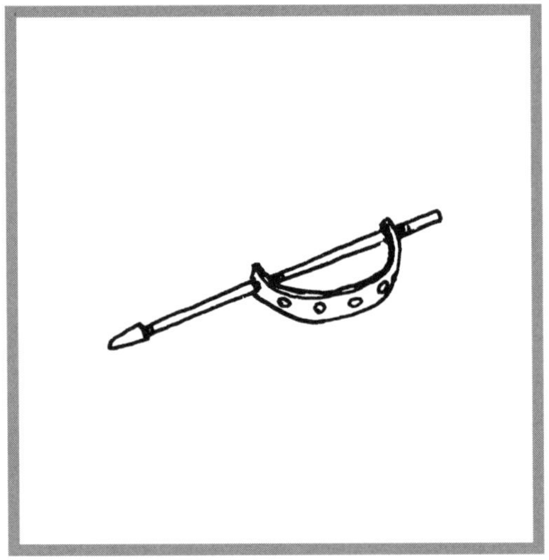

331

Typing aid
Hand-held stick
Adjustable loop either hand

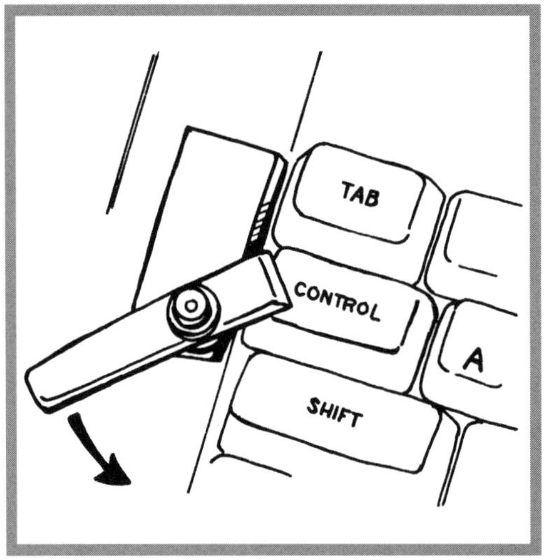

332

Typing aid
Lever key-lockdown
Allows multiple key use

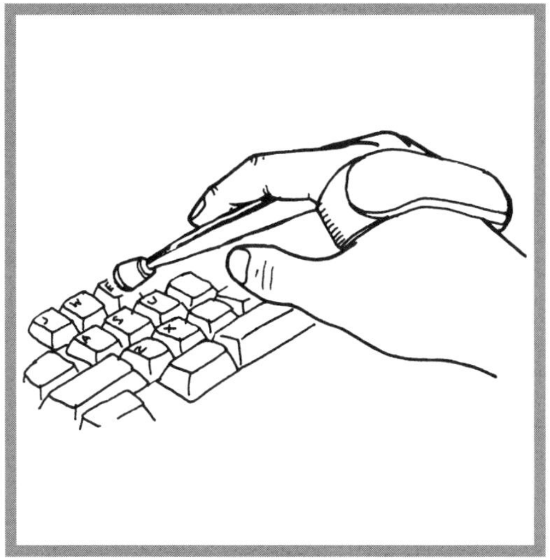

Typing aid
Stick on palmar loop
For Right hand
Velcro adjustable hand loop

333

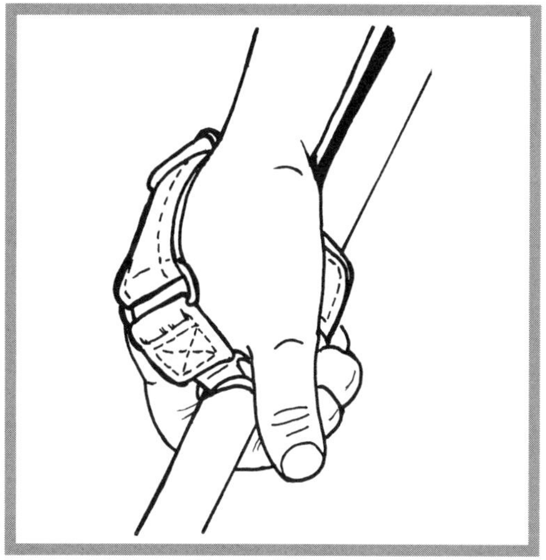

Universal cuff
For broom or similar handle
With rod shaped holder

334

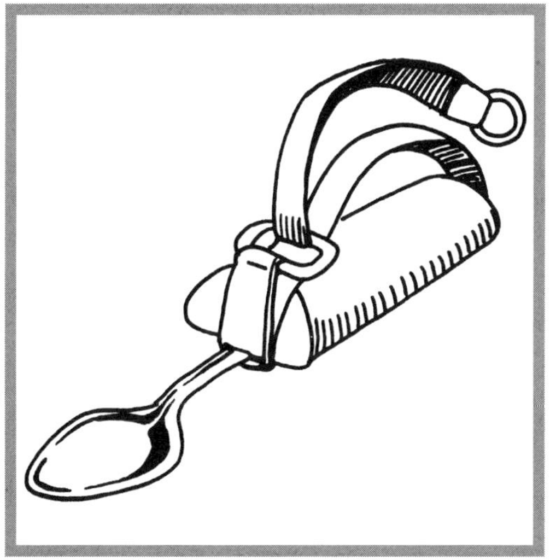

Universal cuff
For either hand
Palmar block with pocket
D-ring velcro close

335

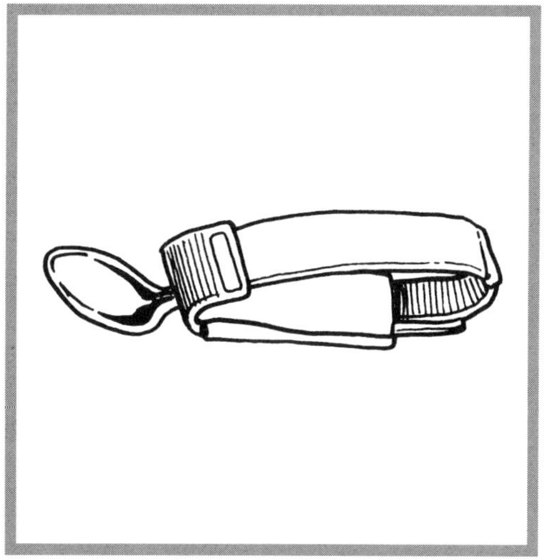

Universal cuff
For either hand
Palmar cuff w pocket
D-ring velcro close

336

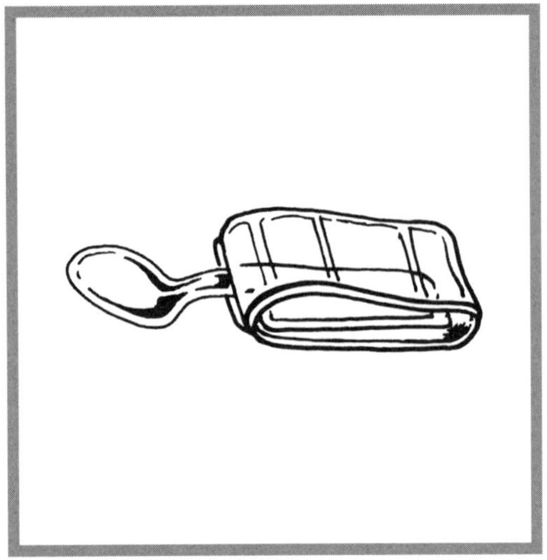

Universal cuff
For either hand
Palmar cuff with pocket
Elastic band

337

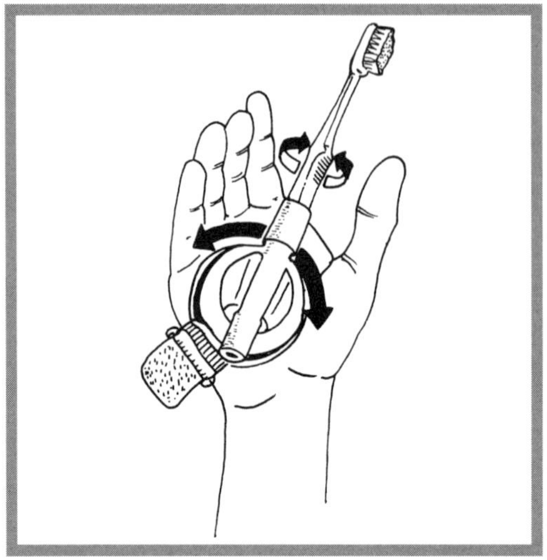

Universal cuff
For either hand
Palmar cuff with pocket
Rotatable pocket

338

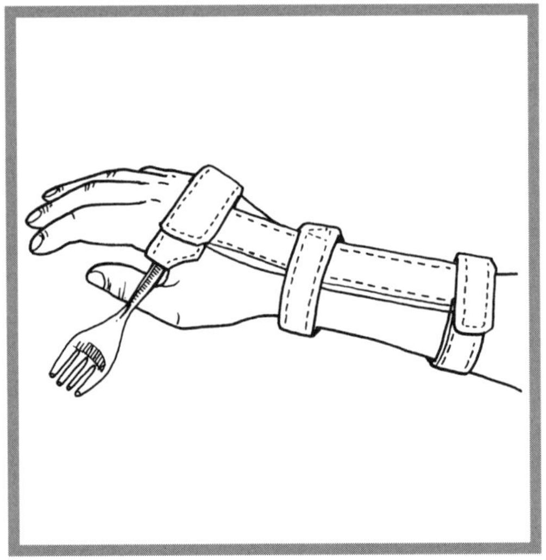

Universal cuff
For Right hand
With wrist support
Velcro closure

339

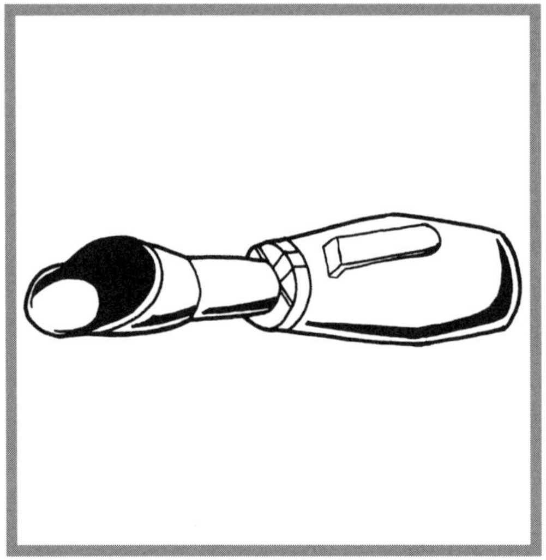

Urinal
Female
Bottle type

340

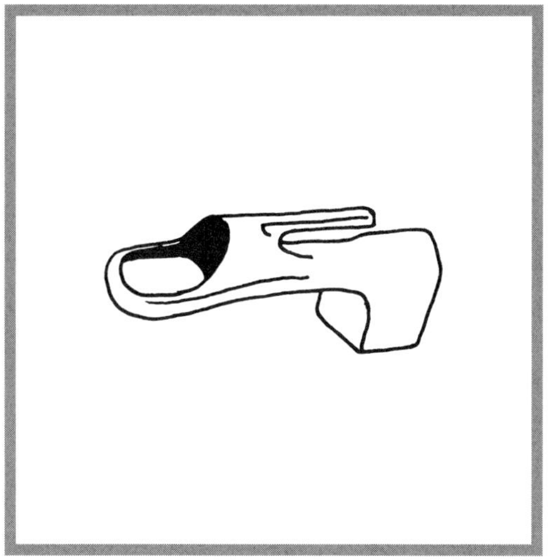

Urinal
Female
For wheelchair use

341

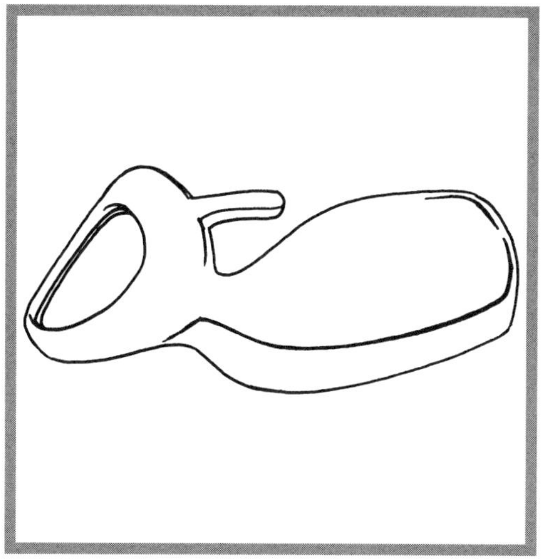

Urinal
Female

342

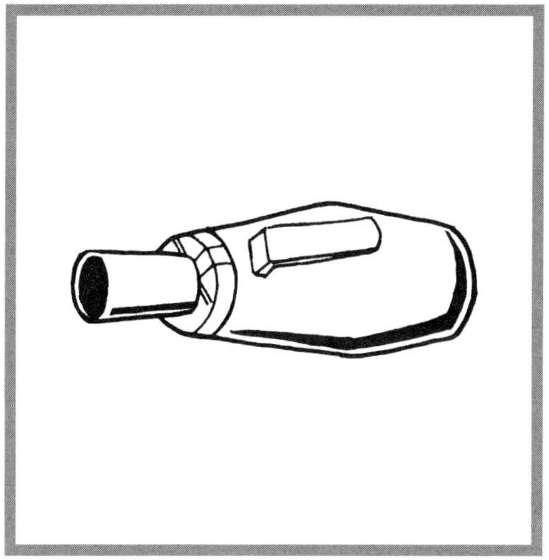

Urinal
Male
Bottle type

343

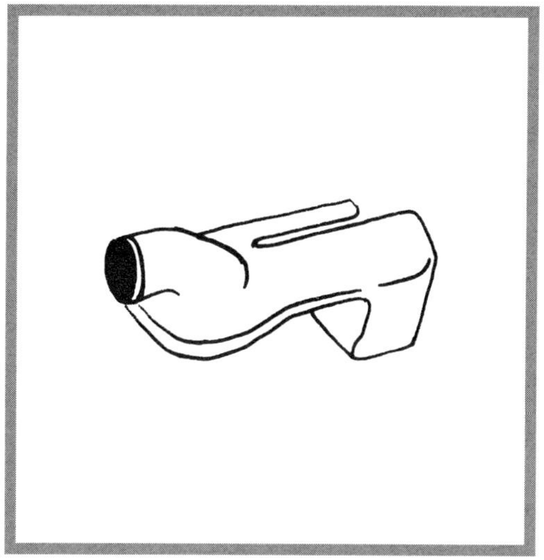

Urinal
Male
For wheelchair use

344

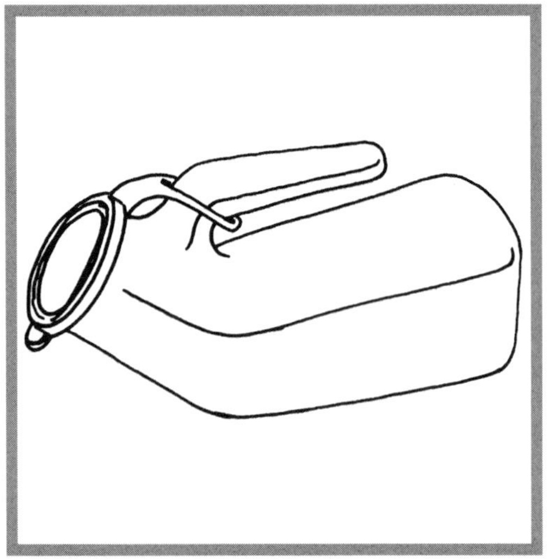

Urinal
Male
Spill-proof
Handle allows hanging

345

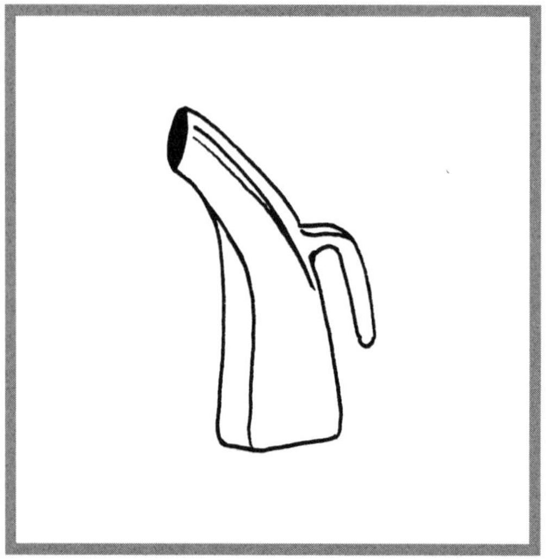

Urinal
Male
Use in seated position

346

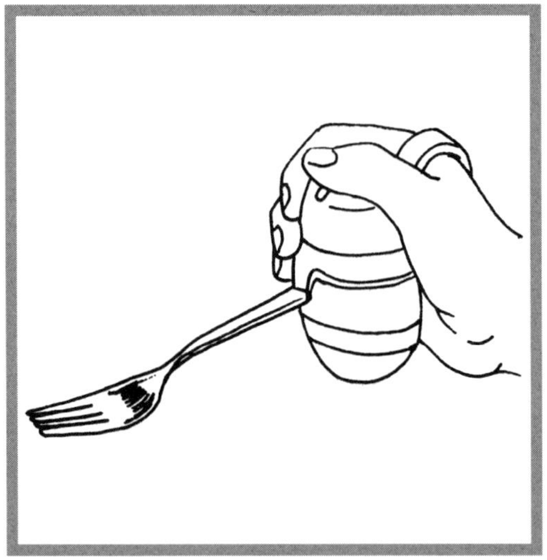

Utensil grip
Palmar ball
Oval grip with palm clip
Fits handle of eating utensil

347

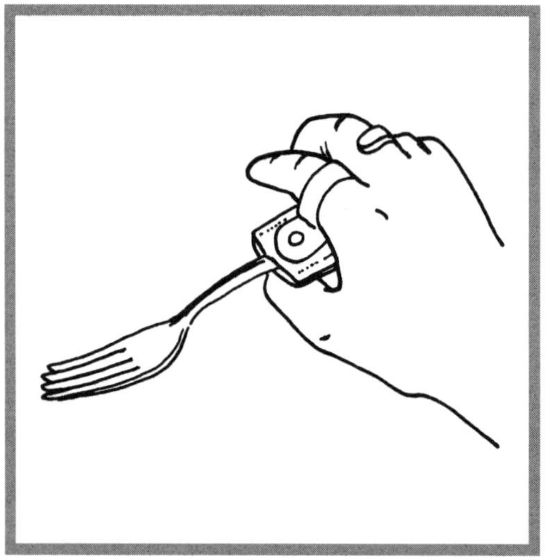

Utensil holder
Palmar block with finger loops
Horizontal pocket

348

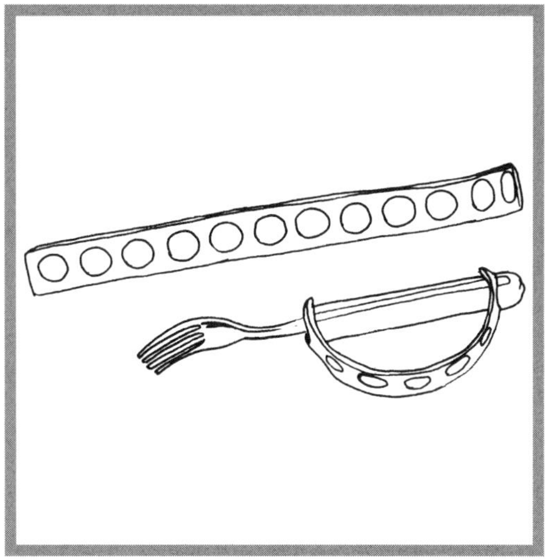

349

Utensil holder
Plastic hand loop

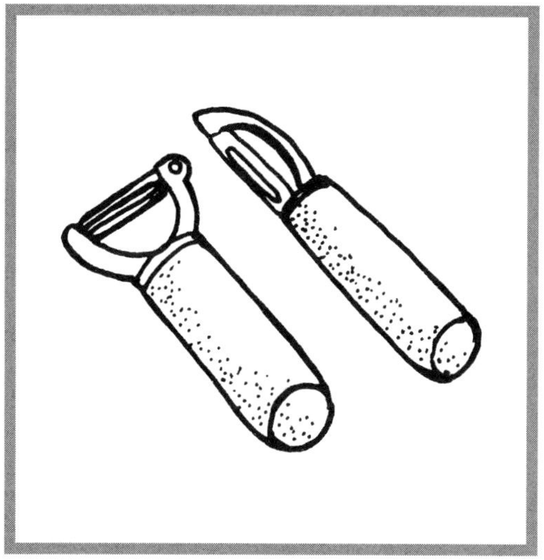

350

Vegetable peeler
Hand held
Manual
Cushion grip handle

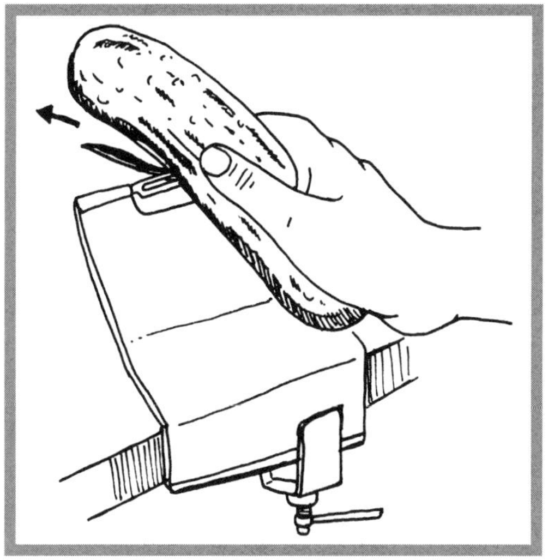

351

Vegetable peeler
One-hand operated
Manual
Clamps to counter

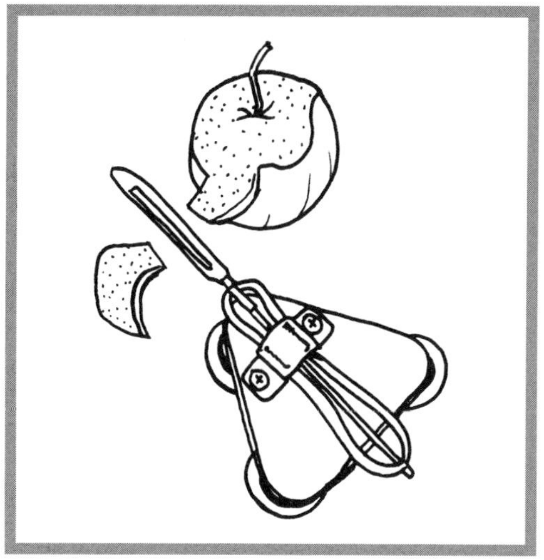

352

Vegetable peeler
One-hand operated
Manual
Suction mounted

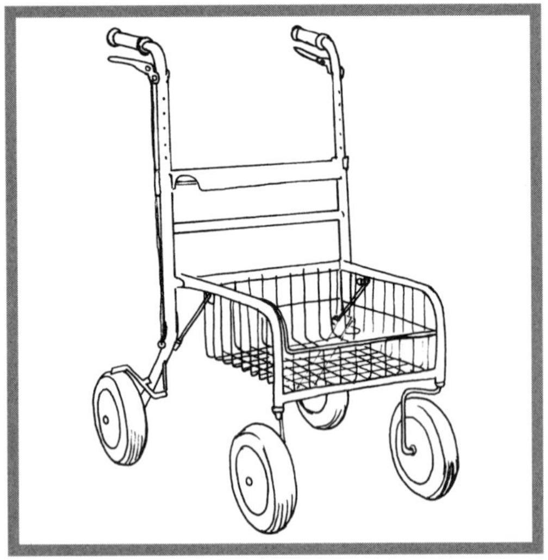

353

Walker
Four wheels
With hand brake

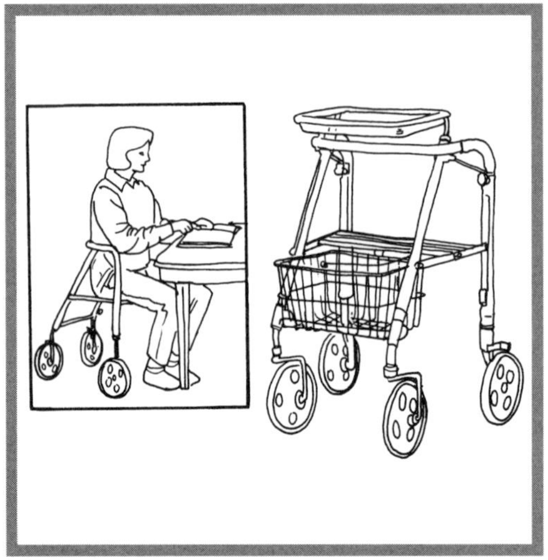

354

Walker
Four wheels
With hand brake
With seat

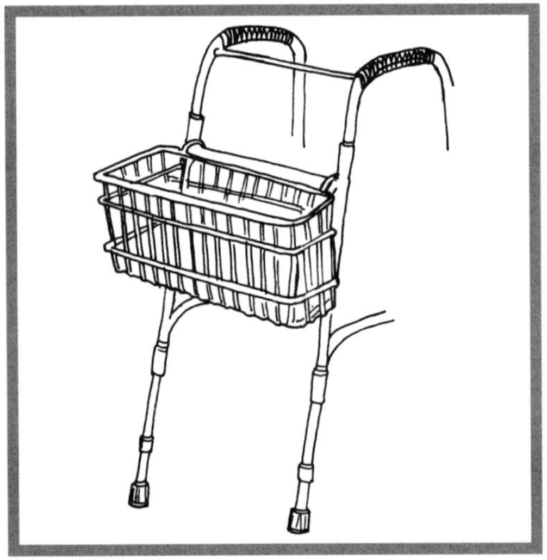

355

Walker basket
Wire
18 X 7 X 7 inches

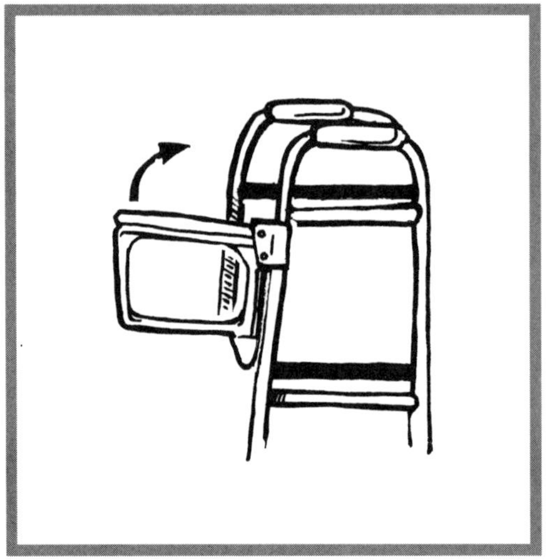

356

Walker standing-assist handle
Clamps to walker frame
Rests on chair for support
Folds against walker

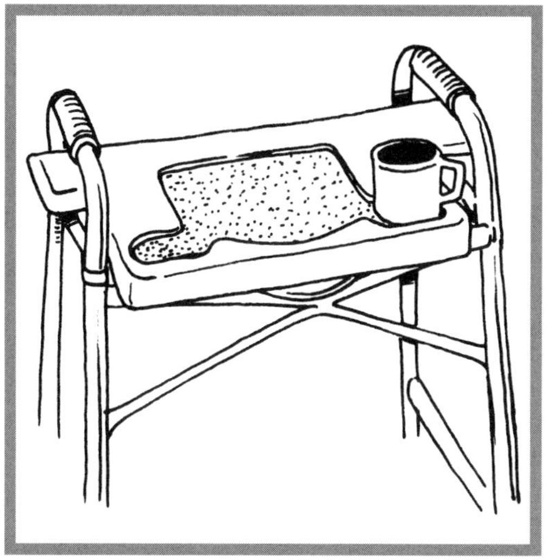

Walker tray
With cup & utensil holder
Slides away forward
With non-skid mat

357

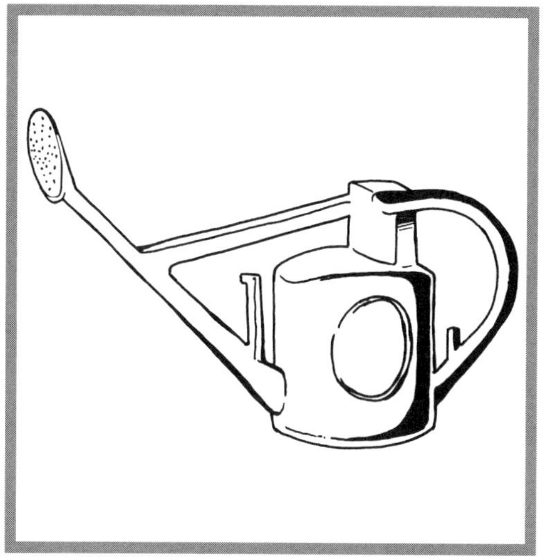

Watering can
Non-spill
Wrap-around handle

358

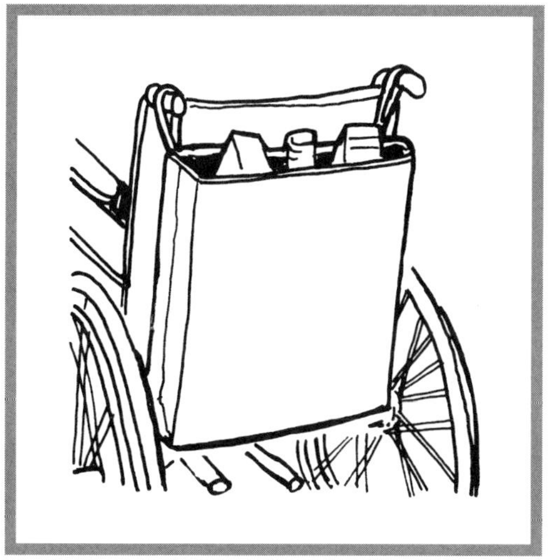

Wheelchair bag
Seat back
Shopping bag

359

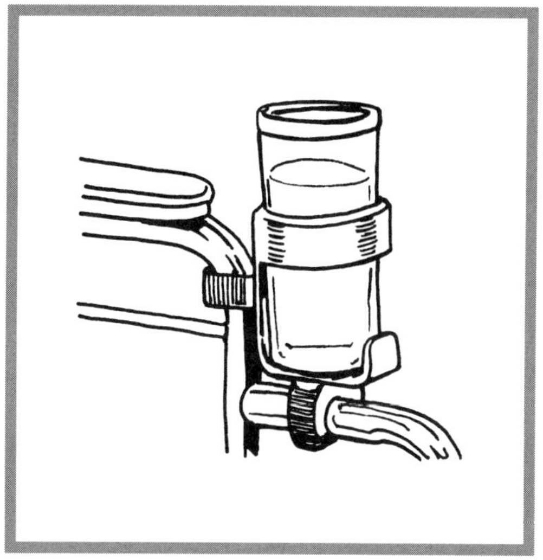

Wheelchair cup holder
For standard arm
Fixed diameter

360

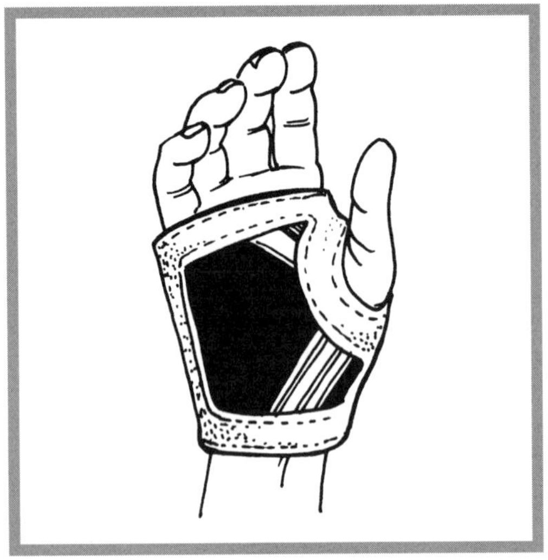

361

Wheelchair gloves fingerless
High-tack soft plastic palm
Closed back cowhide

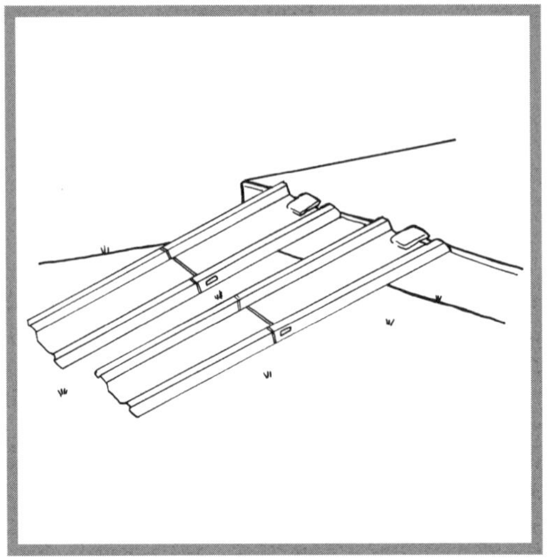

362

Wheelchair ramp
Portable tracks
Folds to 5 feet

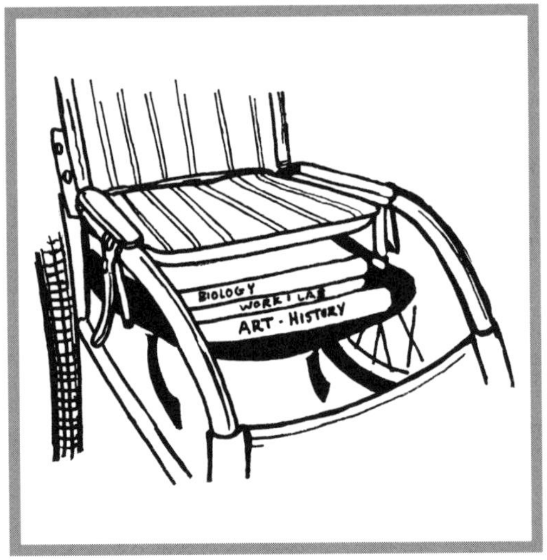

363

Wheelchair shelf
Under seat
12 x 10 x 4-1/2 inches

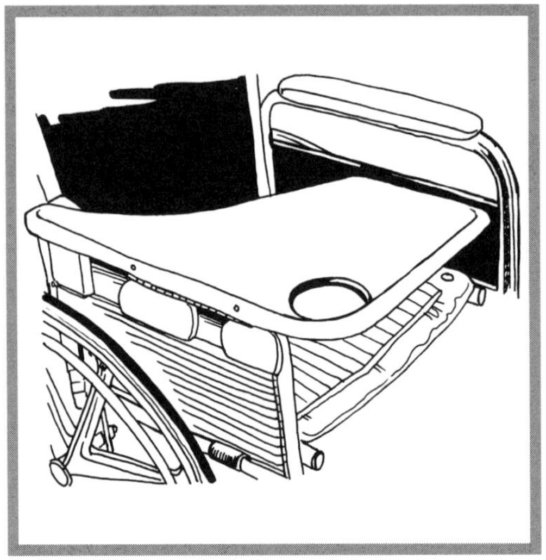

364

Wheelchair tray
Bracket for padded right arm
Flips upward
Half tray

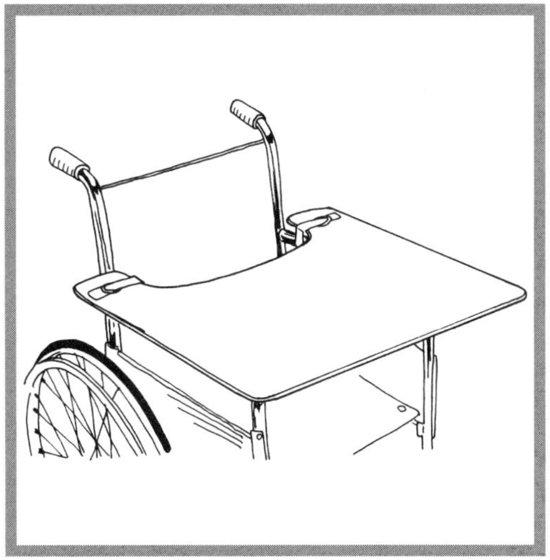

Wheelchair tray
For regular arm
Masonite
D-ring velcro straps

365

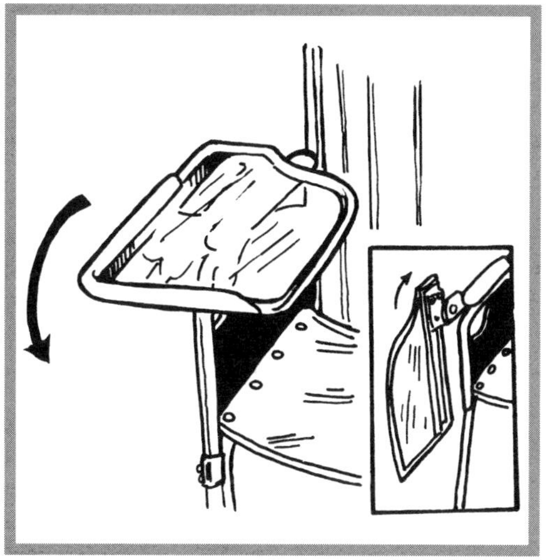

Wheelchair tray
Makes desk arm
Swings away and down

366

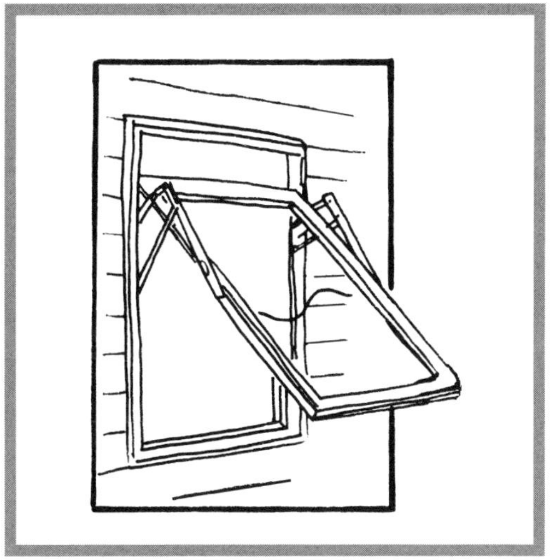

Window
Hinged for 180 degree rotation
High thermal rating
Projecting style

367

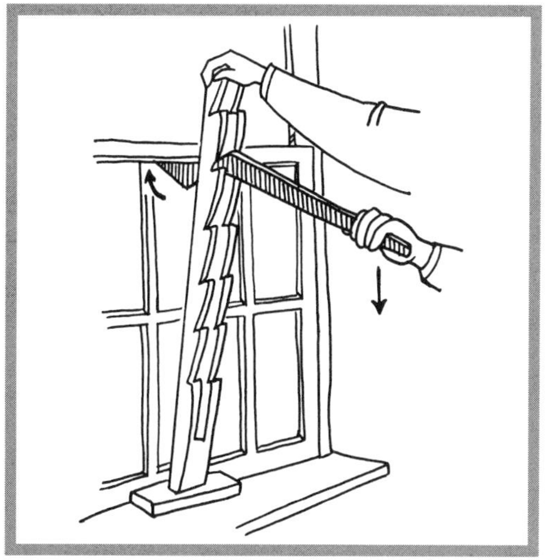

Window jack
Lever operated
For double-hung window

368

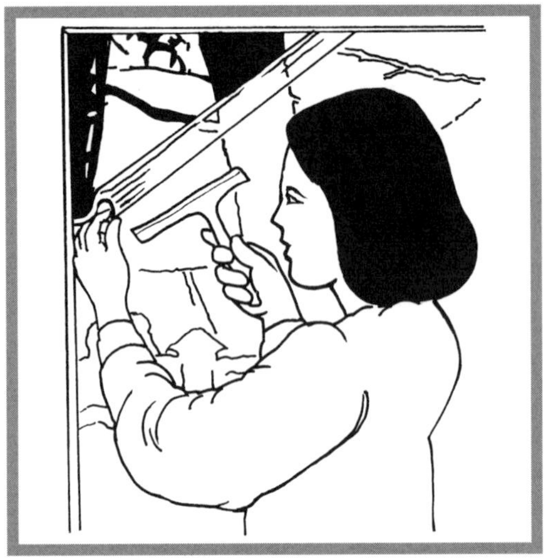

Window tint film
Removable
36 x 54 inch sheet
To reduce glare

369

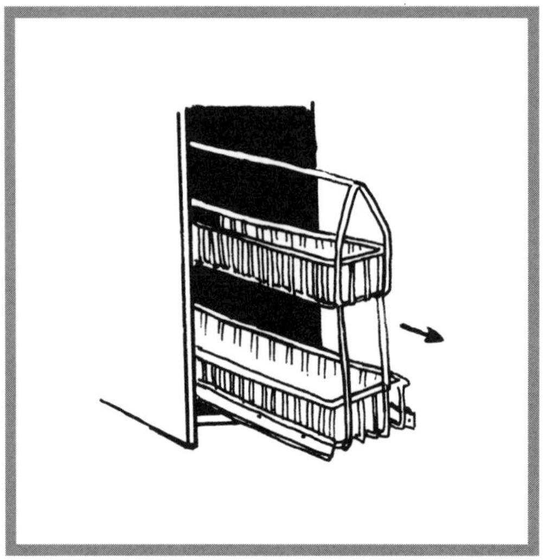

Wire rack basket
In-cabinet base
Sliding

370

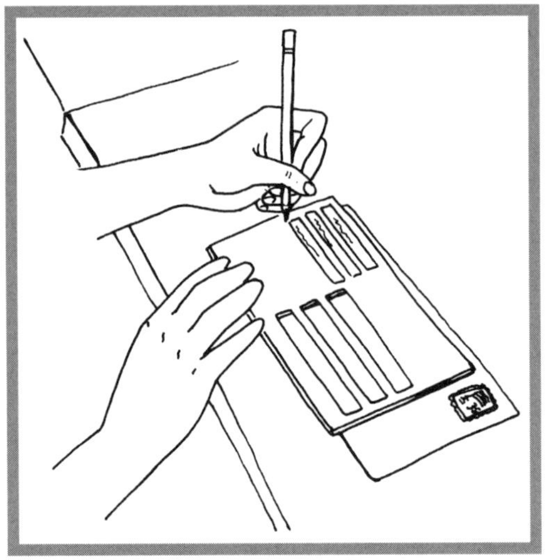

Writing aid
Guide slot
For #10 envelopes

371

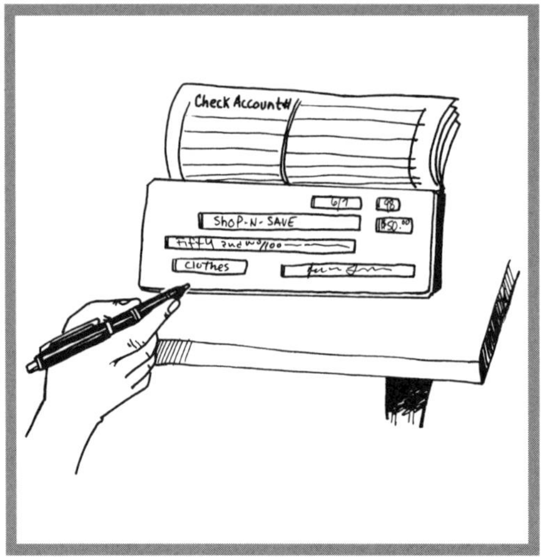

Writing aid
Guide slot
For checks

372

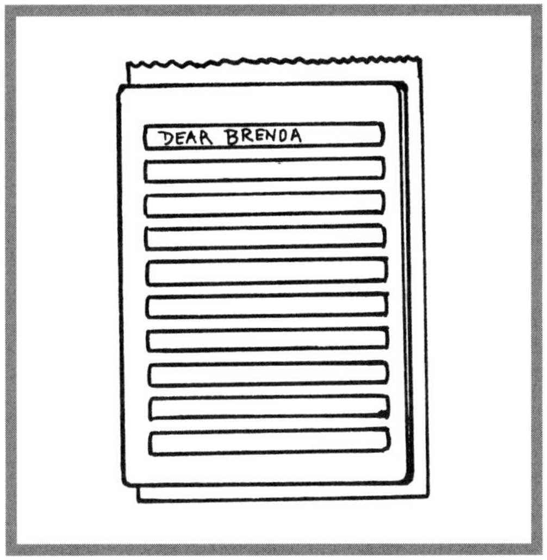

373

Writing aid
Guide slot
Letter writing
Plastic template

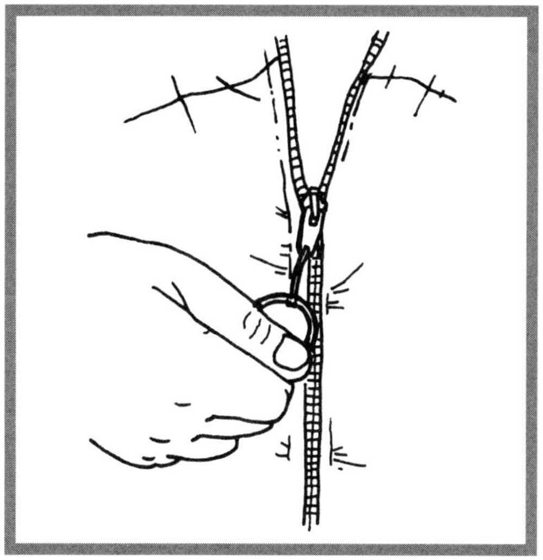

374

Zipper pull
1 inch diameter ring
Clip attaches to zipper

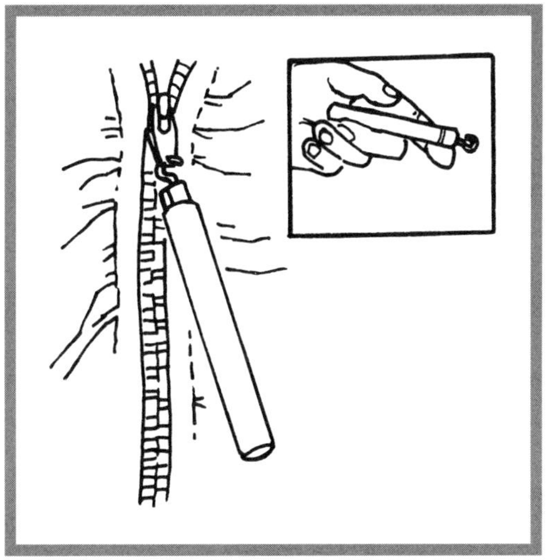

375

Zipper pull
Short wooden handle
Cup hook attaches to zipper

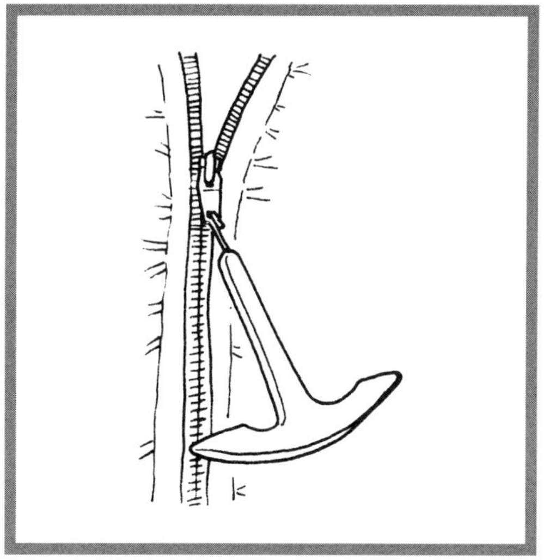

376

Zipper pull
T-handle
Hook attaches to zipper

Generic Names Index

Address book, Large print, not further specified
Address book, Large print, Spiral bound, not further specified
Adjustable bed, Electric & remote control, Raise head and/or flex knees, Dual king size
Adjustable bed, Electric & remote control, Raise head and/or flex knees, Extra long dual king size
Adjustable bed, Electric & remote control, Raise head and/or flex knees, Extra long full size
Adjustable bed, Electric & remote control, Raise head and/or flex knees, Extra long twin size
Adjustable bed, Electric & remote control, Raise head and/or flex knees, Full size
Adjustable bed, Electric & remote control, Raise head and/or flex knees, Long twin size
Adjustable bed, Electric & remote control, Raise head and/or flex knees, not further specified
Adjustable bed, Electric & remote control, Raise head and/or flex knees, Queen size
Adjustable bed, Electric & remote control, Raise head and/or flex knees, Twin size
Adjustable bed, Manual crank, Raise head and/or flex knees, Extra long twin size
Adjustable bed, Manual crank, Raise head and/or flex knees, not further specified
Adjustable bed, Manual non-crank, Raise head and/or flex knees, Adjust by body movement
Adjustable bed, Manual non-crank, Raise head and/or flex knees, not further specified
Adult diaper, see, Incontinence shield washable, Incontinence shield disposable
Alarm clock, 0.5 inch LED display, Vibrating & sound, Battery powered
Alarm clock, 0.5 inch LED display, Vibrating & sound, not further specified
Alarm clock, 0.6 inch LED display, Sound/light alarms, AC but no AC outlet
Alarm clock, 0.6 inch LED display, Sound/light alarms, AC with AC outlet
Alarm clock, 0.6 inch LED display, Sound/light alarms, not further specified
Alarm clock, 1.8 inch LED display, Electronic beep alarm, AC with AC outlet
Alarm clock, 1.8 inch LED display, Electronic beep alarm, not further specified
Alarm clock, 1.8 inch LED display, Vibrating & sound, AC with AC outlet
Alarm clock, 1.8 inch LED display, Vibrating & sound, not further specified
Alarm clock, 5 inch dial with hands, Vibrating & sound, Battery powered
Alarm clock, 5 inch dial with hands, Vibrating & sound, not further specified
Alarm clock, Large LED display, Electronic beep alarm, AC but no AC outlet
Alarm clock, Large LED display, Electronic beep alarm, not further specified
Alarm clock, Talking and display of time, Beep & rooster crow alarm, Battery powered
Alarm clock, Talking and display of time, Beep & rooster crow alarm, not further specified
Alarm clock, Talking and display of time, Voice alarm, Battery powered
Alarm clock, Talking and display of time, Voice alarm, not further specified
Alarm clock radio, 1.8 inch LED display, Radio & buzzer alarm, AC but no AC outlet
Alarm clock radio, 1.8 inch LED display, Radio & buzzer alarm, not further specified
Alarm watch, Talking and digital time, Voice and rooster crow alarm, Battery powered
Alerting device, 80 decibel horn low frequency, Sound activated, not further specified
Alerting device, 80 decibel horn low frequency, Sound activated, Send & receive units
Alerting device, Bed shaker, Receives alarm or phone sound, not further specified
Alerting device, Bed shaker, Receives alarm or phone sound, Sound activated
Alerting device, Bed shaker & light, Receives AC from alarm clock, not further specified
Alerting device, Bed shaker & light, Receives AC from alarm clock, Plugs into clock AC
Alerting device, Bed shaker & light, Receives alarm or phone sound, not further specified
Alerting device, Bed shaker & light, Receives alarm or phone sound, Sound activated
Alerting device, Coded flashing light, Doorbell remote with button, not further specified
Alerting device, Coded flashing light, Doorbell remote with button, Send & receive units
Alerting device, Coded flashing light, Doorbell remote with button, Sending unit only
Alerting device, Electronic distance sensor, Actuates by 15 foot distance, Battery operated rechargeable
Alerting device, Flashes any lamp, Sound activated remote, not further specified
Alerting device, Flashes any lamp, Sound activated remote, Receiving unit only
Alerting device, Flashes any lamp, Sound activated remote, Send & receive units
Alerting device, Light and vibration, Sound activated remote, not further specified
Alerting device, Light and vibration, Sound activated remote, Send & receive units
Alerting device, Wrist receiver, Sound activated remote, not further specified
Alerting device, Wrist receiver, Sound activated remote, Send & receive units
Amplified phone, see, Phone with amplifier
Analog clock, see, Wall clock, with hands
Apple peeler, One-hand operated, Removes only the skin, AC powered
Apple peeler/corer, One-hand operated, Crank operated, not further specified
Apple peeler/corer, One-hand operated, Crank operated, White Mountain type

Appliance knob turner, see, Knob turner
Appliance knobs, Large, Original, From some manufacturers
Appliance knobs, Large, Replacement, From some manufacturers
Appliance knobs, Large, Replacement, not further specified
Appliance labels, Braille, Original, From some manufacturers
Appliance labels, Large print, Original, From some manufacturers
Appliance labels, Large print, Replacement, From some manufacturers
Appliance labels, Large print, Replacement, not further specified
Appliance rollers, Adjust about 18 to 28 inches, Hold about 1000 pounds, To move appliances
Apron hoop, Flexible, Slides onto apron, To replace ties
Armchair, Wicker, No front rung or panel, not further specified
Armchair, Wicker, No front rung or panel, With forward arms
Armchair, Wood frame, No front rung or panel, not further specified
Armchair, Wood frame, No front rung or panel, With forward arms
Artificial larynx, Adjustable pitch, On/off switch, Battery powered
Ashtray for wheelchair, see, Wheelchair ashtray
Ashtray mounting lug, For wheelchair, For plastic ash tray, not further specified
Ashtray mounting lug, For wheelchair, not further specified
Attention signaler, see, Personal alerting device
Automatic page turner, see, Page turner, book holder
Auxiliary handle, For garden tools and similar, Is a side branch with grip, Clamp-on
Auxiliary handle, For garden tools and similar, Is a side branch with grip, not further specified

---

Back cushion, Posture curve, Detachable lumbar roll, Elastic strap
Back cushion, Posture curve, Detachable lumbar roll, not further specified
Back cushion, Posture curve, Integral lumbar roll, Contoured foam
Back cushion, Posture curve, Integral lumbar roll, not further specified
Back cushion, Shoulder support, Integral lumbar roll, Narrow back frame
Back cushion, Shoulder support, Integral lumbar roll, not further specified
Back scrubber, Requires two hands, Webbing loops, not further specified
Back scrubber, Requires two hands, Webbing loops, Terrycloth
Bag closer, One-hand operated, Pull-through closure, not further specified
Bag closer, One-hand operated, Pull-through closure, Wall mount
Bag opener, Hand held pinch operated, For plastic bags, not further specified
Bag opener, Hand held pinch operated, For plastic bags, With magnet hanger
Bag opener, Wall mounted, Safety blade, not further specified
Bag opener, Wall mounted, Safety blade, Use standard razor blades
Basket for cart, For utility cart, Wire, 12 inches deep
Basket for cart, For utility cart, Wire, 6 inches deep
Basket for cart, For utility cart, Wire, not further specified
Bath bench, 15-inch height, No grips, Drainage holes
Bath bench, 15-inch height, No grips, not further specified
Bath bench, 15-inch height, No grips, Solid seat
Bath bench, 15-inch height, With hand grips, Drainage holes
Bath bench, 15-inch height, With hand grips, not further specified
Bath bench, 15-inch height, With hand grips, Solid seat
Bath bench, 6-inch legs for in-tub, not further specified
Bath bench, 6-inch legs for in-tub, With hand grips, not further specified
Bath bench, 8-inch legs for in-tub, No grips, For very heavy person
Bath bench, 8-inch legs for in-tub, No grips, not further specified
Bath bench, Adjustable height, No grips, Drainage holes
Bath bench, Adjustable height, No grips, not further specified
Bath bench, Adjustable height, No grips, Padded
Bath bench, Adjustable height, not further specified
Bath bench, Adjustable height, With armrests, Cut-out seat
Bath bench, Adjustable height, With armrests, not further specified
Bath bench, Adjustable height, With hand grips, Cut-out seat
Bath bench, Adjustable height, With hand grips, not further specified
Bath bench, Adjustable height 13-19 inch, No grips, not further specified
Bath bench, Adjustable height 13-19 inch, not further specified
Bath bench, Adjustable height 13-19 inch, With hand grips, Drainage holes
Bath bench, Adjustable height 13-19 inch, With hand grips, not further specified
Bath bench, Adjustable height 13-20 inch, With hand grips, 11 x 19 inch seat
Bath bench, Adjustable height 13-20 inch, With hand grips, not further specified
Bath bench, Adjustable height 14-21 inch, No grips, Drainage holes
Bath bench, Adjustable height 14-21 inch, No grips, not further specified
Bath bench, Adjustable height 14-21 inch, No grips, not further specified
Bath bench, Adjustable height 14-21 inch, not further specified
Bath bench, Adjustable height 14-21 inch, With hand grips, Extra wide seat
Bath bench, Adjustable height 14-21 inch, With hand grips, not further specified
Bath bench, Adjustable height 16-23 inch, No grips, not further specified
Bath bench, Adjustable height 16-23 inch, No grips, Padded seat
Bath bench, Fixed height, not further specified
Bath bench, Fixed height, With hand grips, Fits across tub edge
Bath bench, Fixed height, With hand grips, not further specified
Bath bench, Fixed height with hand grips, Fits across tub edge, For very heavy person
Bath bench, Fixed height with hand grips, For very heavy person, not further specified

Bath bench, Suspends lower than tub rim, No arms or back, not further specified
Bath bench, Suspends lower than tub rim, No arms or back, Rests on tub rim
Bath brush, Break resistant handle, not further specified
Bath brush, Break resistant handle, Soap pocket in brush, not further specified
Bath brush, Curved handle, Fixed head, Grooved grip
Bath brush, Curved handle, Fixed head, Head in line with handle
Bath brush, Curved handle, Fixed head, not further specified
Bath brush, Curved handle, Handle adjustable with heat, not further specified
Bath brush, Curved handle, Handle adjustable with heat, Wire coil brush
Bath brush, Long handle, Adjustable head, not further specified
Bath brush, Long handle, Adjustable head, Ridged grip
Bath brush, Long handle, Brush on shaft, Small wedge sponge tip
Bath brush, Long handle, Head adjusts to 90 degrees, not further specified
Bath brush, Long handle, Head adjusts to 90 degrees, Oval shaped grip
Bath brush, Long handle, not further specified
Bath chair, 15-inch height, not further specified
Bath chair, 15-inch height, With hand grips, not further specified
Bath chair, Adjustable height, Extends & clamps to tub edge, not further specified
Bath chair, Adjustable height, Extends over tub, Adjusts for left/right entry
Bath chair, Adjustable height, No grips, Cut-out seat
Bath chair, Adjustable height, No grips, For very heavy person
Bath chair, Adjustable height, No grips, not further specified
Bath chair, Adjustable height, not further specified
Bath chair, Adjustable height, With armrests, not further specified
Bath chair, Adjustable height, With armrests, Removable cut-out seat
Bath chair, Adjustable height, With hand grips, Cut-out seat
Bath chair, Adjustable height, With hand grips, Drainage holes
Bath chair, Adjustable height, With hand grips, not further specified
Bath chair, Adjustable height 13-19 inch, With hand grips, Drainage holes
Bath chair, Adjustable height 13-19 inch, With hand grips, not further specified
Bath chair, Adjustable height 13-20 inch, With hand grips, 11x19 inch seat
Bath chair, Adjustable height 13-20 inch, With hand grips, not further specified
Bath chair, Adjustable height 14-21 inch, No grips, not further specified
Bath chair, Adjustable height 14-21 inch, not further specified
Bath chair, Adjustable height 14-21 inch, With hand grips, Extra wide seat
Bath chair, Adjustable height 14-21 inch, With hand grips, not further specified
Bath chair, Adjustable height 14-21 inch, With hand grips, not further specified
Bath chair, Adjustable height 16-21 inch, No grips, not further specified
Bath chair, Adjustable height 16-21 inch, No grips, Padded slat seat
Bath chair, Adjustable height 16-23 inch, No grips, not further specified
Bath chair, Adjustable height 16-23 inch, No grips, Padded seat/back
Bath chair, Adjustable height w/ backrest, No grips, not further specified
Bath chair, Adjustable height w/ backrest, No grips, Padded
Bath chair, Fixed height, No grips, Adjustable sling back
Bath chair, Fixed height, No grips, For person to 600 pounds
Bath chair, Fixed height, No grips, not further specified
Bath chair, Fixed height, With hand grips, Drainage holes
Bath chair, Fixed height, With hand grips, not further specified
Bath chair, Suspends lower than tub rim, With back, not further specified
Bath chair, Suspends lower than tub rim, With back, Rests on tub rim
Bath lift, Attaches to tub spout, Capacity up to 200 lbs, Water pressure powered
Bath lift, Chair with transfer arms, Arms fold into tub, not further specified
Bath lift, Chair with transfer extensions, Extensions fold into tub, Battery pack powered
Bath lift, Manual crank, Floor mounted, Coated metal seat
Bath lift, Manual crank, Floor mounted, not further specified
Bath lift backrest, Water inflatable, For tub lift, not further specified
Bath lift backrest, Water inflatable, not further specified
Bath lift seat, Water inflated, Attaches to faucet, Drains to lower the seat
Bath lift seat, Water inflated, Attaches to faucet, not further specified
Bath mat, Suction cup back, 14 X 36 inches, not further specified
Bath mat, Suction cup back, 14 X 36 inches, Terrycloth covered
Bath mat, Suction cup back, 16 X 41 inches, Machine washable
Bath mat, Suction cup back, 16 X 41 inches, not further specified
Bath mat, Suction cup back, 16 X 41 inches, Textured vinyl
Bath mat, Suction cup back, 18 X 28 inches, not further specified
Bath mat, Suction cup back, 18 X 28 inches, With drainage holes
Bath mitt, Hand shaped with thumb, Elastic at wrist, not further specified
Bath mitt, Hand shaped with thumb, Elastic at wrist, Palm soap pocket
Bath mitt, Hand shaped with thumb, Elastic at wrist, Terrycloth/nylon
Bath mitt, Large rectangular, Velcro & D-ring closure, not further specified
Bath mitt, Large rectangular, Velcro & D-ring closure, Terrycloth
Bath mitt, Large square, Velcro & D-ring closure, not further specified
Bath mitt, Large square, Velcro & D-ring closure, Terrycloth
Bath mitt, Medium square, Velcro & D-ring closure, not further specified
Bath mitt, Medium square, Velcro & D-ring closure, Terrycloth
Bath mitt, Small square, not further specified
Bath mitt, Small square, Velcro & D-ring closure, not further specified
Bath mitt, Small square, Velcro & D-ring closure, not further specified
Bath mitt, Small square, Velcro & D-ring closure, Soap pocket

Bath mitt, Small square, Velcro & D-ring closure, Terrycloth
Bath mitt, Square with soap pocket, Velcro & D-ring closure, not further specified
Bath mitt, Square with soap pocket, Velcro & D-ring closure, Terrycloth
Bath mitt/sponge, Hand shaped with thumb, not further specified
Bath mitt/sponge, Hand shaped with thumb, Velcro & D-ring closure, Large opening
Bath mitt/sponge, Hand shaped with thumb, Velcro & D-ring closure, not further specified
Bath mitt/sponge, Hand shaped with thumb, Velcro & D-ring closure, not further specified
Bath seat, see also, Bath bench
Bath seat, see also, Bath chair
Bath sponge with handle, Contoured sponge, 14 inch handle, Heat-adjustable handle
Bath sponge with handle, Contoured sponge, 15 1/2 inch handle, Bendable wire handle
Bath sponge with handle, Contoured sponge, 18 inch handle, Heat-adjustable handle
Bath sponge with handle, Contoured sponge, 18 inch handle, not further specified
Bath sponge with handle, Contoured sponge, 22 inch handle, Heat-adjustable handle
Bath sponge with handle, Contoured sponge, 22 inch handle, not further specified
Bath sponge with handle, Contoured sponge, 24 inch handle, Bendable wire handle
Bath sponge with handle, Contoured sponge, 24 inch handle, not further specified
Bath sponge with handle, Loofa sponge, 24 inch handle, not further specified
Bath sponge with handle, Loofa sponge, 24 inch handle, Wood removable handle
Bath sponge with handle, Round sponge, 14 inch handle, Heat-adjustable handle
Bath sponge with handle, Round sponge, 22 inch handle, Heat-adjustable handle
Bath sponge with handle, Soap pocket, 12 inch handle, not further specified
Bath sponge with handle, Soap pocket, 12 inch handle, Standard handle
Bath sponge with handle, Standard sponge, 12 inch bendable handle, Built-up handle
Bath sponge with handle, Standard sponge, 12 inch bendable handle, not further specified
Bath sponge with handle, Standard sponge, 14 inch handle with palm clip, For no-thumb palmar grip
Bath sponge with handle, Standard sponge, 14 inch handle with palm clip, not further specified
Bath sponge with handle, Standard sponge, 18 inch handle, Heat-adjustable handle
Bath sponge with handle, Standard sponge, 18 inch handle, not further specified
Bath sponge with handle, Standard sponge, 18 inch handle, Standard handle
Bath sponge with handle, Standard sponge, handle with hand loops, not further specified
Bath sponge with handle, Wedge sponge, 8 inch handle, not further specified
Bath sponge with handle, Wedge sponge, 8 inch handle, Wooden handle
Bath transfer bench, Adjustable height, Extends over tub, not further specified
Bath transfer bench, Adjustable height, No grips, Clamps to tub wall
Bath transfer bench, Adjustable height, No grips, not further specified
Bath transfer bench, Adjustable height, No grips or back, Fits across tub edge
Bath transfer bench, Adjustable height, No grips or back, not further specified
Bath transfer bench, Adjustable height, With back bar, Fits over tub edge
Bath transfer bench, Adjustable height, With back bar, not further specified
Bath transfer bench, Adjustable height, With padded back bar, Fits across tub edge
Bath transfer bench, Adjustable height, With padded back bar, not further specified
Bath transfer bench, Fixed height, With hand rail, Fits across tub edge
Bath transfer bench, Fixed height, With hand rail, not further specified
Bath transfer chair, Adjustable height, Backrest & right-or-left arm, Clamps to tub edge
Bath transfer chair, Adjustable height, Backrest & right-or-left arm, Fits over tub edge
Bath transfer chair, Adjustable height, Backrest & right-or-left arm, not further specified
Bath transfer chair, Adjustable height, Backrest & right-or-left arm, Suction cups on legs
Bath transfer chair, Adjustable height, Hand rail and back, Fits across tub edge
Bath transfer chair, Adjustable height, Hand rail and back, not further specified
Bath transfer chair, Adjustable height, Right-or-left arm, Clamps to tub edge
Bath transfer chair, Adjustable height, Right-or-left arm, not further specified
Bath transfer chair, Adjustable height, With back & arms, Fits over tub edge
Bath transfer chair, Adjustable height, With back & arms, not further specified
Bath transfer chair, Adjustable height, With back & arms, Snap off/rotating seat
Bath transfer chair, Adjustable height, With backrest, not further specified
Bath transfer chair, Adjustable height, With backrest, Suction cups on legs
Bath/shower bench, Non-adjustable 22 inch, Holds 500 pounds, not further specified
Bath/shower bench, Non-adjustable 22 inch, Holds 500 pounds, Rubber feet
Bathroom scale, 1 inch display, LCD display, not further specified
Bathroom scale, 2 inch display numbers, Red LED display, 300 pound capacity
Bathroom scale, 2 inch display numbers, Red LED display, not further specified
Bathroom scale, 7 inch display, Dial display, Black on white numbers
Bathroom scale, 7 inch display, Dial display, not further specified

Bathroom scale, 8 inch display, Dial display, not further specified
Bathroom scale, 8 inch display, Dial display, White on black numbers
Bathroom scale, Extra large display, Dial display, 325 pound capacity
Bathroom scale, Extra large display, Dial display, not further specified
Bathroom scale, Read-out at chest level, 2 inch digital display, Non-illuminated
Bathroom scale, Read-out at chest level, 2 inch digital display, not further specified
Bathroom scale, Read-out at chest level, Dial display, 325 pound capacity
Bathroom scale, Read-out at chest level, Dial display, not further specified
Bathroom scale, Read-out at chest level, Open dial display, Braille dot numbers
Bathroom scale, Read-out at chest level, Open dial display, not further specified
Bathroom scale, Read-out at waist level, Dial display, Capacity up to 300 pounds
Bathroom scale, Recalls previous weight, Voice-synthesized output, No visual display
Bathroom scale, Recalls previous weight, Voice-synthesized output, not further specified
Bathroom scale, With wheelchair platform, Digital display to 580 pounds, not further specified
Bathroom scale, With wheelchair platform, Digital display to 580 pounds, Side ramp & guard rail
Bathtub cabinet, see, Bathtub side opening
Bathtub caddy, Coated wire rack, Adjusts to 32 inches, not further specified
Bathtub caddy, Coated wire rack, Adjusts to 32 inches, Over tub edges
Bathtub caddy/bookholder, Adjustable width, Fits over tub edge, Coated wire
Bathtub caddy/bookholder, Adjustable width, Fits over tub edge, not further specified
Bathtub enclosure, Trackless tub door, Wall mounted, 55.5-60 inch opening
Bathtub enclosure, Trackless tub door, Wall mounted, not further specified
Bathtub headrest, Suction base, not further specified
Bathtub headrest, Suction base, Terry covered foam, not further specified
Bathtub insert, Supported on tub rim, Makes tub shallow, not further specified
Bathtub insert, Supported on tub rim, Makes tub shallow, Requires plumbing
Bathtub temperature controller, Replaces bathtub spout, Auto shut off at 114 degrees, not further specified
Bathtub temperature controller, Replaces bathtub spout, Auto shut off at 114 degrees, With restart button
Bathtub that rotates, Horizontal rotation, Fixed seat, Tub rotates upright
Bathtub tube, see, Bathtub that rotates
Bathtub whirlpool, Fits over tub edge, Side jet, AC powered
Bathtub whirlpool, Fits over tub edge, Side jet, Battery powered
Bathtub whirlpool, Fits over tub edge, Side jet, not further specified
Bathtub whirlpool, Panel in tub bottom, Air bubble jets, AC powered
Bathtub whirlpool, Panel in tub bottom, Air bubble jets, Battery powered
Bathtub whirlpool, Panel in tub bottom, Air bubble jets, not further specified
Bathtub with side opening, Door entry, Elevated 18 inches, Fiberglass
Bathtub with side opening, Door entry, Elevated 18 inches, not further specified
Bathtub with side opening, Door entry, Floor level entry, Fiberglass
Bathtub with side opening, Door entry, Floor level entry, not further specified
Battery 12 volt, Operates appliances, Screw terminal, Deep discharge
Battery 12 volt, Operates appliances, Screw terminal, not further specified
Battery 6-volt, Standard square, Coil terminals, not further specified
Battery 6-volt, Standard square, not further specified
Battery 6-volt, Standard square, Screw terminals, not further specified
Beaker holder, see, Cup handle
Beaker holder, see, Cup holder/handle
Bean bags for game, For use hook velcro target, With loop velcro, not further specified
Beard/mustache trimmer, 5 position guide, Electric, not further specified
Beard/mustache trimmer, 5 position guide, Electric, Rechargeable battery powered
Bed adjustable, see, Adjustable bed
Bed arising aid, Mounted on bedboard, Fixed handle, Steel
Bed arising aid, Mounted on bedframe, Mounts to metal bed frame, Steel
Bed arising aid, Swing-out grab loop, 360 degree swing, Install to bed frame
Bed arising aid, Swing-out grab loop, 360 degree swing, not further specified
Bed board, For adjustable beds, 3-part hinged, Hardwood plywood
Bed board, For adjustable beds, 3-part hinged, not further specified
Bed board, For adjustable beds, Horizontal flexible, not further specified
Bed board, For adjustable beds, Horizontal flexible, Slatted plywood
Bed jacket, Wide armholes, Wide shoulders, Machine washable
Bed jacket, Wide armholes, Wide shoulders, not further specified
Bed ladder, see, Bed pull-up
Bed pad, Home size, 5 inch foam, not further specified
Bed pad, Home size, 5 inch foam, Pillow for heels
Bed pad, Hospital bed size, 5 inch foam, not further specified
Bed pad, Hospital bed size, 5 inch foam, Pillow for heels
Bed pad, Twin size, Eggcrate foam, not further specified
Bed pad, Twin size, not further specified
Bed pad, Twin size full length, Cotton/polyester, not further specified
Bed pad, Twin size full length, Cotton/polyester, Waterproof
Bed pan, Contoured, Plastic, Front/side handles
Bed pan, Contoured, Plastic, not further specified
Bed pan, Contoured, Plastic, Unisex

Bed pan, Contoured, Stainless steel, No handles
Bed pan, Contoured, Stainless steel, not further specified
Bed pan, Wedge shape, Plastic, Loop handle
Bed pan, Wedge shape, Plastic, not further specified
Bed pan, Wedge shaped, Plastic, Female
Bed pan, Wedge shaped, Plastic, not further specified
Bed pelvic lift aid, Inflatable on waterproof fabric, Foot pump, Designed bedpan
Bed protector, see, Mattress protector
Bed pull-up, Ladder type, 4 plastic rungs, 8 foot length
Bed pull-up, Ladder type, 4 plastic rungs, not further specified
Bed pull-up, Ladder type, 4 webbing loops, not further specified
Bed pull-up, Ladder type, 5 plastic rungs, 55 inches long
Bed pull-up, Ladder type, 5 plastic rungs, 7 feet long
Bed pull-up, Ladder type, 5 plastic rungs, not further specified
Bed pull-up, Ladder type, not further specified
Bed rail, Adjustable width, Pull button, not further specified
Bed rail, Adjustable width, Pull button, Secured by crossbars
Bed rail, Adjustable width 24-40 inch, Spring loaded button, not further specified
Bed rail, Adjustable width 24-40 inch, Spring loaded button, Secured by crossbars
Bed rail, Adjustable width 24-44 inch, Spring loaded button, not further specified
Bed rail, Adjustable width 24-44 inch, Spring loaded button, Secured by crossbars
Bed rail, Fixed 60 inch length, Tubular rail, not further specified
Bed rail, Fixed 60 inch length, Tubular rail, Secured by crossbars
Bed rail, Fixed width, Mesh center, not further specified
Bed rail, Fixed width, Mesh center, Secured by crossbars
Bed rail, Telescoping length, Pull button, not further specified
Bed rail, Telescoping length, Pull button, Side rail only
Bed rail curtain, 36 inch length, Cushioned over rail, 7x12 inch vinyl window
Bed rail curtain, 36 inch length, Cushioned over rail, Laps over side rails
Bed rail curtain, 36 inch length, Cushioned over rail, not further specified
Bed rail curtain, 36 inch length, Cushioned over rail, not further specified
Bed rail curtain, 48 inch length, Cushioned over rail, 7x12 inch vinyl window
Bed rail curtain, 48 inch length, Cushioned over rail, Laps over side rails
Bed rail curtain, 48 inch length, Cushioned over rail, not further specified
Bed rail curtain, 62 inch length, Cushioned over rail, 7x12 inch vinyl window
Bed rail curtain, 62 inch length, Cushioned over rail, Laps over side rails
Bed rail curtain, 62 inch length, Cushioned over rail, not further specified
Bed rail curtain, 72 inch length, Cushioned over rail, 7x12 inch vinyl window
Bed rail curtain, 72 inch length, Cushioned over rail, Laps over side rails
Bed rail curtain, 72 inch length, Cushioned over rail, not further specified
Bed rail extender, Adjustable 44 to 63 inches, Extends crossbars, not further specified
Bed rail extender, Adjustable 44 to 63 inches, not further specified
Bed rail half length, Adjusts to fit all beds, 15 inch height, not further specified
Bed rail half length, Adjusts to fit all beds, not further specified
Bed rail half length, Fixed 40 inch length, Tubular rail, not further specified
Bed rail half length, Fixed 40 inch length, Tubular rail, Secured by crossbars
Bed rail pad, see, Bed rail curtain
Bed shaker & light, see, Alerting device, bed shaker & light
Bed specs, see, Prism glasses, not over regular glasses
Bed table, see, Overbed table
Bed wedge, 12 inch elevation, For legs or head, not further specified
Bed wedge, 12 inch elevation, not further specified
Bed wedge, 7 inch elevation, For legs or head, not further specified
Bed wedge, 7 inch elevation, not further specified
Belliclamp, see, Jar holder, hands free
Bib, Tied neck, Disposable plastic, 2 inch catch pocket
Bib, Tied neck, Disposable plastic, not further specified
Bib, Tied neck, Vinyl, 18 x 26 inches
Bib, Tied neck, Vinyl, 18x36 inch crumb catcher
Bib, Tied neck, Vinyl, not further specified
Bib, Velcro neck closure, Terry/vinyl, 18 x 27 inches
Bib, Velcro neck closure, Terry/vinyl, not further specified
Bib, Velcro neck closure, Terrycloth, 18 x 26 inches
Bib, Velcro neck closure, Terrycloth, 18 x 36 inches
Bib, Velcro neck closure, Terrycloth, 3 inch crumb catcher
Bib, Velcro neck closure, Terrycloth, not further specified
Bib, Velcro neck closure, Terrycloth/vinyl, not further specified
Bib, Velcro neck closure, Terrycloth/vinyl, Reversible
Bib holder, Clip attachment, Nylon cord, Holder with no bib
Bib holder, Clip attachment, Nylon cord, not further specified
Bible, Large print, Various versions, not further specified
Bidet, Floor mounted, not further specified
Bidet, Floor mounted, Plumbed, not further specified
Bidet arm, Fits in toilet bowl, Water with air dry, not further specified
Bidet arm, Fits in toilet bowl, Water with air dry, Plumbed
Bidet basin, Basin on toilet rim, not further specified

Bidet basin, Basin on toilet rim, Not plumbed, not further specified
Bidet basin, Basin on toilet rim, Not plumbed, Spout and soap tray
Bidet basin, Basin on toilet rim, Plumbed, not further specified
Bidet hose, Use over toilet, 120 degree bent head, Control on wall
Bidet hose, Use over toilet, 120 degree bent head, not further specified
Bidet/sitz bath, Basin on toilet rim, Hand held spray, Connects to faucet
Bidet/sitz bath, Basin on toilet rim, Hand held spray, not further specified
Bidet/sitz bath, Basin on toilet rim, Pour-fill, Lift to empty
Bidet/sitz bath, Basin on toilet rim, Pour-fill, not further specified
Big button phone, see, Phone with big buttons
Billiard ..., see, Pool ...
Bingo call numbers, Braille & visual, Raised numbers, In plastic case
Bingo call numbers, Braille & visual, Raised numbers, not further specified
Bingo cards, Braille & visual, Raised numbers, 7X10 inches
Bingo cards, Braille & visual, Raised numbers, 8X9 inches
Bingo cards, Braille & visual, Raised numbers, not further specified
Bingo cards, Large bold numbers, 5/8 inch numbers, 7X7 inches
Bingo cards, Large bold numbers, 5/8 inch numbers, not further specified
Biocurve pen, see, Pen, contoured
Blanket support, For feet, Adjustable frame, Held under mattress
Blanket support, For feet, Adjustable frame, not further specified
Blender, Hand held, Light weight, 2-speed AC powered
Blender, Hand held, Light weight, not further specified
Blouse, Pull-over, Long sleeve, Cotton/polyester
Blouse, Pull-over, Long sleeve, not further specified
Blouse, Pull-over, Long sleeve, Polyester
Blouse, Pull-over, Short raglan sleeve, Cotton/polyester
Blouse, Pull-over, Short raglan sleeve, not further specified
Blouse, Pull-over, Short raglan sleeve, Polyester
Blouse, Pull-over, Short sleeve, not further specified
Blouse, Pull-over, Short sleeve, Polyester
Blouse, Velcro closure, Long sleeve, not further specified
Blouse, Velcro closure, Long sleeve, Polyester
Body pillow, Body length support, Polyester fill, Machine wash
Body pillow, Body length support, Polyester fill, not further specified
Body pillow case, For body pillow, Polyester/cotton, Machine wash
Body pillow case, For body pillow, Polyester/cotton, not further specified
Bolster, see, Positioning cushion
Bolster pillow, see, Body pillow
Book end, Clips to wood/steel shelf, not further specified
Book holder, Bed/table easel type, Adjustable angle/width, Adjustable plexiglas tray
Book holder, Bed/table easel type, Adjustable angle/width, not further specified
Book holder, Clamp-on easel, Adjustable arm, not further specified
Book holder, Clamp-on easel, Adjustable arm, Velcro page holders
Book holder, Clamp-on easel, Holds 4 pound book, Adjustable lexan and aluminum
Book holder, Clamp-on easel, Holds 4 pound book, not further specified
Book holder, Desktop easel type, 45 degree angle, Bars for positioning
Book holder, Desktop easel type, 45 degree angle, not further specified
Book holder, Desktop easel type, 45 degree angle, Page holding pins
Book holder, Desktop easel type, 6 adjustable angles/heights, Aluminum/masonite
Book holder, Desktop easel type, 6 adjustable angles/heights, not further specified
Book holder, Desktop easel type, Adjustable angle, 11 x 19 inch surface
Book holder, Desktop easel type, Adjustable angle, not further specified
Book holder, Desktop easel type, Adjustable angle, Page holding pins
Book holder, Desktop easel type, Adjustable angle, Spring loaded levers
Book holder, Desktop easel type, Adjustable angle/height, not further specified
Book holder, Desktop easel type, Adjustable angle/height, Spring loaded levers
Book holder, Desktop easel type, Adjustable angle/width, Adjustable plexiglas tray
Book holder, Desktop easel type, Adjustable angle/width, not further specified
Book holder, Desktop easel type, Adjustable height, Foam lined ledge
Book holder, Desktop easel type, Adjustable height, not further specified
Book holder, Desktop easel type, Adjustable height, Page holding pins
Book holder, Desktop easel type, Adjustable height/width, not further specified
Book holder, Desktop easel type, Adjustable height/width, Page holding pins
Book holder, Desktop easel type, Adjusts to 5 angles, not further specified
Book holder, Desktop easel type, Adjusts to 5 angles, Page holding pins
Book holder, Desktop easel type, Adjusts to any angle, not further specified
Book holder, Desktop easel type, Adjusts to any angle, Spring loaded levers
Book holder, Desktop easel type, Fixed angle, Adjustable wire frame
Book holder, Desktop easel type, Fixed angle, Folds flat to store
Book holder, Desktop easel type, Fixed angle, not further specified
Book holder, Desktop easel type, Fixed angle, Page holding pins
Book holder, Overhead easel, Adjustable angle/height, not further specified
Book holder, Overhead easel, Adjustable angle/height, Overhead & lap desk
Book holder, Overhead easel, Adjustable angle/height, Overhead only
Book holder, Overhead easel, Adjustable height 14-25 inch, not further specified
Book holder, Overhead easel, Adjustable height 14-25 inch, Overhead only
Book holder, Overhead easel, Adjustable height/page bars, not further specified

Book holder, Overhead easel, Adjustable height/page bars, Overhead only
Book holder, Portable work desk, Adjusts to 10 angles, Closes as case
Book holder, Portable work desk, Adjusts to 10 angles, not further specified
Book holder, see, Page turner, book holder
Book holder, Tabletop, Wedge design, Lip at bottom edge
Book holder, Tabletop, Wedge design, not further specified
Book holder, Tray on floor stand, Adjusts to any angle, Acrylic tray
Book holder, Tray on floor stand, Adjusts to any angle, not further specified
Book holder pins, Replacement pins, For bottom of holder, not further specified
Book holder pins, Replacement pins, not further specified
Book holder/writer, Desktop easel type, 20-degree angle, Clip holds writing
Book holder/writer, Desktop easel type, 20-degree angle, not further specified
Bookmark, Holds book open, Leather strip, not further specified
Bookmark, Holds book open, Leather strip, Weighted ends
Bottle brush, Double nylon brush, Suction base, 16 inch diameter base
Bottle brush, Double nylon brush, Suction base, 6 inch diameter base
Bottle brush, Double nylon brush, Suction base, not further specified
Bottle brush, Nylon brush, Suction base, 12 inch stem
Bottle brush, Nylon brush, Suction base, not further specified
Bottle brush head, Replacement, not further specified
Bottle handle, For 1 or 2 liter, Replaces screw top, not further specified
Bottle handle, For 1 or 2 liter bottle, Replaces screw top, Lever opens lid
Bowl for eating, High-sided, 1/2 to 1.75 inches high, Dishwasher safe
Bowl for eating, High-sided, 1/2 to 1.75 inches high, not further specified
Bowl for eating, High-sided, 7.5 inch dim 1.75 high, Melamine
Bowl for eating, High-sided, 7.5 inch dim 1.75 high, not further specified
Bowl for eating, High-sided scoop, 6.5 inch diameter 2.75 high, Neoprene foam bottom
Bowl for eating, High-sided scoop, 6.5 inch diameter 2.75 high, not further specified
Bowl for eating, High-sided scoop, 6.6 inch diameter, Melamine
Bowl for eating, High-sided scoop, 6.6 inch diameter, not further specified
Bowl for eating, High-sided scoop, 7.75 inch diameter, Melamine
Bowl for eating, High-sided scoop, 7.75 inch diameter, not further specified
Bowl for eating, High-sided scoop, Dinner size, Neoprene foam bottom
Bowl for eating, High-sided scoop, Dinner size, not further specified
Bowl for eating, High-sided scoop, Large bowl, Neoprene foam bottom
Bowl for eating, High-sided scoop, Large bowl, not further specified
Bowl for eating, High-sided scoop, Medium bowl, Neoprene foam bottom
Bowl for eating, High-sided scoop, Medium bowl, not further specified
Bowl for eating, High-sided scoop, Medium bowl, Removable non-skid base
Bowl for eating, High-sided scoop, Small bowl, Non-skid base
Bowl for eating, High-sided scoop, Small bowl, not further specified
Bowl for eating, Scoop, Oval, Extra thick plastic
Bowl for eating, Scoop, Oval, not further specified
Bowl for eating, Scoop back, High back 11 inch oval, Non-skid base
Bowl for eating, Scoop back, High back 11 inch oval, not further specified
Bowl for eating, Scoop back, High back 8 inch oval, Break-resist plastic
Bowl for eating, Scoop back, High back 8 inch oval, not further specified
Bowl for eating, Scoop back, Vertical back 11 inch oval, Melamine
Bowl for eating, Scoop back, Vertical back 11 inch oval, not further specified
Bowl for eating, Scoop back, Vertical back 8 inch oval, Melamine
Bowl for eating, Scoop back, Vertical back 8 inch oval, not further specified
Bowl for eating, Scoop side, 5.5X6.6 inch oval, Melamine
Bowl for eating, Scoop side, 5.5X6.6 inch oval, not further specified
Bowl for eating, Scoop side, 7 inch diameter, Melamine
Bowl for eating, Scoop side, 7 inch diameter, not further specified
Bowl for eating, With inner lip, 5.5 inch diameter, Microwave safe
Bowl for eating, With inner lip, 5.5 inch diameter, not further specified
Bowl for eating, With inner lip, 6.5 inch diameter, Ceramic
Bowl for eating, With inner lip, 6.5 inch diameter, not further specified
Bowl for eating, With inner lip, 9 inch diameter, not further specified
Bowl for eating, With inner lip, 9 inch diameter, Suction base
Box top opener, Hand held, not further specified
Box top opener, Hand held, Push/turn/lift required, Built-up handle
Box top opener, Hand held, Push/turn/lift required, not further specified
Bra, Front hook closure, Cotton/polyester, Full fitting
Bra, Front hook closure, Cotton/polyester, not further specified
Bra, Front hook closure, Nylon/spandex, Longline
Bra, Front hook closure, Nylon/spandex, not further specified
Bra, Front hook closure, Nylon/spandex, Posture support
Bra, Front velcro closure, not further specified
Bra, Front velcro closure, Soft nylon, not further specified
Bracelet fastener, One-hand operated, Clips hold bracelet, not further specified
Bracelet fastener, One-hand operated, Clips hold bracelet, Plastic base
Bracket for remote control, For wheelchair, not further specified
Bracket for remote control, not further specified
Braille labeler, Plier grip, 1/4 and 1/2 inch tape, not further specified
Braille labeler, Plier grip, not further specified
Build-up material, see, Handle build-up material
Bulb planter, see, Garden bulb planter

Burglar alarm, see, Intruder alarm
Butter cutter, see, Eating aid, butter cutter
Button & zipper aid, Built-up handle, Grooved cylinder handle, Metal loop & zipper hook
Button & zipper aid, Built-up handle, Grooved cylinder handle, not further specified
Button & zipper aid, Built-up handle, Rubber grip, Metal loop & zipper hook
Button & zipper aid, Built-up handle, Rubber grip, not further specified
Button & zipper aid, Palm clip handle, C-shaped clip, Metal loop & zipper hook
Button & zipper aid, Palm clip handle, C-shaped clip, not further specified
Button & zipper aid, Palm clip on handle, Adjustable metal cuff, Metal loop zipper hook
Button & zipper aid, Palm clip on handle, Adjustable metal cuff, not further specified
Button & zipper aid, Palm clip on handle, Adjustable metal straps, Metal loop & zipper hook
Button & zipper aid, Palm clip on handle, Adjustable metal straps, not further specified
Button & zipper aid, Straight handle, Foam grip, Metal loop & zipper hook
Button & zipper aid, Straight handle, Foam grip, not further specified
Button & zipper aid, Straight handle, Rubber grip, Metal loop & zipper hook
Button & zipper aid, Straight handle, Rubber grip, not further specified
Button & zipper aid, Straight handle, Wood and rubber grip, Metal loop & zipper hook
Button & zipper aid, Straight handle, Wood and rubber grip, not further specified
Button & zipper aid, Straight handle, Wooden handle, Metal loop & zipper hook
Button & zipper aid, Straight handle, Wooden handle, not further specified
Button extender, Elastic loop, For cuff and collar, not further specified
Button extender, Elastic loop, not further specified
Button extender, Metal spring loop, For cuff and collar, not further specified
Button extender, Metal spring loop, not further specified
Button hook, 20 inch straight handle, For limited elbow extension, Metal button loop
Button hook, 20 inch straight handle, For limited elbow extension, not further specified
Button hook, Built-up handle, Adjustable finger rings, Metal button loop
Button hook, Built-up handle, Adjustable finger rings, not further specified
Button hook, Built-up handle, Plastic handle, Metal button loop
Button hook, Built-up handle, Plastic handle, not further specified
Button hook, Built-up handle, Rubber grip, Metal button loop
Button hook, Built-up handle, Rubber grip, not further specified
Button hook, Built-up handle, Rubber handle, Metal button hook
Button hook, Built-up handle, Rubber handle, Metal button loop
Button hook, Built-up handle, Rubber handle, not further specified
Button hook, Built-up handle, Weighted 8 ounces, Metal button loop
Button hook, Built-up handle, Weighted 8 ounces, not further specified
Button hook, Knob handle, Wood handle, Metal button hook
Button hook, Knob handle, Wood handle, Metal button loop
Button hook, Knob handle, Wood handle, not further specified
Button hook, Straight handle, Plastic, Metal button hook
Button hook, Straight handle, Plastic, not further specified
Button hook, Straight handle, Wood handle, Metal button loop
Button hook, Straight handle, Wood handle, not further specified
Button hook, Suction cup mounted, For one-hand use, Metal button loop
Button hook, Suction cup mounted, For one-hand use, not further specified
Button hook, Suction cup mounted, For one-hand use, Wire button hook
Button hook, Tapered handle, Wood handle, Large wire hook
Button hook, Tapered handle, Wood handle, not further specified

Cabinet door lock/latch, Plastic spring latch, Allows partial opening, not further specified
Cabinet door lock/latch, With magnetic key, No external knob, not further specified
Cabinet door lock/latch, With magnetic key, not further specified
Cabinet door opener, see, Car door opener
Caddy, see, Holder by purpose, As Shower caddy
Calculator, Large keys & display, Adjustable display angle, not further specified
Calculator, Large keys & display, Adjustable display angle, Solar/battery operated
Calculator, Large keys & display, Talking, Battery powered
Calculator, Large keys & display, Talking, not further specified
Calculator, Large non-slip keys, Large display, not further specified
Calculator, Large non-slip keys, Large display, Solar/battery operated
Calculator, Standard display, Talking, Battery powered
Calculator, Standard display, Talking, not further specified
Calendar, Braille, Raised black numbers, Magnetic as for refrigerator
Calendar, Braille, Raised black numbers, not further specified
Call signal, see, Alerting device
Camera rest, For Recreation belt, not further specified
Camisole, Adjustable straps, Cotton/polyester, not further specified
Camisole, Adjustable straps, not further specified
Camisole, Adjustable straps, Nylon, not further specified
Can opener, One-hand operated/countertop, Can held on hand-raised stand, AC powered
Can opener, One-hand operated/countertop, Can held on hand-raised stand, not further specified
Can opener, One-hand operated/hand held, Auto stop squeeze but no-press, Cordless rechargeable

Can opener, One-hand operated/hand held, Auto stop squeeze but no-press, not further specified
Can opener, One-hand operated/hand held, Right hand thumb press lever, Cordless rechargeable
Can opener, One-hand operated/hand held, Right hand thumb press lever, not further specified
Can opener, One-hand operated/hand held, Uncrimps rim, AC powered
Can opener, One-hand operated/hand held, Uncrimps rim, Cordless rechargeable
Can opener, One-hand operated/hand held, Uncrimps rim, not further specified
Can opener, One-hand operated/wall mount, Can held on hand-raised stand, Hand cranked
Can opener, One-hand operated/wall mount, Can held on hand-raised stand, not further specified
Can opener base, Lifts can to can opener, Clamp is raised by hand, not further specified
Can opener base, Lifts can to can opener, Clamp is raised by hand, Suction cup feet
Can opener/knife sharpener, Countertop, Power can piercing, AC powered
Can opener/knife sharpener, Countertop, Power can piercing, not further specified
Can tab & twist-cap opener, Two hands needed to operate, For pop/soda bottles and cans, not further specified
Cane holder, Adjustable clip-on, Hooks cane on table edge, not further specified
Cane holder, Adjustable clip-on, not further specified
Cane holder, Adjustable clip-on, Presses below table, not further specified
Cane ice tip, 4-point, Retractable, not further specified
Cane ice tip, 4-point, Retractable, Over cane tip
Cane ice tip, 4-point, Retractable with wire handle, not further specified
Cane ice tip, 4-point, Retractable with wire handle, Replaces cane tip
Cane ice tip, 5-point, Retractable, not further specified
Cane ice tip, 5-point, Retractable, Over cane tip
Cane ice tip, 5-point, Retractable, Replaces cane tip
Cane ice tip, Single point, Folding, not further specified
Cane ice tip, Single point, Folding, Over cane tip
Car door opener, Hand held, For button or pull, Lightweight
Car door opener, Hand held, For button or pull, not further specified
Car door opener, Hand held, For button or pull, Vinyl coating
Car door opener, Hand held, For button or pull, Y-shaped
Car door opener, Hand held, For pull-up handle, not further specified
Car door opener, Hand held, For push button, not further specified
Car door opener, Hand held, not further specified
Car door opener, see, Cupboard door opener
Carbon monoxide alarm, see, Gas detector alarm, carbon monoxide
Card ..., see, Playing card ...
Card shuffler, see, Playing card shuffler
Carpet saver runner, Non-skid backing, Absorbent fabric, For flat surface & for stair
Carpet saver runner, Non-skid backing, Absorbent fabric, not further specified
Carpet sweeper, Manual, 180 degree arc handle, Lightweight
Carpet sweeper, Manual, 180 degree arc handle, not further specified
Carpet sweeper, Manual, 180 degree arc handle, not further specified
Carpet sweeper, Manual, 180 degree arc handle, not further specified
Carpet sweeper, Manual, not further specified
Carrying aid, Shoulder strap, With hook, Adjustable length
Carrying aid, Shoulder strap, With hook, not further specified
Carrying bag, see, Walker bag
Cart, see, Utility cart, Garden cart
Cart, Two wheel folding, Capacity up to 100 pounds, Non-marring tires
Cart flatbed, see, Flatbed cart
Cassette tape player, Raised tactile markings, With headphone jacks, Battery powered
Cassette tape recorder/player, Raised tactile markings, With headphone jacks, Battery powered
Cassette tape recorder/player, Variable speed, With headphone jacks, Battery powered
Catapult, see, Chair rising aid
Catheter, see, Urinal, male ... sheath
Cathing mirror, see, Mirror self inspection
Ceiling brush, Telescoping handle, Detachable brush, not further specified
Ceiling brush, Telescoping handle, Detachable brush, Weight 3 pounds
Ceiling fan, Remote controlled, 4 lights, 5 blade
Ceiling fan, Remote controlled, 4 lights, not further specified
Ceiling fan, Remote controlled, not further specified
Chair, Straight or standard, No front rung or panel, not further specified
Chair, Straight or standard, not further specified
Chair catapult, see, Chair rising aid
Chair leg extender, Adjustable height, Sleeves with spacers, not further specified
Chair leg extender, Adjustable height, Sleeves with spacers, Plastic
Chair leg extender, Fixed 3 inch extension, Sleeves with spacers, not further specified
Chair leg extender, Fixed 3 inch extension, Sleeves with spacers, Plastic
Chair rising aid, Pneumatic lift seat, Settings to 300 pounds, 17 x 17 x 3-1/2 inches
Chair rising aid, Pneumatic lift seat, Settings to 300 pounds, not further specified
Chair rising aid, Spring loaded seat, Padded, Carrying handle
Chair rising aid, Spring loaded seat, Padded, not further specified
Chair rising aid, Wooden frame with handgrips, Fits over chair, Adjustable size
Chair rising aid, Wooden frame with handgrips, Fits over chair, not further specified
Chair with power lift, Power reclining, Positions upright to reclining, not further specified

Chair with power lift, Power reclining, Positions upright to reclining, With footrest
Checker Set, Large rubber pieces, Brightly colored, not further specified
Checker set, Tactile & visual, Raised/recessed squares, not further specified
Checker set, Tactile & visual, Raised/recessed squares, Red and black checkers
Cheese slicer, Spatulate with cutting slot, 90 degree handle, Dishwasher safe
Cheese slicer, Spatulate with cutting slot, 90 degree handle, not further specified
Chinese checker set, Large peg pieces, Hardwood board, not further specified
Chinese checker set, Large peg pieces, Hardwood board, With instructions
Cigarette holder, Adjustable palm clip, Cigarette held by clip, not further specified
Cigarette holder, Adjustable palm clip, not further specified
Clock, Liquid crystal display, 1.5 inch diameter overall, not further specified
Clock, Liquid crystal display, 1.5 inch diameter overall, Velcro mount
Clock wall mounted, see, Wall clock
Closed caption decoder, TV/VCR/cable/satellite, Can connect to TV directly, not further specified
Closed caption decoder, TV/VCR/cable/satellite, not further specified
Closed caption decoder, VCR/cable/satellite, No direct TV connection, not further specified
Closed caption decoder, VCR/cable/satellite, not further specified
Closet carousel, Wire rack system, Motorized rotating, 10 sections/10 rods
Closet carousel, Wire rack system, Motorized rotating, 16 sections/16 rods
Closet carousel, Wire rack system, Motorized rotating, 9 sections/15 rods
Closet carousel, Wire rack system, Motorized rotating, not further specified
Closet carousel, Wire rack system, Motorized rotating, Various numbers sections/rods
Closet rod, Lowered on droppers, Auxiliary, not further specified
Closet rod, Lowered on droppers, Auxiliary, Suspends from regular rod
Closet rod, Raises & lowers, Electrical, AC powered
Closet rod, Raises & lowers, Electrical, not further specified
Closet rod, Raises & lowers, Manual/mechanical, not further specified
Closet rod, Raises & lowers, not further specified
Clothes hamper, Under-cabinet mount, Organizer type, not further specified
Clothes hamper, Under-cabinet mount, Organizer type, Sliding extra deep
Clothes hook rack, Six clothes hooks, Hangs over door
Clothes rod, Three loop type rods, On tension pole, Portable
Clothes rod, With shoe shelf, On two tension poles, Portable
Clothes rod basket, Hangs from top rod, Creates lower storage, For seated use
Clothespins, Press-down type, No squeeze required, not further specified
Clothespins, Press-down type, not further specified
Coffee maker, Automatic shut-off, Timer to turn off, Limits the heating interval
Coffee maker, Automatic shut-off, Timer to turn off, not further specified
Comb, 19 inch handle, Adjustable angle, Handle folds to 8 inches
Comb, 19 inch handle, Adjustable angle, not further specified
Comb, 20 inch handle, Adjustable angle, Bendable handle
Comb, 20 inch handle, Adjustable angle, not further specified
Comb, Built-up handle, 1.25 inch foam handle, not further specified
Comb, Built-up handle, 1.5 inch foam handle, not further specified
Comb, Built-up handle, not further specified
Comb, Long handle, Adjustable angle, Built up handle grip
Comb, Long handle, Adjustable angle, Grooved handle
Comb, not further specified
Comb, Weighted handle 8 ounce, not further specified
Comb hair lift, see, Hair lift comb
Commode, Adjustable 17-22 inches high, With back and arms, not further specified
Commode, Adjustable 17-22 inches high, With back and arms, Wood frame painted
Commode, Adjustable 19-23 inches high, With back and arms, Extra wide
Commode, Adjustable 19-23 inches high, With back and arms, not further specified
Commode, Adjustable 19-23 inches high, With back and drop arms, not further specified
Commode, Adjustable 19-23 inches high, With back and drop arms, With lid
Commode, Adjustable 19-23 inches high, With side rails and back, Holds up to 200 pounds
Commode, Adjustable 19-23 inches high, With side rails and back, not further specified
Commode, Adjustable height, Backless with arms, 3-way with lid
Commode, Adjustable height, Backless with arms, not further specified
Commode, Adjustable height, Backless with drop arms, not further specified
Commode, Adjustable height, Backless with drop arms, With lid
Commode, Adjustable height, With arms, 3 way with lid
Commode, Adjustable height, With arms, not further specified
Commode, Adjustable height, With back and arms, Aluminum tube frame
Commode, Adjustable height, With back and arms, not further specified
Commode, Adjustable height, With back and arms, With lid
Commode, Adjustable height, With back and arms, With transfer seat on right
Commode, Adjustable height, With back and drop arms, not further specified
Commode, Adjustable height, With back and drop arms, Padded seat
Commode, Adjustable height, With side rails & rail back, No lid
Commode, Adjustable height, With side rails no back, No lid

Commode, Adjustable height, With side rails no back, not further specified
Commode, Adjustable height, With side rails no back, Slants forward
Commode, Fixed height, Removable back and arms, not further specified
Commode, Fixed height, Removable back and arms, Rolling and folds
Commode, Fixed height, With back and arms, Chair look-alike
Commode, Fixed height, With back and arms, Holds 250 pounds
Commode, Fixed height, With back and arms, not further specified
Commode, Fixed height, With back and arms, Rolling
Commode, Fixed height, With back and arms, Rolling & padded
Commode, Fixed height, With back and arms, Wide padded seat
Commode, Wide and fixed height, With back and arms, For extremely heavy person
Commode, Wide and fixed height, With back and arms, not further specified
Commode pail, 5 quart capacity, Plastic, Fits most commodes
Commode pail, 5 quart capacity, Plastic, not further specified
Commode pail, For shower chair/commode, not further specified
Commode pail, not further specified
Commode pail liners, Disposable, not further specified
Commode pail liners, Disposable, Self-sealing, not further specified
Commode/bath chair, Adjustable height, Back and arms, not further specified
Commode/bath chair, Adjustable height, Back and arms, Padded adjustable back
Commode/bath chair, Adjustable height, No grips, not further specified
Commode/bath chair, Adjustable height, No grips, Open seat front
Commode/bath chair, Fixed height, Back and arms, Lightweight plastic resin
Commode/bath chair, Fixed height, Back and arms, not further specified
Commode/bath transfer seat, Adjustable height & backrest, Back & movable arm, not further specified
Commode/bath transfer seat, Adjustable height & backrest, Back & movable arm, Padded seat and back
Commode/bath transfer seat, Adjustable height & backrest, not further specified
Commode/bath transfer seat, Adjustable height & backrest, Swing arm, not further specified
Commode/bath transfer seat, Adjustable height & backrest, With back and arms, not further specified
Commode/bath transfer seat, Adjustable height & backrest, With back and arms, Smooth hard surface
Commode/bath transfer seat, Adjustable height & backrest, With back and fixed arms, not further specified
Commode/bath transfer seat, Adjustable height & backrest, With back and fixed arms, Padded
Commode/shower chair, Adjustable height, Back and arms, Cut-out padded seat
Commode/shower chair, Adjustable height, Back and arms, not further specified
Commode/shower chair, Fixed height, Back & arms, not further specified
Commode/shower chair, Fixed height, Back & arms, Rolling
Communication aid, Fabric covered cork board, 24 x 18 inches, Built-in hanger
Communication aid, Fabric covered cork board, 24 x 36 inches, Built-in hanger
Communication aid, Visual board with stickers, Everyday life topics, Indexed
Communication aid, Visual board with stickers, Everyday life topics, not further specified
Computer cart, Wheelchair accessible, 5 inch locking casters, not further specified
Computer cart, Wheelchair accessible, 5 inch locking casters, Privacy panels
Computer software, Character recognition, Speech synthesizer, not further specified
Computer software, Character recognition, Speech synthesizer, Reads typewriter & dot matrix
Computer software, Screen enlarger, 2 power, not further specified
Computer software, Screen enlarger, 2 power, Uses DOS operating system
Computer software, Screen enlarger, 2X to 16X zoom, not further specified
Computer software, Screen enlarger, 2X to 16X zoom, Requires EGA or VGA graphics
Computer software, Screen enlarger, 5 power, not further specified
Computer software, Screen enlarger, 5 power, Requires DOS with 512K RAM
Computer workstation, Bi-level adjustable height, Mouse arm support, 43 X 36 inch surface
Cookbook, Large print, Easel style, not further specified
Cookbook, Large print, not further specified
Cookbook rack, Under-cabinet mount, Spring hinge mount, Lowers into position
Cookbook rack, Under-cabinet mount, Spring hinge mount, not further specified
Corner guard, Clear soft plastic, Covers sharp corners, not further specified
Corner guard, Clear soft plastic, Covers sharp corners, Various sizes
Corner guard, Rubber, Covers sharp corners, not further specified
Corner guard, Rubber, Covers sharp corners, Various sizes
Cosmetic mirror, see, Makeup mirror
Crescent blade knife, see, Table/kitchen knife, crescent blade
Cribbage board, not further specified
Cribbage board, With raised hole markers, not further specified
Croakie, see, Eyeglass retainer, strap
Crock pot, see, Slow cooker
Crossword puzzles, Large print, not further specified
Crossword puzzles, not further specified
Crutch armrests, Imitation lamb's-wool, Attaches with velcro, not further specified
Crutch handgrips, Imitation lamb's-wool, Attaches with velcro, not further specified
Cup, Hook handle, Lid with spout, Clear polycarbonate
Cup, Hook handle, Lid with spout, not further specified
Cup, see also, Mug
Cup, Single cup handle, Lid with spout, not further specified
Cup, Single cup handle, No lid, Non-skid bottom
Cup, Single cup handle, No lid, not further specified

Cup, Single cup handle, not further specified
Cup base, For Tumbler vacuum control, 5 inch diameter, Non-tip
Cup base, For Tumbler vacuum control, 5 inch diameter, not further specified
Cup base non-slip, For various cups, High-tack soft plastic, Disk fastens to cup
Cup base non-slip, For various cups, High-tack soft plastic, not further specified
Cup flow button, For Tumbler vacuum control, Flow regulator, not further specified
Cup holder, Weighted, Holds cups/tumblers, not further specified
Cup holder, Weighted, Holds cups/tumblers, Spring attached lid
Cup holder carousel, Under-cabinet mount, Manual revolving, 8 cups
Cup holder carousel, Under-cabinet mount, Manual revolving, not further specified
Cup holder wire rack, Under-cabinet mount, Sliding, 12 cups
Cup holder wire rack, Under-cabinet mount, Sliding, not further specified
Cup holder/handle, Attaches to table, Cup has hook handle, Non-spill lid
Cup holder/handle, Attaches to table, Cup has hook handle, not further specified
Cup holder/handle, Hand loop and ledge grip, Fixed diameter, not further specified
Cup holder/handle, Hand loop and ledge grip, Fixed diameter, Oversized handle
Cup holder/handle, Hook handle, Adjustable diameter, not further specified
Cup holder/handle, Hook handle, Adjustable diameter, Oversized handle
Cup lid with spout, For cup holder/handle, not further specified
Cup lid with spout, For Tumbler vacuum control, Replacement lid, not further specified
Cup lid with spout, not further specified
Cupboard door opener, Hand held, Hook type, not further specified
Cupboard door opener, Hand held, Hook type, S-shaped
Cupboard door opener, see also, Car door opener
Cupboard lock, Magnetic key release, not further specified
Cupboard lock, not further specified
Curling iron with brush, Cool tip, Swivel cord, 30 second heat-up
Curling iron with brush, Cool tip, Swivel cord, not further specified
Cutting board, see also, Sandwich board
Cutting board, With colander, For over-sink, Side storage area
Cutting board, With spikes, For over-sink, Flat top
Cutting board, With spikes, Suction cup feet, Flat top
Cutting board, With spikes, Suction cup feet, not further specified
Cutting board, With spikes, Suction cup feet, With juice grooves
Cutting board, With spikes & corner guard, For over-sink, Flat top
Cutting board, With spikes & corner guard, For over-sink, No handles
Cutting board, With spikes & corner guard, For over-sink, not further specified
Cutting board, With spikes & corner guard, For over-sink, Plastic coated handles
Cutting board, With spikes & corner guard, Rubber feet, not further specified
Cutting board, With spikes & corner guard, Suction cup base, Flat polyethylene
Cutting board, With spikes & corner guard, Suction cup base, not further specified
Cutting board, With spikes & corner guard, Suction cup base, With handle
Cutting board, With spikes & raised rim, Plain bottom, Hardwood
Cutting board, With spikes & raised rim, Plain bottom, not further specified
Cutting board, With spikes & raised rim, Suction cup base, Maple
Cutting board, With spikes & raised rim, Suction cup base, not further specified
Cutting board, With spikes & raised rim, Suction cup base, Plastic
Cutting board, With spikes and jar vice, Suction cup base, For one-hand use
Cutting board, With spikes and jar vice, Suction cup base, not further specified
Cutting board kit, Pins/guards/suction cups, not further specified
Cutting board kit, Pins/guards/suction cups, To convert wooden board, not further specified
Cutting board spikes, 2-inch long stainless, not further specified
Cutting board spikes, not further specified
Cutting frame, Base with adjustable width, not further specified
Cutting frame, Base with adjustable width, Without knife, not further specified
Cutting frame, Two hands needed to operate, Gripping jaws/squeeze handles, not further specified
Cutting frame, Two hands needed to operate, Gripping jaws/squeeze handles, Steel
Cutting frame/knife, Base with adjustable width, With knife, 120 degree knife handle
Cutting frame/knife, Base with adjustable width, With knife, not further specified
Cutting frame/knife, Base with adjustable width, With serrated knife, 120 degree knife handle
Cutting frame/knife, Base with adjustable width, With serrated knife, not further specified

---

Decubitus cushion cover, Large, Denim, not further specified
Decubitus cushion cover, Large, not further specified
Decubitus cushion cover, Medium, Denim, not further specified
Decubitus cushion cover, Medium, not further specified
Decubitus cushion cover, Small, Denim, not further specified
Decubitus cushion cover, Small, not further specified
Dental floss, For dental flosser, not further specified
Dental floss, For dental flosser, Unwaxed, not further specified
Dental floss, For dental flosser, Waxed, not further specified
Dental flosser, Fits Universal cuff, not further specified

Dental flosser, Fits Universal cuff, Use turn-round cuff, not further specified
Dental flosser, Hand held, Fork shape, not further specified
Dental flosser, Hand held, Fork shape, Plastic
Dental flosser, Stand mounted, not further specified
Dental flosser, Stand mounted, With floss spool, not further specified
Dental plaque remover, see, Plaque remover
Denture brush, One-hand operated, Scrub brush type, not further specified
Denture brush, One-hand operated, Scrub brush type, Suction cup base
Denture brush, One-hand operated, Tooth brush type, not further specified
Denture brush, One-hand operated, Tooth brush type, Suction cup base
Dibble, see, Garden bulb planter
Dice, With raised dots, Large size, not further specified
Dice, With raised dots, not further specified
Dice set, With raised dots, Standard size, not further specified
Disabled parking sign, Magnetic, Place on vehicle door, not further specified
Dish brush, One-hand operated, Rounded bristles, not further specified
Dish brush, One-hand operated, Rounded bristles, Suction cup base
Dolly, see, Cart
Dominoes, With raised dots, Black dots on white, not further specified
Dominoes, With raised dots, not further specified
Door, Interior passage, Folding, Bi-fold
Door, Interior passage, Folding, not further specified
Door, Interior passage, Sliding, not further specified
Door, Interior passage, Sliding, Outside the wall
Door, Interior passage, Sliding, Pocket in wall
Door entry bathtub, see, Bathtub, door entry
Door hinge offset, see, Offset door hinge
Door intercom, see, Entry monitor
Door jam (not jamb) or jammer, see, Door stop
Door knob gripper, Spoke grip, Fits standard knob, not further specified
Door knob gripper, Spoke grip, not further specified
Door knob gripper, Textured grip, not further specified
Door knob gripper, Textured grip, Stretches over knob, not further specified
Door knob lever, 2-1/2 inch lever, Grips with gaskets, Adjustable with heat gun
Door knob lever, 2-1/2 inch lever, Grips with gaskets, not further specified
Door knob lever, 3 inch lever, Screw fastened, 2-1/2 inch diameter knob
Door knob lever, 3 inch lever, Screw fastened, 2-3/4 inch diameter knob
Door knob lever, 3 inch lever, Screw fastened, not further specified
Door knob lever, 3 inch lever, Screw fastened, not further specified
Door knob lever, 4 inch lever, Grips with gaskets, Fits various knobs
Door knob lever, 4 inch lever, Grips with gaskets, not further specified
Door knob lever, 4-1/2 inch lever, Soft rubber slip-on, Fits standard knobs
Door knob lever, 4-1/2 inch lever, Soft rubber slip-on, not further specified
Door knob lever, 4.5 inch lever, Portable, Fits 2-inch diameter knob
Door knob lever, 4.5 inch lever, Portable, not further specified
Door knob lever, Extension, Soft rubber slip-on, Fits various knobs
Door knob lever, Extension, Soft rubber slip-on, not further specified
Door knob lever, Extension luminous, Soft rubber slip-on, Fits various knobs
Door knob lever, Extension luminous, Soft rubber slip-on, not further specified
Door knock sensor, Knock activated, Flashing light signal, not further specified
Door knock sensor, Knock activated, Flashing light signal, Not remote
Door knock sensor, Knock activated, Flashing light signal, With remote receiver
Door latch, Adjustable magnetic grip, No external knob, not further specified
Door lock light, Attach above keyhole, Battery operated, not further specified
Door lock light, Attach above keyhole, not further specified
Door opener, see, Door operator
Door opening alarm, Doorstop type, Sound signal, Battery powered
Door opening alarm, Doorstop type, Sound signal, not further specified
Door opening alarm, see also, Intruder alarm
Door operator, For door/gate up to 60 pounds, Closing operation only, Spring mechanism
Door operator, Electric, Door mounted button, AC powered
Door operator, Electric, Door mounted button, not further specified
Door operator, Electric, Wall plate-button, AC powered
Door operator, Electric, Wall plate-button, not further specified
Door operator, For sliding glass door, Remote control, Motion detector option
Door operator, Push/pull operation, Actuates latch, Manual-mechanical
Door operator, Push/pull operation, Actuates latch, not further specified
Door Operator, With remote control, Kit includes manual latch, Requires compressed air source
Door peephole, Wide angle, In hole in door, Requires drilling
Door screen, Retracting/rolling, not further specified
Door screen, Retracting/rolling, Zero swing area, not further specified
Door stop, Wedges under knob, Steel pole, not further specified
Door stop, Wedges under knob, Steel pole, Wide rubber foot
Door threshold ramp, not further specified
Door threshold ramp, One-sided, 1 inch high, 12 inches wide
Door threshold ramp, One-sided, 1 inch high, not further specified
Door threshold ramp, One-sided, 1/4 inch high, 2 to 3 inches wide
Door threshold ramp, One-sided, 1/4 inch high, not further specified
Door threshold ramp, Replaces threshold, 1 inch high, 28 inches wide

Faucet turner, Clamps onto knob faucet grip, Wrench handle, not further specified
Faucet turner, Clamps onto knob faucet grip, Wrench handle, Stainless steel
Faucet turner, Clamps to knob or crosshead, Long and short lever options, Chromed
Faucet turner, Clamps to knob or crosshead, Long and short lever options, not further specified
Faucet turner, Hooks onto cross-head taps, Wrench handle, Molded plastic
Faucet turner, Hooks onto cross-head taps, Wrench handle, not further specified
Faucet turner, Hooks onto single handle tap, Wrench handle, Molded plastic
Faucet turner, Hooks onto single handle tap, Wrench handle, not further specified
Faucet turner, Screw clamp to crosshead tap, Wrench handle, not further specified
Faucet turner, Screw clamp to crosshead tap, Wrench handle, Wood
Faucet turner, Spring loaded pins, L-handle, not further specified
Faucet turner, Spring loaded pins, L-handle, Plastic
Faucet turner, Spring loaded pins, T-handle, not further specified
Faucet turner, Spring loaded pins, T-handle, Plastic
Feeding cup, see, Tumbler with vacuum control
Feeding tumbler, see, Tumbler with vacuum control
Fingernail brush, Suction cup base, not further specified
Fingernail brush, Suction cup base, Plastic, not further specified
Fingernail clipper, Mounted on base, Large lever operated, not further specified
Fingernail clipper, Mounted on base, Large lever operated, With emery board holder
Fingernail clipper, Non-skid feet, Weight stabilized, With 4 inch file
Fingernail clipper, One-hand operation, Clips by pressing on base, not further specified
Fingernail clipper, One-hand operation, Clips by pressing on base, With emery board holder
Fingernail clipper, Suction cup base, Weight stabilized, not further specified
Fingernail clipper, Suction cup base, Weight stabilized, With emery boards
Fingernail clipper, With finger-positioning guide, Pinch operated, not further specified
Fingernail clipper, With finger-positioning guide, Pinch operated, With thumb/finger rings
Fingernail file, Suction cup base, Abrasive cloth, not further specified
Fingernail file, Suction cup base, not further specified
Fingernail scissors, Plier handle, Self opening, End loop
Fingernail scissors, Plier handle, Self opening, not further specified
Fire Escape Ladder, Reaches 12 feet, Capacity up to 600 lbs, Aluminum and plastic
Fire Escape Ladder, Reaches 24 feet, Capacity up to 600 lbs, Aluminum and plastic
Fire extinguisher, Hand held under 5 pounds, All classes of fire, not further specified
Fire extinguisher, Hand held under 5 pounds, All classes of fire, With wall bracket
Fire extinguisher, In-range hood, Automatic, Heat sensitive
Fire extinguisher, In-range hood, Automatic, not further specified
Fireplace screen, Wrap around, 32 inches high x 39 x 7, Black
Fireplace screen, Wrap around, 32 inches high x 39 x 7, not further specified
Firewood cart, 16 inch wheels, Holds 200 pounds, not further specified
Firewood cart, 16 inch wheels, Holds 200 pounds, Tubular frame
Flashlight, Lithium battery long-life, Twist-on switch, Knurled body
Flashlight, Snaps to cane/walker, Twist to switch on, Battery powered
Flatbed cart, Rubber casters, Folding handle, not further specified
Flatbed cart, Rubber casters, Folding handle, Up to 240 pounds
Flatbed cart heavy duty, Rubber casters, Folding handle, not further specified
Flatbed cart heavy duty, Rubber casters, Folding handle, Up to 440 pounds
Flatware, Built-up handles, Adjustable finger rings, Can add weights
Flatware, Built-up handles, Adjustable finger rings, not further specified
Flatware, Built-up handles, Angled for Left hand use, Molded plastic handles
Flatware, Built-up handles, Angled for Left hand use, not further specified
Flatware, Built-up handles, Angled for Left hand use, Spoon & fork only
Flatware, Built-up handles, Angled for Right hand use, Molded plastic handles
Flatware, Built-up handles, Angled for Right hand use, not further specified
Flatware, Built-up handles, Angled for Right hand use, Spoon & fork only
Flatware, Built-up handles, Collar at handle base, Contoured handles
Flatware, Built-up handles, Collar at handle base, not further specified
Flatware, Built-up handles, Curved for arthritis, not further specified
Flatware, Built-up handles, Curved for arthritis, Polypropylene handles
Flatware, Built-up handles, Hard plastic coated heads, 1 inch diameter handles
Flatware, Built-up handles, Hard plastic coated heads, not further specified
Flatware, Built-up handles, Hard plastic coated heads, Oval handles
Flatware, Built-up handles, Hard plastic coated heads, Rubberized handles
Flatware, Built-up handles, Indented for Left hand use, not further specified
Flatware, Built-up handles, Indented for Right hand use, not further specified
Flatware, Built-up handles, Knife is serrated, not further specified
Flatware, Built-up handles, Knife is serrated, Oval handles
Flatware, Built-up handles, not further specified
Flatware, Built-up handles, Right angle knife, 1 inch diameter foam handles
Flatware, Built-up handles, Right angle knife, not further specified
Flatware, Built-up handles, Soft plastic coated heads, 1 inch diameter handles
Flatware, Built-up handles, Soft plastic coated heads, not further specified
Flatware, Built-up handles, Standard heads, 1 inch diameter foam handles

Flatware, Built-up handles, Standard heads, 1-1/2 inch foam handles
Flatware, Built-up handles, Standard heads, 1-1/2 inch soft foam handles
Flatware, Built-up handles, Standard heads, 1-3/8 inch soft foam handles
Flatware, Built-up handles, Standard heads, 1-5/16 inch handles
Flatware, Built-up handles, Standard heads, 8 ounce weighted handles
Flatware, Built-up handles, Standard heads, Adjustable finger grips
Flatware, Built-up handles, Standard heads, Adjustable finger rings
Flatware, Built-up handles, Standard heads, Firm foam handles
Flatware, Built-up handles, Standard heads, not further specified
Flatware, Built-up handles, Standard heads, Rubberized handles
Flatware, Built-up handles, Standard heads, Solid plastic handles
Flatware, Coated tube handles, Knife with right angle rocker blade, not further specified
Flatware, Coated tube handles, Standard heads, 1 inch diameter
Flatware, Coated tube handles, Standard heads, 1-1/2 inch diameter
Flatware, Coated tube handles, Standard heads, 1-1/4 inch diameter
Flatware, Coated tube handles, Standard heads, not further specified
Flatware, Drop head handles, Swivel heads adjustable stops, not further specified
Flatware, Drop head handles, Swivel heads adjustable stops, Stainless steel
Flatware, Extension handles, Adjustable angles, 10 inches long
Flatware, Extension handles, Adjustable angles, not further specified
Flatware, Handle separable from heads, Interchangeable heads, not further specified
Flatware, Handle separable from heads, Interchangeable heads, Teaspoon fork knife tablespoon
Flatware, Long coated tube handles, Standard heads, 1 inch diameter
Flatware, Long coated tube handles, Standard heads, not further specified
Flatware, On horizontal palm clips, Standard heads, Adjustable coated clips
Flatware, On horizontal palm clips, Standard heads, not further specified
Flatware, On vertical palm clip, Hard plastic coated heads, Adjustable clip
Flatware, On vertical palm clip, Hard plastic coated heads, not further specified
Flatware, On vertical palm clips, Standard heads, Adjustable coated clips
Flatware, On vertical palm clips, Standard heads, not further specified
Flatware, With thumb/forefinger grips, Adjustable grips, not further specified
Flatware, With thumb/forefinger grips, Adjustable grips, Plastic coated grips
Flo-Trol cup, see, Tumbler with vacuum control
Floor cart, Ball bearing wheels, 5 inch wooden handle, not further specified
Floor cart, Ball bearing wheels, 5 inch wooden handle, Rubber back stop
Floor cart, Ball bearing wheels, Extended hinged handle, not further specified
Floor cart, Ball bearing wheels, Extended strap or cord handle, not further specified
Floor cart, Nylon casters, 15 inches square, not further specified
Floor cart, Nylon casters, 15 inches square, Wood
Floor chair and mattress, Folds out, Unfolded lies directly on floor, Folded makes low armless chair
Floor trivet, see, Floor cart
Floss(er), see, Dental floss(er)
Fluorescent light tube, 15 watts equivalent to 54 watt, Globe shape, 9000 hour bulb
Fluorescent light tube, 15 watts equivalent to 54 watt, Globe shape, not further specified
Fluorescent light tube, 15 watts equivalent to 54 watt, Tapered capsule, 9000 hour bulb
Fluorescent light tube, 15 watts equivalent to 54 watt, Tapered capsule, not further specified
Fluorescent light tube, 18 watts equivalent to 75 watt, Tapered capsule, 9000 hour bulb
Fluorescent light tube, 18 watts equivalent to 75 watt, Tapered capsule, not further specified
Fluorescent light tube, 27 watt equivalent to 100 watt, Rod shape, 9000 hour bulb
Fluorescent light tube, 27 watt equivalent to 100 watt, Rod shape, not further specified
Fluorescent light tube, Cool white, not further specified
Fluorescent light tube, Cool white, Various sizes, not further specified
Fluorescent light tube, Daylight simulation, not further specified
Fluorescent light tube, Daylight simulation, Various sizes, not further specified
Fluorescent light tube, Warm white, not further specified
Fluorescent light tube, Warm white, Various sizes, not further specified
Fluorescent tube/ballast, 13 watts equivalent to 54 watt, Rod shape tube, 45000 hour ballast
Fluorescent tube/ballast, 13 watts equivalent to 54 watt, Rod shape tube, not further specified
Foam tubing, Handle adapter, 1/2 inch ID x 1-1/2 OD, 1 yard long
Foam tubing, Handle adapter, 1/2 inch ID x 1-1/2 OD, not further specified
Foam tubing, Handle adapter, 1/2 inch ID x 1-1/4 OD, 1 yard long
Foam tubing, Handle adapter, 1/2 inch ID x 1-1/4 OD, 2 yards long
Foam tubing, Handle adapter, 1/2 inch ID x 1-1/4 OD, not further specified
Foam tubing, Handle adapter, 1/2 inch ID x 1-3/8 OD, not further specified
Foam tubing, Handle adapter, 1/2 inch ID x 1-3/8 OD, Slips onto utensil handle
Foam tubing, Handle adapter, 1/2 inch ID x 2 OD, 1 yard long
Foam tubing, Handle adapter, 1/2 inch ID x 2 OD, not further specified
Foam tubing, Handle adapter, 1/4 inch ID x 1 OD, 1 yard long
Foam tubing, Handle adapter, 1/4 inch ID x 1 OD, not further specified
Foam tubing, Handle adapter, 1/4 inch ID X 1-1/2 OD, 1 yard long
Foam tubing, Handle adapter, 1/4 inch ID X 1-1/2 OD, not further specified
Foam tubing, Handle adapter, 1/4 inch ID X 1-1/4 OD, 1 yard long
Foam tubing, Handle adapter, 1/4 inch ID X 1-1/4 OD, 2 yard long
Foam tubing, Handle adapter, 1/4 inch ID X 1-1/4 OD, not further specified

Foam tubing, Handle adapter, 1/4 inch ID X 3/4 OD, 1 yard long
Foam tubing, Handle adapter, 1/4 inch ID X 3/4 OD, not further specified
Foam tubing, Handle adapter, 1/8 inch ID X 1-1/4 OD, 2 yards long
Foam tubing, Handle adapter, 1/8 inch ID X 1-1/4 OD, not further specified
Foam tubing, Handle adapter, 3/4 inch ID X 2-1/4 OD, 1 yard long
Foam tubing, Handle adapter, 3/4 inch ID X 2-1/4 OD, not further specified
Foam tubing, Handle adapter, 3/8 inch ID X 1 OD, 1 foot long
Foam tubing, Handle adapter, 3/8 inch ID X 1 OD, not further specified
Foam tubing, Handle adapter, 3/8 inch ID X 1-1/4 OD, 1 yard long
Foam tubing, Handle adapter, 3/8 inch ID X 1-1/4 OD, 3 inches long
Foam tubing, Handle adapter, 3/8 inch ID X 1-1/4 OD, not further specified
Foam tubing, Handle adapter, 3/8 inch ID X 1-1/8 OD, 1 foot long
Foam tubing, Handle adapter, 3/8 inch ID X 1-1/8 OD, 1 yard long
Foam tubing, Handle adapter, 3/8 inch ID X 1-1/8 OD, not further specified
Foam tubing, Handle adapter, 3/8 inch ID X 1-3/8 OD, 1 yard long
Foam tubing, Handle adapter, 3/8 inch ID X 1-3/8 OD, not further specified
Foam tubing, Handle adapter, 3/8 inch ID X 1-3/8 OD, Oval cross section
Foam tubing, Handle adapter, 3/8 inch ID X 1-7/8 OD, 1 yard long
Foam tubing, Handle adapter, 3/8 inch ID X 1-7/8 OD, not further specified
Foam tubing, Handle adapter, 4 sizes in a kit, not further specified
Foam tubing, Handle adapter, 5/8 inch ID X 1-1/8 OD, 1 foot long
Foam tubing, Handle adapter, 5/8 inch ID X 1-1/8 OD, not further specified
Foam tubing, Handle adapter, 6 assorted sizes, 1 foot long each
Foam tubing, Handle adapter, 6 assorted sizes, not further specified
Foam tubing, Handle adapter, 7 assorted sizes, Each 1 yard long
Foam tubing, Handle adapter, 7 assorted sizes, not further specified
Foam tubing, Handle adapter, not further specified
Foam tubing, Handle adapter, Various diameters, not further specified
Foam tubing, Handle adapter, Various diameters, Various lengths
Food bumper, see, Food guard for plate
Food Chopper, For vegetables/nuts etc., Auto chopping-blade rotation, Push-down operation
Food chopper knife, Top palmar handle, 2 crescent blades, Blades parallel to handle
Food chopper knife, Top palmar handle, 2 crescent blades, not further specified
Food grater, One-hand operated, Suction cup base, Fine/coarse grater
Food grater, One-hand operated, Suction cup base, Interchangeable graters
Food grater, One-hand operated, Suction cup base, not further specified
Food guard for plate, Clips inside plate, 6 to 8 inch plate, not further specified
Food guard for plate, Clips inside plate, 6 to 8 inch plate, Stainless steel
Food guard for plate, Clips inside plate, 8 to 10 inch plate, not further specified
Food guard for plate, Clips inside plate, 8 to 10 inch plate, Stainless steel
Food guard for plate, Clips inside plate, 9 to 11 inch plate, not further specified
Food guard for plate, Clips inside plate, 9 to 11 inch plate, Stainless steel
Food guard for plate, Clips inside plate, 9 to 11 inch plate, White plastic
Food guard for plate, Clips inside plate, Any size plate, Flexible white plastic
Food guard for plate, Clips inside plate, Any size plate, not further specified
Food guard for plate, Clips inside plate, Scooping contour top, not further specified
Food guard for plate, Clips inside plate, Scooping contour top, White plastic
Food guard for plate, Snaps around rim, 6 to 8 inch plate, Clear plastic
Food guard for plate, Snaps around rim, 6 to 8 inch plate, not further specified
Food guard for plate, Snaps around rim, 8 to 10 inch plate, Clear plastic
Food guard for plate, Snaps around rim, 8 to 10 inch plate, not further specified
Food guard for plate, Snaps around rim, 9 to 11 inch plate, Clear plastic
Food guard for plate, Snaps around rim, 9 to 11 inch plate, not further specified
Food guard for plate, Snaps around rim, Any size plate, Clear plastic tapered ends
Food guard for plate, Snaps around rim, Any size plate, not further specified
Food guard for plate, Snaps around rim, not further specified
Food mixer, Counter stand, 1-1/2 & 4 quart bowls, 12 speed
Food mixer, Counter stand, 1-1/2 & 4 quart bowls, not further specified
Foot brush, With sponge tip, Brush at lower edge, Adjusts with heat gun
Foot brush, With sponge tip, Brush at lower edge, not further specified
Foot brush, With wedge sponge tip, Brush at lower edge, Long handle
Foot brush, With wedge sponge tip, Brush at lower edge, not further specified
Foot brush sponge, not further specified
Foot brush sponge, Replacement tip, not further specified
Foot brush sponge, Replacement tip, not further specified
Foot brush sponge, Replacement tip, Wedge tip, not further specified
Foot rest, For shower chair, Folding, not further specified
Foot rest, For shower chair, not further specified
Foot rest, Free standing, Adjustable tilt, Padded wood
Forearm crutch cuff, Imitation lamb's-wool, Attaches with velcro, not further specified
Forearm crutch handgrips, Imitation lamb's-wool, Attaches with velcro, not further specified
Fork, Built-up handle, 3 large tines, not further specified
Fork, Built-up handle, 3 large tines, Tapered handle
Fork, Built-up handle, Angled for Left hand, Adjustable finger rings
Fork, Built-up handle, Angled for Left hand, not further specified
Fork, Built-up handle, Angled for Right hand, 7 ounce weighted handle
Fork, Built-up handle, Angled for Right hand, Adjustable finger rings

Fork, Built-up handle, Angled for Right hand, not further specified
Fork, Built-up handle, Angled for Right hand, Weighted 9 inch long handle
Fork, Built-up handle, Curved for Left hand, not further specified
Fork, Built-up handle, Curved for Left hand, Tapered handle
Fork, Built-up handle, Curved for Right hand, 9 inches long with large head
Fork, Built-up handle, Curved for Right hand, not further specified
Fork, Built-up handle, Curved for Right hand, not further specified
Fork, Built-up handle, Indented for Left hand, not further specified
Fork, Built-up handle, Indented for Left hand, Vinyl handle
Fork, Built-up handle, Indented for Right hand, not further specified
Fork, Built-up handle, Indented for Right hand, Vinyl handle
Fork, Built-up handle, Large head, Arched handle
Fork, Built-up handle, Large head, not further specified
Fork, Built-up handle, Large tines, not further specified
Fork, Built-up handle, Large tines, Polypropylene handle
Fork, Built-up handle, not further specified
Fork, Built-up handle, Plastic coated tines, 1 inch diameter handle
Fork, Built-up handle, Plastic coated tines, not further specified
Fork, Built-up handle, Standard head, 1 inch foam handle
Fork, Built-up handle, Standard head, 1-1/2 inch foam handle
Fork, Built-up handle, Standard head, 1-1/2 inch soft foam handle
Fork, Built-up handle, Standard head, 1-1/4 inch tapered foam handle
Fork, Built-up handle, Standard head, 1-3/8 inch foam handle
Fork, Built-up handle, Standard head, 1-5/16 inch foam handle
Fork, Built-up handle, Standard head, 8 ounce weighted ridged grip
Fork, Built-up handle, Standard head, Adjustable finger rings
Fork, Built-up handle, Standard head, Curved handle for arthritis
Fork, Built-up handle, Standard head, Handle indented for fingers
Fork, Built-up handle, Standard head, not further specified
Fork, Built-up handle, Standard head, Oval handle
Fork, Built-up handle, Standard head, Oval lightweight handle
Fork, Built-up handle, Standard head, Ridged handle
Fork, Built-up handle, Standard head, Slim polycarbonate handle
Fork, Built-up handle, Standard head, Weighted & adjustable rings
Fork, Built-up handle, Swivel head, Adjustable finger rings
Fork, Built-up handle, Swivel head, not further specified
Fork, Built-up handle, Swivel head, Weighted 1-1/8 inch diameter
Fork, Built-up handle, Swivel head with stops, not further specified
Fork, Built-up handle, Swivel head with stops, Oval plastic handle
Fork, Built-up tube handle, Standard head, 7 ounce weighted handle
Fork, Built-up tube handle, Standard head, 8 ounce weighted handle
Fork, Built-up tube handle, Standard head, not further specified
Fork, Built-up tube handle, Swivel head no stops, 1 inch diameter
Fork, Built-up tube handle, Swivel head no stops, not further specified
Fork, Coated tube handle, Standard head, 1 inch diameter handle
Fork, Coated tube handle, Standard head, 1-1/2 inch diameter handle
Fork, Coated tube handle, Standard head, 1-1/4 inch diameter handle
Fork, Coated tube handle, Standard head, not further specified
Fork, Detachable handle, Head only, Interchangeable handles
Fork, Detachable handle, Head only, not further specified
Fork, Drop head handle, Swivel head adjustable stop, Flat handle
Fork, Drop head handle, Swivel head adjustable stop, not further specified
Fork, Drop head handle, Swivel head adjustable stop, Stainless steel
Fork, Drop head handle, Swivel head no stops, Flat handle
Fork, Drop head handle, Swivel head no stops, not further specified
Fork, Horizontal palm clip, Adjustable angle to clip, not further specified
Fork, Horizontal palm clip, Adjustable angle to clip, not further specified
Fork, Horizontal palm clip, Adjustable angle to clip, Plastic coated metal clip
Fork, Horizontal palm clip, Adjustable angle to clip, Plastic coated tines
Fork, Moldable handle, not further specified
Fork, Moldable handle, Shaped with heat gun, not further specified
Fork, On horizontal palm clip, Adjustable angle to clip, not further specified
Fork, On horizontal palm clip, Adjustable angle to clip, Semi-rigid plastic clip
Fork, On vertical palm clip, Adjustable angle to clip, Bendable steel clip
Fork, On vertical palm clip, Adjustable angle to clip, not further specified
Fork, On vertical palm clip, Adjustable angle to clip, Plastic coated head
Fork, see also, Kitchen fork
Fork, see for other characteristics, Flatware, (by functional characteristic)
Fork, Side cutter, For Left hand use, not further specified
Fork, Side cutter, For Left hand use, Semi-sharp edge right tine
Fork, Side cutter, For Right hand use, not further specified
Fork, Side cutter, For Right hand use, Semi-sharp edge left tine
Fork, With thumb/forefinger grip, Standard head, Adjustable plastic coated grip
Fork, With thumb/forefinger grip, Standard head, not further specified
Fork extension handle, Adjustable angle, Thumb screw lock, 10 inches long
Fork extension handle, Adjustable angle, Thumb screw lock, 10 inches long & weighted
Fork extension handle, Adjustable angle, Thumb screw lock, 15 inches long
Fork extension handle, Adjustable angle, Thumb screw lock, 15 inches long & weighted
Fork extension handle, Adjustable angle, Thumb screw lock, not further specified
Fork/cutter combination, Built-up square handle, Spring-mounted push-down head, not further specified

Fork/cutter combination, Built-up square handle, Spring-mounted push-down head, Rectangular cutting blade
Fracture pan, see, Bed pan, wedge shaped
Freestyle bed, see, Adjustable bed, manual non-crank
Freezer failure alarm, Light flash & beep, Tape mounted, Battery powered
Fruit picker, Long handle, Extends up to 8 feet, not further specified
Fruit picker, Long handle, Extends up to 8 feet, Wire basket and raker claws
Fruit/vegetable peeler, Vibrating blade, Electric, not further specified
Fruit/vegetable peeler, Vibrating blade, Electric, Stands on counter
Frying pan, Cool outside, Electric, not further specified
Frying pan, Cool outside, not further specified
Furniture glides, For heavy furniture, For all floor types, Capacity 110 pounds per glide
Futon, Cotton over foam core, Polyester/cotton cover, not further specified
Futon, Cotton over foam core, Polyester/cotton cover, Use with frame
Futon frame, 3 position/self-lock, Full size, Hardwood slats
Futon frame, 3 position/self-lock, Full size, not further specified
Futon frame, 3 position/self-lock, Queen size, Hardwood slats
Futon frame, 3 position/self-lock, Queen size, not further specified
Futon frame, 3 position/self-lock, Twin size, Hardwood slats
Futon frame, 3 position/self-lock, Twin size, not further specified
Game, 25 inch round target w velcro, Scoring points labeled, 6 fuzzy balls included
Garbage bag caddy, see, Trash bag holder
Garden armchair, Slatted back, Rounded seat, curved back, Wood construction
Garden bag caddy, Two 6 inch wheels, Folding tubular frame, Holds 33 gallon bag
Garden Bench, 4 feet long, Rounded seat, curved back, Wood construction
Garden Bench, 5 feet long, Rounded seat, curved back, Wood construction
Garden bulb planter, T-handle, 34 inches long, not further specified
Garden bulb planter, T-handle, 34 inches long, With foot treads
Garden cart, 20 inch pneumatic tires, Aluminum folding, 300 pound capacity
Garden cart, 20 inch pneumatic tires, Aluminum folding, not further specified
Garden cart, 20 inch pneumatic wheels, One-piece plastic, 300 pound capacity
Garden cart, 20 inch semi-pneumatic wheels, One-piece plastic, 200 pound capacity
Garden cart, Heavy-duty flotation tires, One-piece plastic, 700 pound capacity
Garden cart, Large rear wheels, Steel frame plywood, 400 pound capacity
Garden cart, Large rear wheels, Steel frame plywood, not further specified
Garden cart, Large rear wheels, With rear end gate, 300 pound capacity
Garden cart, Large rear wheels, With rear end gate, not further specified
Garden hose caddy, Long handle, 8 inch wheels, not further specified
Garden hose caddy, Long handle, 8 inch wheels, Stores 250 feet of hose
Garden hose hanger, see, Hose hanger
Garden hose wand, 34 inch extension, With shut-off valve, not further specified
Garden rake, Adjustable width, 52 inch long handle, Rubberized handle
Garden sod cutter, 54 inch long Handle, 4 wide inch chopper blade, 1-1/4 inch diameter handle
Garden tools, Lightweight, not further specified
Garden tools, Lightweight, Trowel/scratcher, not further specified
Garden tools, Short handles, Rake & shovel & hoe, For wheelchair use
Garden tools, Short handles, Rake & shovel & hoe, not further specified
Garden workseat, 10 inch wheels, Seat 18 inches high, not further specified
Garden workseat, 10 inch wheels, Seat 18 inches high, Swivel seat
Garden workseat, 7 inch wheels, Capacity to 250 pounds, With storage tray
Garden workseat, Semi-pneumatic wheels, Seat 15 inches high, 360 degree swivel seat
Garden workseat, Wide tires, Seat 10 inches high, not further specified
Garden workseat, Wide tires, Seat 10 inches high, With storage trays
Garden workseat, Wide tires, Seat 18 inches high, Capacity up to 400 pounds
Garden workseat, Wide wheels, Seat 11 inches high, With storage tray
Garden workseat, Wide wheels, Seat 12 inches high, With storage
Garden workseat tray, Mounts under seat, not further specified
Garment rack on tension pole, Floor to ceiling mount, Swinging arms, 3 arms hold clothes
Garment rack on tension pole, Floor to ceiling mount, Swinging arms, not further specified
Gas detector, Carbon monoxide, Spot turns dark, Requires periodic inspection
Gas detector alarm, Carbon monoxide, 85 decibel sound, AC powered
Gas detector alarm, Carbon monoxide, 85 decibel sound, not further specified
Gas detector alarm, Carbon monoxide, Strobe light & sound, AC powered
Gas detector alarm, Carbon monoxide, Strobe light & sound, not further specified
Gas detector alarm, Natural and propane, 85 decibel sound, not further specified
Gas detector alarm, Natural and propane, Strobe light & sound, AC powered
Gas detector alarm, Natural and propane, Strobe light & sound, not further specified
Gas detector alarm, Natural gas and propane, 85 decibel sound, AC powered
Goblet, Tall wide stem grip, Break resistant, not further specified
Goblet, Tall wide stem grip, not further specified
Gown for lounging, Snap back, Long sleeve, not further specified
Gown for lounging, Snap back, Long sleeve, Unisex/flannel

Gown for lounging, Snap back, not further specified
Gown for lounging, Snap back, Short sleeve, not further specified
Gown for lounging, Snap back, Short sleeve, Various colors
Gown for lounging, Tie back, Long sleeve, not further specified
Gown for lounging, Tie back, Long sleeve, Unisex
Gown for lounging, Tie back, Long sleeve, Various colors
Gown for lounging, Tie back, not further specified
Gown for lounging, Tie back, Short sleeve, not further specified
Gown for lounging, Velcro front closure, 3/4 sleeve, not further specified
Gown for lounging, Velcro front closure, 3/4 sleeve, Various colors
Grab bar, Accessory for bath seat, not further specified
Grab bar, Hinged wall mounted, Horizontal loop bar, 24 inch textured
Grab bar, Hinged wall mounted, Horizontal loop bar, Adjustable horizontal/vertical
Grab bar, Hinged wall mounted, Horizontal loop bar, not further specified
Grab bar, Hinged wall mounted, Horizontal single bar, 28 inch textured
Grab bar, Hinged wall mounted, Horizontal single bar, 30 inch smooth
Grab bar, Hinged wall mounted, Horizontal single bar, Adjustable horizontal/vertical
Grab bar, Hinged wall mounted, Horizontal single bar, not further specified
Grab bar, not further specified
Grab bar, Portable suction cup mounted, Rod handle perpendicular, Designed for steadying only
Grab bar, Portable suction cup mounted, Single loop, Designed for steadying only
Grab bar, Tub edge cam clamp, Bi-level, Flowing molded shape
Grab bar, Tub edge cam clamp, Bi-level, not further specified
Grab bar, Tub edge cam-action clamp, Double bi-level step shaped, not further specified
Grab bar, Tub edge cam-action clamp, Double bi-level step shaped, Tubular joined by crossbar
Grab bar, Tub edge cam-action clamp, Single level, not further specified
Grab bar, Tub edge cam-action clamp, Single level, Tubular
Grab bar, Tub edge screw clamp, Bi-level loop with crossbar, 18 inches high tubular
Grab bar, Tub edge screw clamp, Bi-level loop with crossbar, not further specified
Grab bar, Tub edge screw clamp, Bi-level step shaped, 14 inches high tubular
Grab bar, Tub edge screw clamp, Bi-level step shaped, 18 inches high tubular
Grab bar, Tub edge screw clamp, Bi-level step shaped, not further specified
Grab bar, Tub edge screw clamp, Single level, not further specified
Grab bar, Tub edge screw clamp, Single level, Tubular textured grip
Grab bar, Tub edge screw clamp, Single level U shape, 6 inches high tubular
Grab bar, Tub edge screw clamp, Single level U shape, 7 inches high tubular
Grab bar, Tub edge screw clamp, Single level U shape, not further specified
Grab bar, Wall, Single loop grip, 10 inches long textured
Grab bar, Wall, Single loop grip, Folds upward against wall
Grab bar, Wall, Single loop grip, not further specified
Grab bar, Wall, Straight, 12 inches long smooth
Grab bar, Wall, Straight, 16 inches long smooth
Grab bar, Wall, Straight, 24 in long smooth
Grab bar, Wall, Straight, 24 inches long textured grip
Grab bar, Wall, Straight, 32 inches long smooth
Grab bar, Wall, Straight, 32 inches long textured grip
Grab bar, Wall, Straight, not further specified
Grab bar, Wall, Tri loop grip, 25 inches long
Grab bar, Wall, Tri loop grip, not further specified
Grab bar, Wall, Two arms 90 degree angle left, 16 x 32 inches smooth
Grab bar, Wall, Two arms 90 degree angle left, not further specified
Grab bar, Wall, Two arms 90 degree angle right, 16 x 32 inches smooth
Grab bar, Wall, Two arms 90 degree angle right, not further specified
Grab bar, Wall, Two arms at 110 degree angle, 13 inches long each arm smooth
Grab bar, Wall, Two arms at 110 degree angle, not further specified
Grab bar, Wall, Two arms at 90 degree angle, 25 x 30 inches smooth
Grab bar, Wall, Two arms at 90 degree angle, not further specified
Grab bar mounting kit, 2.5 inch #14 screws, For stud mounting, not further specified
Grab bar mounting kit, Screws w/toggle nuts, 1/4 inch-20 x 3 1/2 inch, For hollow wall mounting
Grab bar mounting kit, Screws with expansion shield, 1/4 inch hole 2 inch bolt, For solid walls
Grab bar support, For hinged wall mounted bar, Provides a leg to the floor, 40 inch high
Grab bar support, For hinged wall mounted bar, Provides a leg to the floor, not further specified
Grab pole, Vertical, Tension mount floor to ceiling, not further specified
Grab pole, Vertical, Tension mount floor to ceiling, Portable
Grab pole connector, Corner piece, For vertical pole, 21 inch
Grab pole connector, Corner piece, For vertical pole, not further specified
Grab pole connector, End piece, For vertical pole, 18 inch
Grab pole connector, End piece, For vertical pole, not further specified
Grab pole handrail, Horizontal, For vertical pole, 18 inches long
Grab pole handrail, Horizontal, For vertical pole, 24 inches long
Grab pole handrail, Horizontal, For vertical pole, not further specified
Grab pole system, Vertical poles, Tension mount floor to ceiling, A set with connectors
Grasping cuff, see, Sport grasping cuff
Grass shears, 4 inch cutting head, 28 inch extension handle, Cordless rechargeable
Grass/weed shears, Stand-up handle, Squeeze operation, Carbon steel blades

Grass/weed shears, Stand-up handle, Squeeze operation, not further specified
Green Mountain peeler, see, Apple peeler/corer
Gun holder one-hand, Supports gun forearm, Car window mount, Hunting use legally restricted
Gutter cleaner, Garden hose powered, not further specified
Gutter cleaner, Garden hose powered, Telescoping handle, not further specified
Gutter flusher, see, Gutter cleaner, Garden hose powered
Gutter rake, Curved fork, Extendible handle, 4 to 7 feet long
Gutter rake, Curved fork, Extendible handle, not further specified
Gutter scoop, Polyethylene scoop, Extendible handle, not further specified
Gutter scoop, Polyethylene scoop, not further specified

Hair brush, 16 inch built-up handle, Adjustable angle, not further specified
Hair brush, Built-up handle, Adjustable angle, 1-1/4 inch diameter
Hair brush, Built-up handle, Adjustable angle, Natural bristles
Hair brush, Built-up handle, Adjustable angle, not further specified
Hair brush, Built-up handle, Adjustable angle, Nylon bristles
Hair brush, Built-up handle, Washable foam handle, 1-1/2 inch diameter
Hair brush, Built-up handle, Washable foam handle, not further specified
Hair brush, Velcro hand strap, D-ring closure, not further specified
Hair brush, Velcro hand strap, D-ring closure, Stiff bristles
Hair brush, With velcro hand strap, D-ring closure, not further specified
Hair brush, With velcro hand strap, D-ring closure, Soft bristles
Hair brush and comb, Built-up handle, Adjustable angle, Interchangeable comb/brush
Hair brush and comb, Built-up handle, Adjustable angle, not further specified
Hair dryer, Hand-held, Compact, Dual voltage 110-220
Hair dryer, Hand-held, Compact, not further specified
Hair dryer, Hands free, Adjustable bonnet on stand, 2 heat settings
Hair dryer, Hands free, Adjustable bonnet on stand, 4 heat settings
Hair dryer, Hands free, Adjustable bonnet on stand, not further specified
Hair dryer, Hands free, Blower with no bonnet, 2 heat & 2 speed settings
Hair dryer, Hands free, Blower with no bonnet, not further specified
Hair dryer, One-hand operation, Wall mounted, AC powered
Hair lift comb, 11 inch handle, Spaced prongs, not further specified
Hair lift comb, 11 inch handle, Spaced prongs, Velcro hand strap
Hair lift comb, With cuff for hand, Velcro D-ring closure, not further specified
Hair pick, see, Hair lift comb
Hair trimmer, 5 position guide, not further specified
Hair trimmer, 5 position guide, Rechargeable battery powered, not further specified
Hair trimmer, Trimming only, Battery powered, not further specified
Hair trimmer, Trimming only, not further specified
Hairdryer holder, Universal bracket, Suction cup mount, Portable
Hand brush, Suction cup base, Base with finger grooves, Hook for hanging
Hand brush, Suction cup base, not further specified
Hand brush, Suction cup base, Short bristles, not further specified
Handle build-up material, 2 part epoxy, Dishwasher safe, not further specified
Handle build-up material, 2 part epoxy, not further specified
Handle build-up material, Pre-mixed, Dishwasher safe, 4 ounce can beige
Handle build-up material, Pre-mixed, Dishwasher safe, 4 ounce can gray
Handle build-up material, Pre-mixed, Dishwasher safe, not further specified
Handle build-up material, Thermoplastic, Pellets, Self-cohering when heated
Handle grip, Adjusts 1/8 to 3/8 inch, Built-up vinyl, not further specified
Handle grip, Adjusts 1/8 to 3/8 inch, Built-up vinyl, Uses set screws
Hanger extension, For clothes hanger, From rod to standard hanger, For seated use
Hanger extension, Hanger with extension rod, Hangs from rod, For seated use
Headphone, For TV/stereo, Sender & receiver, Infrared transmitter
Headphone, For TV/stereo, Sender & receiver, not further specified
Hedge shears, 32 inch handles, 8 inch steel blades, horizontal cut
Hedge shears, 32 inch handles, 8 inch steel blades, vertical cut
Heel/ankle cover, Imitation lamb's-wool, Attaches with velcro, not further specified
High-tack soft plastic, Trade name Dycem, not further specified
Hinge door offset, see, Offset door hinge
Home security system, Keypad control, Fire/break-in alarm, Calls police/emergency number
Home security system, Keypad control, Fire/break-in alarm, not further specified
Homecare lifter, see, Transfer lift system
Hook and loop closure, see, velcro ...
Hose coupler, Quick-connect, No twisting required, For garden hose
Hose coupler, Quick-connect, No twisting required, not further specified
Hose guide, Swiveling, Stake in ground, 4 guides
Hose guide, Swiveling, Stake in ground, not further specified
Hose guide, Swiveling, Stake in ground, One guide
Hose hanger, Wall mount, Stores 150 feet hose, For garden hose
Hose hanger, Wall mount, Stores 150 feet hose, not further specified
Hose reel, Wall mount, Stores 150 feet hose, Detachable reel
Hose reel, Wall mount, Stores 150 feet hose, not further specified
Hydrocushion, see, Bath tub lift

Ice cube tray, Enclosed bottle style, Small cubes, not further specified

Illuminated light switch, Replaces standard switch, Is night light when turned off, not further specified
Incontinence alarm, Bed, Pad sensor, Battery powered
Incontinence alarm, Bed, Pad sensor, not further specified
Incontinence brief men's, Full brief with fly, Light absorbent not waterproof, Machine washable
Incontinence brief men's, Full brief with fly, Light absorbent not waterproof, not further specified
Incontinence garment, see, Incontinence brief or, Incontinence pant
Incontinence pad disposable, Use in incontinence pants, Heavy absorbent, Fits in liner pouch
Incontinence pad disposable, Use in incontinence pants, Heavy absorbent, not further specified
Incontinence pad disposable, Use in incontinence pants, Light absorbent, Fits in liner pouch
Incontinence pad disposable, Use in incontinence pants, Light absorbent, not further specified
Incontinence pad disposable, Use in regular underwear, Light absorbent, Adheres to underwear
Incontinence pad disposable, Use in regular underwear, Light absorbent, not further specified
Incontinence pants open net, Elastic waist, With pad holder, not further specified
Incontinence pants open net, Elastic waist, With pad holder, Women's medium
Incontinence pants washable, Elastic waist, Flannel lined, Full side coverage
Incontinence pants washable, Elastic waist, Flannel lined, not further specified
Incontinence pants washable, Elastic waist, Light absorbent no lining, Full side coverage
Incontinence pants washable, Elastic waist, Light absorbent no lining, not further specified
Incontinence pants with pouch, Adhesive tab closure at sides, With pad holder pouch, Full side coverage
Incontinence pants with pouch, Adhesive tab closure at sides, With pad holder pouch, not further specified
Incontinence pants with pouch, Adhesive tab closure at sides, With pad holder pouch, Open sides
Incontinence pants with pouch, Elastic waist, With pad holder pouch, Full side coverage
Incontinence pants with pouch, Elastic waist, With pad holder pouch, Men's extra large 44-48
Incontinence pants with pouch, Elastic waist, With pad holder pouch, Men's large 44-42
Incontinence pants with pouch, Elastic waist, With pad holder pouch, Men's medium 34-36
Incontinence pants with pouch, Elastic waist, With pad holder pouch, Men's small 32-34
Incontinence pants with pouch, Elastic waist, With pad holder pouch, not further specified
Incontinence pants with pouch, Elastic waist, With pad holder pouch, Vinyl coating flannel lining
Incontinence pants with pouch, Elastic waist, With pad holder pouch, Women's medium
Incontinence seatpad, For chair, Disposable, not further specified
Incontinence seatpad, For chair, not further specified
Incontinence seatpad, For wheelchair, not further specified
Incontinence seatpad, For wheelchair, Washable, not further specified
Incontinence shield disposable, Adhesive tab side closure, Heavy absorbent waterproof, Full side coverage
Incontinence shield disposable, Adhesive tab side closure, Heavy absorbent waterproof, not further specified
Incontinence shield disposable, With waist band no sides, Heavy absorbent waterproof, Elastic edges at legs
Incontinence shield disposable, With waist band no sides, Heavy absorbent waterproof, Elastic straps waist & sides
Incontinence shield disposable, With waist band no sides, Heavy absorbent waterproof, not further specified
Incontinence shield disposable, With waist band no sides, Light absorbent waterproof, Elastic edges at legs
Incontinence shield disposable, With waist band no sides, Light absorbent waterproof, not further specified
Incontinence shield disposable, With waist band no sides, Medium absorbent waterproof, Elastic edges at legs
Incontinence shield disposable, With waist band no sides, Medium absorbent waterproof, not further specified
Incontinence shield washable, Pin closure, Machine washable, Full side coverage
Incontinence shield washable, Pin closure, Machine washable, not further specified
Incontinence shield washable, Snap closure, Machine washable, Full side coverage
Incontinence shield washable, Snap closure, Machine washable, not further specified
Intercom, FM radio wireless 3 channel, Set of sender and receiver, AC powered
Intercom receiver unit, FM radio wireless 3 channel, Receiver only, AC powered
Intruder alarm, Interrupted-beam, Sound signal, Battery powered
Intruder alarm, Interrupted-beam, Sound signal, not further specified
Intruder alarm, Motion activated, 110 decibel siren, Battery powered
Intruder alarm, Motion activated, 110 decibel siren, not further specified
Intruder alarm, Motion activated, Actuates lighting, AC powered
Intruder alarm, Motion activated, Actuates lighting, Installed in socket
Intruder alarm, Motion activated, Actuates lighting, not further specified
Intruder alarm, Motion activated, Actuates lighting, Plug-in with light
Intruder alarm, Motion activated, Actuates sound, AC powered with adapter
Intruder alarm, Motion activated, Actuates sound, Battery powered
Intruder alarm, Motion activated, Wireless transmitter only, Battery powered
Intruder alarm, Receiving unit only, For driveway alert, not further specified

Intruder alarm, Receiving unit only, not further specified
Intruder alarm, see also, Door opening alarm
Intruder alarm, Sound-activated, Turns on light, In light socket
Intruder alarm, Sound-activated, Turns on light, not further specified
Intruder alarm, Transmitter only, For driveway alert, not further specified
Intruder alarm, Transmitter only, not further specified
Intruder alarm sense/transmit, Motion activated, Wireless transmitter only, Battery powered
Intruder alarm system, see, Home security system
Intruder alarm/light, Motion activated, Actuates lighting, AC powered
Intruder alarm/light, Motion activated, Actuates lighting, AC powered hardwired
Intruder alarm/light, Motion activated, Actuates lighting, not further specified
Iron, Automatic shut-off, Timer to turn off, Limits heat interval
Iron, Automatic shut-off, Timer to turn off, not further specified
Ironing board, Folds away, Mounts to cabinet sides, Requires 37 inch surface
Ironing board, Folds away, Wall mounted, Requires 48 inch surface
Ironing board, Over-door mount, Folds up to door, 32 x 12 inch board
Ironing board, Over-door mount, Folds up to door, not further specified
Ironing board organizer, Wall mounted, Basket & hook, Holds board & iron
Ironing board organizer, Wall mounted, Basket & hook, not further specified

---

Jar holder, Hands free, Frame with wooden ram, Push with body
Jar opener, Gripped in hand, Non-slip sheet, not further specified
Jar opener, Gripped in hand, Non-slip sheet, Smooth surface
Jar opener, Gripped in hand, Non-slip sheet, Textured surface
Jar opener, One-hand operation, Mounted cam gripper, not further specified
Jar opener, One-hand operation, Mounted cam gripper, Under cabinet mount
Jar opener, One-hand operation, Mounted wedge gripper, Folding wall mount
Jar opener, One-hand operation, Mounted wedge gripper, not further specified
Jar opener, One-hand operation, Mounted wedge gripper, Rigid wall mount
Jar opener, One-hand operation, Mounted wedge gripper, Under cabinet mount
Jar opener, Two hands needed to operate, Band wrench, 7 inch handle
Jar opener, Two hands needed to operate, Band wrench, not further specified
Jar opener, Two hands needed to operate, Lever wrench, not further specified
Jar opener, Two hands needed to operate, Lever wrench, With handle
Jar opener, Two hands needed to operate, Wedge grip, Gripped in hand
Jar opener, Two hands needed to operate, Wedge grip, not further specified
Jar opener motorized, One-hand operation, Cone gripper, Under cabinet mount
Jar/bottle holder, Gripped-in-hand rubber cone, Portable or permanent mount, 1 to 4 inch jars
Jar/bottle holder, Gripped-in-hand rubber cone, Portable or permanent mount, not further specified
Jar/bottle holder, One-hand operation, Rubber base cone grippers, 1 to 4 inch jars
Jar/bottle holder, One-hand operation, Rubber base cone grippers, not further specified
Jar/bottle holder, Rubber gripper, Portable or permanent mount, 1 to 4 inch jars
Jar/bottle holder, Rubber gripper, Portable or permanent mount, not further specified
Jar/bottle opener, Electric, Cone gripper, not further specified
Jar/bottle opener, Electric, Cone gripper, Under cabinet mount
Jar/bottle opener, Gripped in hand, not further specified
Jar/bottle opener, Gripped in hand, Rubber dome gripper, not further specified
Jar/bottle opener, Mounted wedge grip, Mounted wedge gripper, not further specified
Jar/bottle opener, Mounted wedge grip, Mounted wedge gripper, Under cabinet mount
Jar/bottle opener, One-hand operation, Mounted cam gripper, not further specified
Jar/bottle opener, One-hand operation, Mounted cam gripper, Under cabinet mount
Jar/bottle opener, One-hand operation, Mounted cone gripper, not further specified
Jar/bottle opener, One-hand operation, Mounted cone gripper, Wall mount
Jar/bottle opener, One-hand operation, Mounted cranked clamp, not further specified
Jar/bottle opener, One-hand operation, Mounted cranked clamp, Wall mount
Jar/bottle opener, One-hand operation, Mounted knurled cam and post, not further specified
Jar/bottle opener, One-hand operation, Mounted knurled cam and post, Under cabinet mount
Jar\bottle opener, One-hand operation, Wedge gripper, Under cabinet mount

---

Key cover set, Color coded jackets, 6 to a package, not further specified
Key cover set, Color coded jackets, not further specified
Key cover with light, Thumb button switch, Color coded-4 colors, Battery powered
Key cover with light, Thumb button switch, Color coded-4 colors, not further specified
Key holder with door opener, Padded handle, 3 keys, not further specified
Key holder with door opener, Padded handle, 3 keys, Opens lift car door handles
Key holder with door opener, Straight handle, One key, not further specified
Key holder with door opener, Straight handle, One key, Opens lift car door handles
Key holder/handle, Curved handle, 1 key, not further specified

Key holder/handle, Curved handle, 2 keys, Adjustable angles
Key holder/handle, Curved handle, 2 keys, not further specified
Key holder/handle, Curved handle, 2 keys, not further specified
Key holder/handle, Curved handle, not further specified
Key holder/handle, Handle notched for fingers, 3 keys, 3-1/2 inches long x 1 inch
Key holder/handle, Handle notched for fingers, 3 keys, not further specified
Key holder/handle, Straight handle, 1 key, Adjustable angle
Key holder/handle, Straight handle, 1 key, not further specified
Key holder/handle, Straight handle, 2 keys, Keys fold away
Key holder/handle, Straight handle, 2 keys, not further specified
Key holder/handle, Straight handle, 2 keys, not further specified
Key holder/handle, Straight handle, 3 keys, Adjustable handle with thong
Key holder/handle, Straight handle, 3 keys, not further specified
Key holder/handle, Straight handle, 4 keys, not further specified
Key holder/handle, Straight handle, 5 keys, Adjustable angle with thong
Key holder/handle, Straight handle, 5 keys, not further specified
Key holder/handle, Straight handle, 8 keys, Adjustable angle
Key holder/handle, Straight handle, 8 keys, not further specified
Key holder/handle, Straight handle, not further specified
Key holder/handle, T-handle, 1 key, not further specified
Key holder/handle, T-handle, 3 keys, 2.5 inches long
Key holder/handle, T-handle, 3 keys, not further specified
Key holder/handle, T-handle, 3 keys, not further specified
Key holder/handle, T-handle, not further specified
Key organizer, Book style, With write-on index, Holds several keys
Key organizer, Book style, With write-on index, not further specified
Key turner, see, Key holder/handle
Keyless entry, see, Entry system, keyless
Kitchen cabinet, Vertical height adjustable, 27 to 39 inch counter height, AC powered
Kitchen cabinet, Vertical height adjustable, 27 to 39 inch counter height, not further specified
Kitchen cabinet, With slide-out work surface, With lazy susan shelves, not further specified
Kitchen cabinet, With slide-out work surface, With lazy susan shelves, Side tambour doors
Kitchen cabinet door, Tambour, Roll-up, not further specified
Kitchen cabinet door, Tambour, Roll-up, Zero door swing area
Kitchen caddy, see, Wire rack
Kitchen carousel, Wire rack system, Shelves rotate vertically, AC powered with battery backup
Kitchen carousel, Wire rack system, Shelves rotate vertically, not further specified
Kitchen fork, Built-up handle, 12 inches long, not further specified
Kitchen knife, 120 degree handle, Serrated blade, Loop handle
Kitchen knife, 120 degree handle, Serrated blade, not further specified
Kitchen knife, 120 degree handle, Straight edge, Loop handle
Kitchen knife, 120 degree handle, Straight edge, not further specified
Kitchen knife, 30 degree handle, Serrated blade, not further specified
Kitchen knife, 90 degree handle, Electric, not further specified
Kitchen knife, 90 degree handle, Electric, Velcro wrist strap
Kitchen knife, 90 degree handle, not further specified
Kitchen knife, 90 degree handle, Serrated blade, not further specified
Kitchen knife, 90 degree handle, Straight edge, 13 inch blade
Kitchen knife, 90 degree handle, Straight edge, 8 inch blade
Kitchen knife, 90 degree handle, Straight edge, not further specified
Kitchen knife, 90 degree handle, Straight edge, not further specified
Kitchen knife, 90-degree handle, Serrated blade, 6 inch blade
Kitchen knife, 90-degree handle, Serrated blade, not further specified
Kitchen knife, Built-up handle, Rolling blade, Guard over blade
Kitchen knife, Built-up handle, Rolling blade, No guard over blade
Kitchen knife, Built-up handle, Rolling blade, not further specified
Kitchen knife, Built-up handle, Straight blade, not further specified
Kitchen knife, Cutout handle, Extra long blade, not further specified
Kitchen knife, Cutout handle, Extra long blade, Stainless steel
Kitchen knife, Cutout handle, Long blade, not further specified
Kitchen knife, Cutout handle, Long blade, Stainless steel
Kitchen knife, Knob handle, Circular blade non-rolling, 3.5 inch
Kitchen knife, Knob handle, Circular blade non-rolling, not further specified
Kitchen knife, Straight handle, Rocker blade, not further specified
Kitchen knife, Straight handle, Rocker blade, Wood handle
Kitchen knife, Straight handle, Rolling blade, 2-1/2 inch
Kitchen knife, Straight handle, Rolling blade, not further specified
Kitchen knife, Straight handle, Wide rocker blade, not further specified
Kitchen knife, Straight handle, Wide rocker blade, Nylon coated handle
Kitchen knife, Top palmar handle, Crescent blade, Blade angle offset from handle
Kitchen knife, Top palmar handle, Crescent blade, Blade parallel to handle
Kitchen knife, Top palmar handle, Crescent blade, not further specified
Kitchen knife rack, Under-cabinet mount, Spring hinge mounted, Lowers into position
Kitchen knife rack, Under-cabinet mount, Spring hinge mounted, not further specified
Kitchen ladle, Built-up handle, 12 inches long, not further specified
Kitchen pot lid, See thru cover, Fits 12 to 13 inch diameter, not further specified
Kitchen pot lid rack, Free standing, Holds 6 pot lids, Countertop or in-cabinet
Kitchen pot lid rack, Free standing, Holds 6 pot lids, not further specified
Kitchen pot lid rack, Under-cabinet, Coated wire rack, not further specified

Light bulb changer, For standard bulbs, Accepts extender, not further specified
Light bulb changer, For standard bulbs, Accepts extender, Suction cup end
Light bulb changer, For std./flood/recessed/track, Accepts extender handle, not further specified
Light bulb changer, For std./flood/recessed/track, With extender handle, not further specified
Light fixture, Adhesive stick-up, Fluorescent, 8 AA batteries
Light fixture, Adhesive stick-up, Fluorescent, Battery powered
Light fixture, Adhesive stick-up, Fluorescent, not further specified
Light fixture, Ceiling, Fluorescent, 2 40 watt bulbs
Light fixture, Ceiling, Fluorescent, 4 20 watt bulbs
Light fixture, Ceiling, Fluorescent, 4 40 watt bulbs
Light fixture, Ceiling, Fluorescent, not further specified
Light fixture, Ceiling, Fluorescent/square, 2 40 watt U bulbs
Light fixture, Ceiling, Fluorescent/square, not further specified
Light fixture, Closet with pull cord, Fluorescent, Battery powered
Light fixture, Closet with pull cord, Fluorescent, not further specified
Light fixture, Cordless wall mount, 5 inch diameter, Battery powered
Light fixture, Under-cabinet, Fluorescent, 1 40 watt tube plug-in
Light fixture, Under-cabinet, Fluorescent, not further specified
Light fixture for stairway, see, Stairway lights
Light switch, see, Wall switch
Light switch dropper, Rod and handle, 14 inch long, For toggle switches
Light switch dropper, Rod and handle, 14 inch long, not further specified
Light switch dropper, Rod and handle, 17 inch long, For toggle switches
Light switch dropper, Rod and handle, 17 inch long, not further specified
Light switch dropper, Rod and handle, Fits over wall switch, For toggle switches
Light switch extender, see, Light switch dropper
Lighted magnifier, see, Magnifier with light
Lighter for fireplace, Long handle, Push button ignition, Butane fueled
Lighter for fireplace, Long handle, Push button ignition, not further specified
Lock for cabinet door, see, Cabinet door lock/latch
Lockset, With lever handle, Replaces knob type, not further specified
Lockset, With lever handle, Replaces knob type, Passage door no lock
Lockset, With lever handle, Replaces knob type, Passage door with lock button
Lockset, With lever handle, Replaces knob type, With code-button lock
Lockset, With lever handle, Replaces knob type, With key lock
Log caddy, see, Firewood cart
Log tongs reacher, 9 inch jaw spread, 35 inch, Leather handgrips
Log tongs reacher, 9 inch jaw spread, 35 inch, not further specified
Luggage cart, Folding, Use upright or flat, not further specified
Luggage cart, Folding, Use upright or flat, Straps to hold load

---

Magazine, For those with disabilities, Provides tips and information, Published quarterly
Magnifier, Bar reading, Power in 1.25X - 2.5X range, Magnifies vertically only
Magnifier, Bar reading, Power in 1.25X - 2.5X range, not further specified
Magnifier, Hand rectangular reading, For object distance 10 inches, Corner handle
Magnifier, Hand rectangular reading, For object distance 10 inches, not further specified
Magnifier, Hand rectangular reading, For object distance 5 inches, not further specified
Magnifier, Hand rectangular reading, For object distance 5 inches, Ribbed corner handle
Magnifier, Hand rectangular reading, Power in 1.25X - 2.5X range, Corner handle
Magnifier, Hand rectangular reading, Power in 1.25X - 2.5X range, Corner handle for Right hand
Magnifier, Hand rectangular reading, Power in 1.25X - 2.5X range, not further specified
Magnifier, Hand rectangular reading, Power in 2.6X - 4X range, Corner handle for Right hand
Magnifier, Hand rectangular reading, Power in 2.6X - 4X range, Corner handle R hand
Magnifier, Hand rectangular reading, Power in 2.6X - 4X range, not further specified
Magnifier, Hand round for detail viewing, Power in 4.1X - 6X range, not further specified
Magnifier, Hand round for detail viewing, Power in 4.1X - 6X range, not further specified
Magnifier, Hand round for detail viewing, Power in 4.1X - 6X range, One 1.75 inch lens
Magnifier, Hand round for detail viewing, Power in 4.1X - 6X range, One aspheric lens
Magnifier, Hand round for detail viewing, Power in 4.1X - 6X range, Wide handle
Magnifier, Hand round for detail viewing, Power in 4.1X - 6X range, With lens cover
Magnifier, Hand round reading, Power in 1.25X - 2.5X range, 5 inch glass lens
Magnifier, Hand round reading, Power in 1.25X - 2.5X range, Handle is a 5X bar magnifier
Magnifier, Hand round reading, Power in 1.25X - 2.5X range, Lightweight frame
Magnifier, Hand round reading, Power in 1.25X - 2.5X range, not further specified
Magnifier, Hand round reading, Power in 1.25X - 2.5X range, With lens cover
Magnifier, Hand round reading, Power in 2.6X - 4X range, Lightweight frame
Magnifier, Hand round reading, Power in 2.6X - 4X range, not further specified
Magnifier, Hand round reading, Power in 2.6X - 4X range, not further specified
Magnifier, Hand round reading, Power in 2.6X - 4X range, Wide handle
Magnifier, Hand round reading, Power in 2.6X - 4X range, With lens cover

Magnifier, Hand/stand reading, Power in 2.6X - 4X range, Hinged to stand
Magnifier, Hand/stand reading, Power in 2.6X - 4X range, not further specified
Magnifier, Illuminated screen display, Table top, Magnifies print photos etc
Magnifier, Loupe for very fine detail, Power in 12.1X - 20X range, Monocle
Magnifier, Loupe for very fine detail, Power in 12.1X - 20X range, not further specified
Magnifier, Loupe for very fine detail, Power in 8.1X - 12X range, Monocle
Magnifier, Loupe for very fine detail, Power in 8.1X - 12X range, not further specified
Magnifier, Neck suspended detail, 8 and 3 inch focal lengths, not further specified
Magnifier, Neck suspended detail, 8 and 3 inch focal lengths, One bifocal lens
Magnifier, Neck suspended detail, Power in 4.1X - 6X range, Neck cord and stand
Magnifier, Neck suspended detail, Power in 4.1X - 6X range, not further specified
Magnifier, Neck suspended detail, Power in 6.1X - 8X range, Hands free for work
Magnifier, Neck suspended detail, Power in 6.1X - 8X range, not further specified
Magnifier, Neck suspended reading, Power in 1.25X - 2.5X range, 7X10 inch sheet lens
Magnifier, Neck suspended reading, Power in 1.25X - 2.5X range, Footed frame
Magnifier, Neck suspended reading, Power in 1.25X - 2.5X range, not further specified
Magnifier, Neck suspended reading, Power in 2.6X - 4X range, Neck cord
Magnifier, Neck suspended reading, Power in 2.6X - 4X range, not further specified
Magnifier, Pocket detail with case, Power in 1.25X - 2.5X range, not further specified
Magnifier, Pocket detail with case, Power in 1.25X - 2.5X range, One 2 inch lens
Magnifier, Pocket detail with case, Power in 2.6X - 4X range, not further specified
Magnifier, Pocket detail with case, Power in 2.6X - 4X range, not further specified
Magnifier, Pocket detail with case, Power in 2.6X - 4X range, One 1.4 inch lens
Magnifier, Pocket detail with case, Power in 2.6X - 4X range, One 50mm square lens
Magnifier, Pocket detail with case, Power in 2.6X - 4X range, One 60mm oval lens
Magnifier, Pocket detail with case, Power in 2.6X - 4X range, One 60mm square lens
Magnifier, Pocket detail with case, Power in 2.6X - 4X range, One lens
Magnifier, Pocket detail with case, Power in 2.6X - 4X range, One round lens
Magnifier, Pocket detail with case, Power in 4.1X - 6X range, not further specified
Magnifier, Pocket detail with case, Power in 4.1X - 6X range, One round lens
Magnifier, Pocket detail with case, Powers 1.25x & 2.5x & 3.75X, 2 folding lenses
Magnifier, Pocket detail with case, Powers 1.25x & 2.5x & 3.75X, not further specified
Magnifier, Pocket detail with case, Powers 3X & 4X & 7X, 2 lenses
Magnifier, Pocket detail with case, Powers 3X & 4X & 7X, not further specified
Magnifier, Pocket detail with case, Powers 3X & 5X & 8X, 2 lenses
Magnifier, Pocket detail with case, Powers 3X & 5X & 8X, not further specified
Magnifier, Pocket detail with case, Powers 4X & 5X & 9X, 2 glass lenses
Magnifier, Pocket detail with case, Powers 4X & 5X & 9X, not further specified
Magnifier, Pocket detail with case, Powers 4X & 6X & 10X, 2 folding lenses
Magnifier, Pocket detail with case, Powers 4X & 6X & 10X, 2 folding lenses
Magnifier, Pocket detail with case, Powers 4X & 6X & 10X, not further specified
Magnifier, Pocket detail with case, Powers 4X & 6X & 10X, not further specified
Magnifier, Pocket detail with case, Powers 4X & 6X & 10X & 20X, 3 folding lenses
Magnifier, Pocket detail with case, Powers 4X & 6X & 10X & 20X, not further specified
Magnifier, Pocket detail with case, Powers 5X & 7X & 12X, 2 aspheric lenses
Magnifier, Pocket detail with case, Powers 5X & 7X & 12X, not further specified
Magnifier, Sheet or flat lens reading, Power in 1.25X - 2.5X range, 2.5x7.25 inches
Magnifier, Sheet or flat lens reading, Power in 1.25X - 2.5X range, 7.5x11.75 inches
Magnifier, Sheet or flat lens reading, Power in 1.25X - 2.5X range, 7x10 inches
Magnifier, Sheet or flat lens reading, Power in 1.25X - 2.5X range, not further specified
Magnifier, Spectacle type, Power in 1.25X - 2.5X range, Adjustable head band
Magnifier, Spectacle type, Power in 1.25X - 2.5X range, not further specified
Magnifier, Spectacle type, Power in 2.6X - 4X range, Adjustable head band
Magnifier, Spectacle type, Power in 2.6X - 4X range, Attaches to glasses
Magnifier, Spectacle type, Power in 2.6X - 4X range, not further specified
Magnifier, Spectacle type, Power in 2.6X - 4X range, Wear like glasses
Magnifier, Stand mounted detail, Power in 1.25X - 2.5X range, 40mm round
Magnifier, Stand mounted detail, Power in 1.25X - 2.5X range, 60mm round
Magnifier, Stand mounted detail, Power in 1.25X - 2.5X range, not further specified
Magnifier, Stand mounted detail, Power in 1.25X - 2.5X range, not further specified
Magnifier, Stand mounted detail, Power in 2.6X - 4X range, 2 inch lens
Magnifier, Stand mounted detail, Power in 2.6X - 4X range, not further specified

Magnifier, Stand mounted detail, Power in 4.1X - 6X range, 1.5 inch aspheric lens
Magnifier, Stand mounted detail, Power in 4.1X - 6X range, 1.75 inch lens
Magnifier, Stand mounted detail, Power in 4.1X - 6X range, not further specified
Magnifier, Stand mounted detail, Power in 4.1X - 6X range, With carrying bag
Magnifier, Stand mounted fine detail, Power in 6.1X - 8X range, not further specified
Magnifier, Stand mounted fine detail, Power in 6.1X - 8X range, Round aspheric lens
Magnifier, Stand mounted fine detail, Power to 20X adjustable, 26mm eyepiece
Magnifier, Stand mounted fine detail, Power to 20X adjustable, not further specified
Magnifier, Stand mounted fine detail, Power to to 15X adjustable, 29mm eyepiece
Magnifier, Stand mounted fine detail, Power to to 15X adjustable, not further specified
Magnifier, Stand mounted reading, Power in 1.25X - 2.5X range, 4 inch lens
Magnifier, Stand mounted reading, Power in 1.25X - 2.5X range, not further specified
Magnifier, Stand mounted reading, Power in 2.6X - 4X range, 4 inch gooseneck
Magnifier, Stand mounted reading, Power in 2.6X - 4X range, not further specified
Magnifier, Stand mounted reading, Power in 2.6X - 4X range, Rectangular tilting
Magnifier, Tripod mounted fine detail, Power in 6.1X - 8X range, not further specified
Magnifier, Tripod mounted fine detail, Power in 6.1X - 8X range, Round
Magnifier with holding clips, Clips hold work parts, Power in 1.25X - 2.5X range, 'helping hand' style
Magnifier with holding clips, Clips hold work parts, Power in 1.25X - 2.5X range, not further specified
Magnifier with light, Edge clamp with adjustable arm, Object distance 12 inches, 40 watt incandescent bulb
Magnifier with light, Edge clamp with adjustable arm, Object distance 12 inches, 60 watt incandescent bulb
Magnifier with light, Edge clamp with adjustable arm, Object distance 12 inches, Circular fluorescent light
Magnifier with light, Edge clamp with adjustable arm, Object distance 12 inches, not further specified
Magnifier with light, Edge clamp with adjustable arm, Object distance 12 inches, not further specified
Magnifier with light, Edge clamp with adjustable arm, Object distance 8 inches, Circular fluorescent light
Magnifier with light, Edge clamp with adjustable arm, Object distance 8 inches, not further specified
Magnifier with light, Floor mounted adjustable arm, Object distance 8 inches, Circular fluorescent light
Magnifier with light, Floor mounted adjustable arm, Object distance 8 inches, High intensity bulb
Magnifier with light, Floor mounted adjustable arm, Object distance 8 inches, not further specified
Magnifier with light, Hand held detail, Power in 4.1X - 6X range, Battery powered
Magnifier with light, Hand held detail, Power in 4.1X - 6X range, not further specified
Magnifier with light, Hand held detail, Power in 4.1X - 6X range, not further specified
Magnifier with light, Hand held detail, Power in 4.1X - 6X range, Square lens battery powered
Magnifier with light, Hand held detail, Powers 2.5X & 5X, Bifocal battery powered
Magnifier with light, Hand held detail, Powers 2.5X & 5X, not further specified
Magnifier with light, Hand held fine detail, Power in 6.1X - 8X range, Battery powered
Magnifier with light, Hand held fine detail, Power in 6.1X - 8X range, not further specified
Magnifier with light, Hand held reading, Power in 1.25X - 2.5X range, AC or battery powered
Magnifier with light, Hand held reading, Power in 1.25X - 2.5X range, Battery powered
Magnifier with light, Hand held reading, Power in 1.25X - 2.5X range, not further specified
Magnifier with light, Hand held reading, Power in 1.25X - 2.5X range, not further specified
Magnifier with light, Hand held reading, Power in 1.25X - 2.5X range, Rectangular
Magnifier with light, Hand held reading, Power in 2.6X - 4X range, Battery powered
Magnifier with light, Hand held reading, Power in 2.6X - 4X range, not further specified
Magnifier with light, Hand held reading, Power in 2.6X - 4X range, not further specified
Magnifier with light, Hand held reading, Power in 2.6X - 4X range, Rectangular
Magnifier with light, Hand held reading, Power in 2.6X - 4X range, Square with wide handle
Magnifier with light, Hand held reading, Powers 2X & 4X, Bifocal AC or battery powered
Magnifier with light, Hand held reading, Powers 2X & 4X, not further specified
Magnifier with light, Hand held reading, Powers 2X & 5X, Bifocal battery powered
Magnifier with light, Hand held reading, Powers 2X & 5X, not further specified
Magnifier with light, Hand held very fine detail, Power in 8.1X - 12X range, Battery powered
Magnifier with light, Hand held very fine detail, Power in 8.1X - 12X range, not further specified
Magnifier with light, Hand held with flashlight, Power in 2.6X - 4X range, 2 C batteries
Magnifier with light, Hand held with flashlight, Power in 2.6X - 4X range, not further specified
Magnifier with light, Hand held with flashlight, Power in 4.1X - 6X range, Battery powered

Magnifier with light, Hand held with flashlight, Power in 4.1X - 6X range, not further specified
Magnifier with light, Pocket detail, Power in 6.1X - 8X range, Battery powered
Magnifier with light, Pocket detail, Power in 6.1X - 8X range, not further specified
Magnifier with light, Pocket microscope type, Power in 8.1X - 12X range, Battery powered
Magnifier with light, Pocket microscope type, Power in 8.1X - 12X range, not further specified
Magnifier with light, Stand mounted adjustable arm, Object distance 12 inches, Battery powered
Magnifier with light, Stand mounted adjustable arm, Object distance 12 inches, Circular fluorescent light
Magnifier with light, Stand mounted adjustable arm, Object distance 12 inches, not further specified
Magnifier with light, Stand mounted adjustable arm, Power in 4.1X - 6X range, Circular fluorescent light
Magnifier with light, Stand mounted adjustable arm, Power in 4.1X - 6X range, not further specified
Magnifier with light, Stand mounted adjustable arm, Power in 6.1X - 8X range, Battery powered
Magnifier with light, Stand mounted adjustable arm, Power in 6.1X - 8X range, not further specified
Magnifier with light, Stand mounted fine detail, Power in 8.1X - 12X range, Battery powered
Magnifier with light, Stand mounted fine detail, Power in 8.1X - 12X range, not further specified
Magnifier with light, Stand mounted reading, Powers 2X & 4X, 3 inch diameter bifocal
Magnifier with light, Stand mounted reading, Powers 2X & 4X, not further specified
Magnifier with light, Stand swivel mounted reading, Power in 1.25X - 2.5X range, AC powered
Magnifier with light, Stand swivel mounted reading, Power in 1.25X - 2.5X range, not further specified
Magnifier with light, Stand with 2 goosenecks, Power in 2.6X - 4X range, 60 watt incandescent bulb
Magnifier with light, Stand with 2 goosenecks, Power in 2.6X - 4X range, Fluorescent light
Magnifier with light, Stand with 2 goosenecks, Power in 2.6X - 4X range, not further specified
Magnifying mirror, Demountable gooseneck on stand, Power 5X, 4-1/2 inches diameter
Magnifying mirror, Demountable gooseneck on stand, Power 5X, not further specified
Magnifying mirror, Gooseneck on 13 inch stand, Power 5X, 4-1/2 inches diameter
Magnifying mirror, Gooseneck on 13 inch stand, Power 5X, not further specified
Magnifying mirror, Gooseneck on stand, Power 2X, 4 inch mirror
Magnifying mirror, Gooseneck on stand, Power 2X, not further specified
Magnifying mirror, Hand held, Plane & power 5X, 1-1/2 inches diameter
Magnifying mirror, Hand held, Plane & power 5X, not further specified
Magnifying mirror, Pivoting wire frame, Plane & magnifying, not further specified
Magnifying mirror, Pivoting wire frame, Plane & magnifying, Stands on frame
Magnifying mirror, see also, Makeup mirror
Magnifying mirror, Suction cup mount, Plane and magnifying, Extends to 30 inches
Magnifying mirror, Suction cup mount, Plane and magnifying, not further specified
Magnifying mirror, Wall mount, Plane and magnifying, Extends to 22 inches
Magnifying mirror, Wall mount, Plane and magnifying, Extends to 30 inches
Magnifying mirror, Wall mount, Plane and magnifying, not further specified
Magnifying mirror, With bracket for standing, Plane & magnifying, not further specified
Magnifying mirror, With bracket for standing, Plane & magnifying, Round
Magnifying mirror, With bracket for standing, Plane & magnifying, With neck bracket
Mailbox signaler, Box floor insert, Light signal, Battery powered
Mailbox signaler, Box floor insert, Light signal, not further specified
Mailbox tray, Box floor insert, not further specified
Mailbox tray, Box floor insert, Rolls in/out, not further specified
Makeup mirror, Lighted, Plane and magnifying, Color corrected light
Makeup mirror, Lighted, Plane and magnifying, Directional light
Makeup mirror, Lighted, Plane and magnifying, not further specified
Makeup mirror, Side arms on base, Adjustable angle, not further specified
Makeup mirror, Side arms on base, not further specified
Mattress, Gel, 35 x 75 inches, 3 sections in cover
Mattress, Gel, 35 x 75 inches, not further specified
Mattress, Gel, 35 x 80 inches, 3 sections in cover
Mattress, Gel, 35 x 80 inches, not further specified
Mattress, Gel, 35 x 84 inches, 3 sections in cover
Mattress, Gel, 35 x 84 inches, not further specified
Mattress, Gel mid section, 35 x 75 x 5 - 1/2 in, 3 sections in cover
Mattress, Gel mid section, 35 x 75 x 5 - 1/2 in, not further specified
Mattress, Gel mid section, 35 x 84 x 5-1/2 in, 3 sections in cover
Mattress, Gel mid section, 35 x 84 x 5-1/2 in, not further specified
Mattress, Gel mid section, 35 x 88 x 5-1/2 in, 3 sections in cover
Mattress, Gel mid section, 35 x 88 x 5-1/2 in, not further specified
Mattress, Layered foam, Full bed size, not further specified
Mattress, Layered foam, Full bed size, Pressure reduction
Mattress, Layered foam, Hospital bed size, not further specified
Mattress, Layered foam, Hospital bed size, Pressure reduction
Mattress, Layered foam, Twin bed size, not further specified
Mattress, Layered foam, Twin bed size, Pressure reduction
Mattress cover, Soft vinyl, Double bed size, not further specified

Mattress cover, Soft vinyl, not further specified
Mattress cover, Soft vinyl, Single size bed, not further specified
Mattress pad, Contoured eggcrate, California king size, not further specified
Mattress pad, Contoured eggcrate, California king size, Single section
Mattress pad, Contoured eggcrate, Full size, 3-section design
Mattress pad, Contoured eggcrate, Full size, not further specified
Mattress pad, Contoured eggcrate, Full size, Single section
Mattress pad, Contoured eggcrate, King size, not further specified
Mattress pad, Contoured eggcrate, King size, Single section
Mattress pad, Contoured eggcrate, Queen size, 3-section design
Mattress pad, Contoured eggcrate, Queen size, not further specified
Mattress pad, Contoured eggcrate, Queen size, Single section
Mattress pad, Contoured eggcrate, Twin size, 3-section design
Mattress pad, Contoured eggcrate, Twin size, not further specified
Mattress pad, Contoured eggcrate, Twin size, Single section
Mattress pad, Foam, Full size 2-1/2 inches thick, not further specified
Mattress pad, Foam, Full size 2-1/2 inches thick, Single section
Mattress pad, Foam, Full size x 2 inches, not further specified
Mattress pad, Foam, Full size x 2 inches, Ribs support head
Mattress pad, Foam, King size 2 inches, not further specified
Mattress pad, Foam, King size 2 inches, Ribs support head
Mattress pad, Foam, King size 2-1/2 in, not further specified
Mattress pad, Foam, King size 2-1/2 in, Single section
Mattress pad, Foam, Queen size 2 inches, not further specified
Mattress pad, Foam, Queen size 2 inches, Rib support head
Mattress pad, Foam, Queen size 2-1/2 in, not further specified
Mattress pad, Foam, Queen size 2-1/2 in, Single section
Mattress pad, Foam, Twin size 2 inch, not further specified
Mattress pad, Foam, Twin size 2 inch, Ribs support head
Mattress pad, Foam, Twin size 2-1/2 in, not further specified
Mattress pad, Foam, Twin size 2-1/2 in, Single section
Mattress pad, Gel, 35 x 75 x 3 inches, 3 sections in cover
Mattress pad, Gel, 35 x 75 x 3 inches, not further specified
Mattress pad, Gel, 35 x 80 x 3 inches, 3 sections in cover
Mattress pad, Gel, 35 x 80 x 3 inches, not further specified
Mattress pad, Gel, 35 x 84 x 3 inches, 3 sections in cover
Mattress pad, Gel, 35 x 84 x 3 inches, not further specified
Mattress pad, Merino wool on synthetic base, Full size, 1-1/4 inch thick
Mattress pad, Merino wool on synthetic base, King size, 1-1/4 inch thick
Mattress pad, Merino wool on synthetic base, Queen size, 1-1/4 inch thick
Mattress pad, Merino wool on synthetic base, Twin size, 1-1/4 inch thick
Mattress protector, Absorbent/waterproof, 24 x 36 inches, Disposable
Mattress protector, Absorbent/waterproof, 24 x 36 inches, not further specified
Mattress protector, Absorbent/waterproof, 27 x 30 inches, Disposable
Mattress protector, Absorbent/waterproof, 27 x 30 inches, not further specified
Mattress protector, Absorbent/waterproof, 35 x 36 inches, Disposable
Mattress protector, Absorbent/waterproof, 35 x 36 inches, not further specified
Mattress protector, Absorbent/waterproof, 70 x 36 inches, Disposable
Mattress protector, Absorbent/waterproof, 70 x 36 inches, not further specified
Mattress protector, Backed cotton pad, Full size, not further specified
Mattress protector, Backed cotton pad, Full size, Washable
Mattress protector, Cellulose/waterproof, 23 x 36 inches, Disposable
Mattress protector, Cellulose/waterproof, 23 x 36 inches, not further specified
Mattress protector, Flannel & rubber, 35 x 54 inches, not further specified
Mattress protector, Flannel & rubber, 35 x 54 inches, Washable
Mattress protector, Flannel & rubber, 36 x 36 inches, not further specified
Mattress protector, Flannel & rubber, 36 x 36 inches, Washable
Mattress protector, Soft vinyl, Full size fitted, not further specified
Mattress protector, Soft vinyl, Full size fitted, Washable
Mattress protector, Soft vinyl, King size fitted, not further specified
Mattress protector, Soft vinyl, King size fitted, Washable
Mattress protector, Soft vinyl, Queen size fitted, not further specified
Mattress protector, Soft vinyl, Queen size fitted, Washable
Mattress protector, Soft vinyl, Twin fitted, not further specified
Mattress protector, Soft vinyl, Twin fitted, Washable
Mattress protector, Vinyl, 66 x 36 inches, not further specified
Mattress protector, Vinyl, 66 x 36 inches, Reversible
Mattress protector, Vinyl zippered cover, Full size fitted, not further specified
Mattress protector, Vinyl zippered cover, Full size fitted, Washable
Mattress protector, Waterproof center, 35 x 36 inches, not further specified
Mattress protector, Waterproof center, 35 x 36 inches, Washable cotton
Medication dispenser, see, Medication manager
Medication manager, 28 bins, Push button release, not further specified
Medication manager, 28 bins, Push button release, Wall mount
Medication manager, Chart kit, Color coded, 80 colored stickers
Medication manager, Chart kit, Color coded, not further specified
Medication manager, Manual compartments, 7 day, Braille & big print
Medication manager, Manual compartments, 7 day, not further specified
Medication manager, Manual compartments, 7 day 4 times/day, Braille & big print

Medication manager, Manual compartments, 7 day 4 times/day, not further specified
Medication manager, Programmable, 7 day 4 times/day, LCD reminder display
Medication manager, Programmable, 7 day 4 times/day, not further specified
Medication manager, Programmable signal, Beeps and resets, 2 storage bins
Medication manager, Programmable signal, Beeps and resets, not further specified
Memo speaker, Motion sensor, not further specified
Memo speaker, Motion sensor, Speaks voice message, not further specified
Message center, Clock with whiteboard, Includes dry-erase pens, not further specified
Message center, Clock/calendar with whiteboard, Includes dry-erase pens, not further specified
Message center, Under-cabinet mount, Spring hinge mount, Lowers into position
Message center, Under-cabinet mount, Spring hinge mount, not further specified
Microwave oven, Compact, Dial timer, 600 watt with turntable
Microwave oven, Compact, Dial timer, not further specified
Microwave oven, Compact, Membrane switches, not further specified
Microwave oven, Compact, Membrane switches, Programmable
Microwave oven, Full size, Membrane switches, not further specified
Microwave oven, Full size, Membrane switches, Programmable
Milk carton handle, For half gallon, Slips over carton, 4 inch handle
Milk carton handle, For half gallon, Slips over carton, not further specified
Milk carton opener, Separates cardboard, Hand held, Lift and rotate
Milk carton opener, Separates cardboard, Hand held, not further specified
Mirror, Car wide rear view, Adhesive, Doubles visual field
Mirror, Car wide rear view, Adhesive, not further specified
Mirror, Car wide rear view, Spring loaded clip, Doubles visual field
Mirror, Car wide rear view, Spring loaded clip, not further specified
Mirror, Clip-on, Panoramic, Provides wide view
Mirror, Over-stove, Wall mount, Adjustable angle
Mirror, Over-stove, Wall mount, not further specified
Mirror, Shower, Shower head mount, Fog-free
Mirror, Shower, Shower head mount, not further specified
Mirror, Suction cup base with stalk, 4-1/2 inches diameter, Extends to 26 inches high
Mirror, Suction cup base with stalk, 4-1/2 inches diameter, Extends to 34 inches high
Mirror, Suction cup base with stalk, 4-1/2 inches diameter, not further specified
Mirror self inspection, Flexible shaft, 8 inch square, 18 x 5 inch base
Mirror self inspection, Flexible shaft, 8 inch square, not further specified
Mirror self inspection, Hand loop, 2-1/2 x 3-1/2 inches, not further specified
Mirror self inspection, Hand loop, 2-1/2 x 3-1/2 inches, Telescoping handle
Mirror self inspection, Hand loop, 4 x 6 inch, Flexible shaft with 2 grips
Mirror self inspection, Hand loop, 4 x 6 inch, not further specified
Mirror self inspection, Hand loop, 4 x 6 inches, Diagonal flexible shaft
Mirror self inspection, Hand loop, 4 x 6 inches, not further specified
Mirror self inspection, Hand loop, 4-1/2 inches square, 12 inch flexible shaft
Mirror self inspection, Hand loop, 4-1/2 inches square, not further specified
Mirror self inspection, Hand loop, 5-1/2 inch square, 12 inch flexible shaft
Mirror self inspection, Hand loop, 5-1/2 inch square, Diagonal flexible shaft
Mirror self inspection, Hand loop, 5-1/2 inch square, not further specified
Mirror self inspection, Hand loop, Oval, Diagonal flexible shaft
Mirror self inspection, Hand loop, Oval, not further specified
Mirror self inspection, Hand/thumb loops, 4 x 6 inch, 12 inch flexible shaft
Mirror self inspection, Hand/thumb loops, 4 x 6 inch, not further specified
Mirror self inspection, Handle with cuff, Plastic mirror, Gooseneck handle
Mirror self inspection, Handle with cuff, Plastic mirror, not further specified
Mirror self inspection, On knee spreaders, 6 x 4 inch pivoting, 9 inch abduction
Mirror self inspection, On knee spreaders, 6 x 4 inch pivoting, not further specified
Mirror self inspection, On knee spreaders, Large, not further specified
Mirror self inspection, On knee spreaders, Medium, not further specified
Mirror self inspection, On knee spreaders, not further specified
Mirror self inspection, On knee spreaders, Pivoting, 11 inch abduction
Mirror self inspection, On knee spreaders, Pivoting, 6-1/4 inch abduction
Mirror self inspection, On knee spreaders, Pivoting, not further specified
Mirror self inspection, On knee spreaders, Small, not further specified
Mirror self inspection, Pivoting shaft, 2 x 3-1/2 inches, 12 inch handle
Mirror self inspection, Pivoting shaft, 2 x 3-1/2 inches, not further specified
Mirror self inspection, Pivots and locks, 8 inches square, In-toilet mount
Mirror self inspection, Pivots and locks, 8 inches square, not further specified
Mirror self inspection, Pivots and locks, 8 inches square, On base
Mittens/gloves combo, Fleece w thinsulate lining, Grip palm surface, Knit cuff
Mixer, see, Food mixer
Mixing bowl, One-hand operated suction base, 7.5 inch diameter, not further specified
Mixing bowl, One-hand operated suction base, 7.5 inch diameter, Polypropylene
Mixing bowl & holder, One hand operated tilt frame, 3 quart, All steel with rubber feet
Mixing bowl & holder, One hand operated tilt frame, 3 quart, not further specified

Mixing bowl set, One hand operated suction base, 6-1/4 & 8 & 9-1/2 inch, not further specified
Mixing bowl set, One hand operated suction base, 6-1/4 & 8 & 9-1/2 inch, Set of three
Moldable material, see, Handle build-up material
Monitoring system for home, Temperature/sound/power-out, Calls preprogram phone numbers, Battery powered
Monitoring system for home, Temperature/sound/power-out, Calls preprogram phone numbers, not further specified
Mop, Sponge small round head, 52 inch handle, 1-1/2 pounds
Mop, Sponge small round head, 52 inch handle, not further specified
Mop, Terry cloth, 52 inch handle, 8 x 15 inch thin head
Mop, Terry cloth, 52 inch handle, not further specified
Mop cover, Terry cloth, For mop terry cloth, 8 x 15 inch thin head
Mop cover, Terry cloth, For mop terry cloth, not further specified
Mop on extension handle, Sponge head with rollers, Handle adjusts to 7 feet, Hinged head
Mug, see also, Tumbler, (if no handle it's a tumbler)
Mug, Short and long loop handles, Interchangeable handles
Mug, Single large handle, Lid with hole, Insulated
Mug, Single large handle, Lid with hole, not further specified
Mug, Single large handle, Lid with hole, not further specified
Mug, Single large handle, Lid with spout, not further specified
Mug, Single large handle, No lid, Insulated
Mug, Single large handle, No lid, not further specified
Mug, Single large handle, Non-spill lid, Insulated
Mug, Single large handle, Non-spill lid, not further specified
Mug, Single large handle, not further specified
Mug, Single large handle, Snap-on lid, Insulated
Mug, Single large handle, Snap-on lid, not further specified
Mug, Single large handle, Weighted with lid, Insulated
Mug, Single large handle, Weighted with lid, not further specified
Mug, Single large handle, Weighted with lid, Tall insulated
Mug, Single large handle, Weighted with lid, Wide base
Mug, T-handle, No lid, not further specified
Mug, T-handle, not further specified
Mug, Two handles, not further specified
Mug, Two handles, Wide base, not further specified
Mug, Two horizontal handles, No lid, Insulated
Mug, Two horizontal handles, No lid, not further specified
Mug, Two large handles, Lid with spout, Clear polycarbonate
Mug, Two large handles, Lid with spout, not further specified
Mug, Two large handles, Lid with spout, Polypropylene
Mug, Two large handles, Lid with spout, Wide base
Mug, Two large handles, No lid, Insulated
Mug, Two large handles, No lid, not further specified
Mug, Two loop handles, Lid with spout, not further specified
Mug, Two loop handles, Lid with spout, Polypropylene
Mug, Two loop handles, No lid, Ceramic
Mug, Two loop handles, No lid, not further specified
Mug, Two soft handles, Lid with hole, not further specified
Mug, Two soft handles, not further specified
Mug cover with spout, For 2 hand mug, not further specified
Mug cover with spout, not further specified
Mug handle build-up strip, Flexible strip, Wrap around, Pencil-thick
Mug handle build-up strip, Flexible strip, Wraps around, not further specified
Mug lid, Anti-splash, For insulated mug, Lid only
Mug lid, Anti-splash, For insulated mug, not further specified
Mug lid with spout, For mug with 2 handles, not further specified
Mug lid with spout, not further specified
Mug with holder, Single large handle, Cover plate, Attaches to table
Mug with holder, Single large handle, Cover plate, not further specified
Mug with holder, Single large handle, not further specified
Mug with holder, Single large handle, Snap-on lid, Clips to wheelchair
Mug with holder, Single large handle, Snap-on lid, not further specified
Mug with holder, Single large handle, Snap-on lid with spout, not further specified
Mug with holder, T and J handles, No lid, Modular
Mug with holder, T and J handles, No lid, not further specified
Mug with vacuum control, Two handles, Lid with spout, Flow control lid
Mug with vacuum control, Two handles, Lid with spout, not further specified
Mug with weighted base, Non-spill lid, 2 part, not further specified
Mug with weighted base, Non-spill lid, not further specified
Music sheet/booklet, Large print, not further specified
Music sheet/booklet, not further specified
Music sheet/booklet, One handed performer, For non-keyboard instrument, not further specified
Music sheet/booklet, One handed performer, For piano/keyboard, not further specified

Nail holder, Pliers-style, With 11 nail holes, Feet at handle end
Nail holder, Pliers-style, With 11 nail holes, not further specified
Natural gas alarm, see, Gas detector alarm, natural and propane
Needle, Self threading, not further specified
Needle, Self threading, Slotted eye, not further specified
Needle threader, Free standing, Lever operated, not further specified
Needle threader, Free standing, not further specified
Needle threader, Hand held, not further specified
Needle threader, Hand held, Wire loop, not further specified

Newspaper holder, Center post strip, Rods support bottom of paper, Clamps to table edge
Newspaper holder, Center post strip, Rods support bottom of paper, not further specified
Night light, Automatic on-off photo sensor, 7 watt incandescent, not further specified
Night light, Automatic on-off photo sensor, 7 watt incandescent, Plug-in
Night light, Automatic on-off photo sensor, Neon bulb, not further specified
Night light, Automatic on-off photo sensor, Neon bulb, Plug-in
Night light, Constant on, Luminous panel equiv 7W light, AC powered plug-in
Night light, Constant on, Two 7 watt incandescent, not further specified
Night light, Constant on, Two 7 watt incandescent, Plug-in
Night light, Light/sound activated, 7 watt incandescent, not further specified
Night light, Light/sound activated, 7 watt incandescent, Plug-in
Night light, Motion detector, 7 watt incandescent, not further specified
Night light, Motion detector, 7 watt incandescent, Plug-in
Night stand, Bedside, not further specified
Night stand, Bedside, Swing-out drawers, not further specified
Nightgown, Women's, Long length, Cotton flannel
Nightgown, Women's, Long length, not further specified
Nightgown, Women's, Waltz length, Brushed nylon
Nightgown, Women's, Waltz length, Cotton flannel
Nightgown, Women's, Waltz length, Cotton/polyethylene
Nightgown, Women's, Waltz length, not further specified
Nightshirt, Men's, Short sleeve, Average size
Nightshirt, Men's, Short sleeve, Big size
Nightshirt, Men's, Short sleeve, Extra tall
Nightshirt, Men's, Short sleeve, not further specified
Non-skid applique, Adhesive backing, For bath tub, not further specified
Non-skid applique, Adhesive backing, For bath tub, Various designs textured
Non-skid coating, General use, Spray on, not further specified
Non-skid coating, General use, Spray on, Removes with alcohol
Non-skid floor cover, Sheet, Self adhesive, not further specified
Non-skid floor cover, Sheet, Self adhesive, Textured surface
Non-skid mat, For rugs, Adhesive back, 10 x 20 inches
Non-skid mat, For rugs, Adhesive back, not further specified
Non-skid mat, General use, 10 in diameter, not further specified
Non-skid mat, General use, 10 in diameter, Round pad
Non-skid mat, General use, 10 x 7 inches, High-tack soft plastic smooth
Non-skid mat, General use, 10 x 7 inches, not further specified
Non-skid mat, General use, 10 x 7.25 inches, High-tack plastic textured
Non-skid mat, General use, 10 x 7.25 inches, not further specified
Non-skid mat, General use, 10 x 7.25 inches, not further specified
Non-skid mat, General use, 10 x 7.5 inches, High-tack soft plastic smooth
Non-skid mat, General use, 10 x 7.5 inches, not further specified
Non-skid mat, General use, 14 x 14 inches, Adhesive back
Non-skid mat, General use, 14 x 14 inches, not further specified
Non-skid mat, General use, 15 x 10.5 inches, High-tack soft plastic
Non-skid mat, General use, 15 x 10.5 inches, not further specified
Non-skid mat, General use, 15 x 18 inches, not further specified
Non-skid mat, General use, 15 x 18 inches adhesive back, High-tack soft plastic
Non-skid mat, General use, 2 x 3 feet, With water dam edges
Non-skid mat, General use, 3 x 10 feet, With water dam edges
Non-skid mat, General use, 3 x 4 feet, With water dam edges
Non-skid mat, General use, 3 x 5 feet, With water dam edges
Non-skid mat, General use, 4 x 10 feet, With water dam edges
Non-skid mat, General use, 4 x 6 feet, With water dam edges
Non-skid mat, General use, 5 inch diameter, High-tack soft plastic
Non-skid mat, General use, 5 inch diameter, not further specified
Non-skid mat, General use, 5.5 inch diameter, High-tack soft plastic textured
Non-skid mat, General use, 5.5 inch diameter, not further specified
Non-skid mat, General use, 7.5 inch diameter, High-tack soft plastic textured
Non-skid mat, General use, 7.5 inch diameter, not further specified
Non-skid mat, General use, 8 inch diameter, High-tack soft plastic
Non-skid mat, General use, 8 inch diameter, not further specified
Non-skid mat, General use, 8 x 72 inches, High-tack soft plastic
Non-skid mat, General use, 8 x 72 inches, not further specified
Non-skid mat, General use, 9.5 x 7.5 inch, High-tack soft plastic
Non-skid mat, General use, 9.5 x 7.5 inch, not further specified
Non-skid mat, Placemat, 10 x 14 inch, High-tack soft plastic
Non-skid mat, Placemat, 10 x 14 inch, High-tack soft plastic textured
Non-skid mat, Placemat, 10 x 14 inch, not further specified
Non-skid matting, For rug, 6 in x 25 feet, not further specified
Non-skid matting, For rug, 6 in x 25 feet, Vinyl mesh
Non-skid matting, For rug to carpet, 3 x 5 feet, not further specified
Non-skid matting, For rug to carpet, 3 x 5 feet, Vinyl mesh
Non-skid matting, For rug to carpet, 4 x 6 feet, not further specified
Non-skid matting, For rug to carpet, 4 x 6 feet, Vinyl mesh
Non-skid matting, For rug to carpet, 6 x 9 feet, not further specified
Non-skid matting, For rug to carpet, 6 x 9 feet, Vinyl mesh
Non-skid matting, For rug to carpet, 8 x 10 feet, not further specified
Non-skid matting, For rug to carpet, 8 x 10 feet, Vinyl mesh
Non-skid matting, For rug to carpet, 9 x 12 feet, not further specified
Non-skid matting, For rug to carpet, 9 x 12 feet, Vinyl mesh

Non-skid matting, For rug to floor, 20 x 40 inches, not further specified
Non-skid matting, For rug to floor, 20 x 40 inches, Vinyl coated net
Non-skid matting, For rug to floor, 24 x 40 feet, not further specified
Non-skid matting, For rug to floor, 24 x 40 feet, Vinyl coated net
Non-skid matting, For rug to floor, 3 feet x 5 feet, not further specified
Non-skid matting, For rug to floor, 3 feet x 5 feet, Vinyl coated net
Non-skid matting, For rug to floor, 4 feet x 6 feet, not further specified
Non-skid matting, For rug to floor, 4 feet x 6 feet, Vinyl mesh
Non-skid matting, For rug to floor, 58 x 96 inches, not further specified
Non-skid matting, For rug to floor, 58 x 96 inches, Vinyl mesh
Non-skid matting, For rug to floor, 6 x 9 feet, not further specified
Non-skid matting, For rug to floor, 6 x 9 feet, Vinyl mesh
Non-skid matting, For rug to floor, 8 x 10 feet, not further specified
Non-skid matting, For rug to floor, 8 x 10 feet, Vinyl mesh
Non-skid matting, For rug to floor, 9 x 12 feet, not further specified
Non-skid matting, For rug to floor, 9 x 12 feet, Vinyl mesh
Non-skid matting, General use, 1 x 12 feet, not further specified
Non-skid matting, General use, 1 x 12 feet, Rubber coated mesh
Non-skid matting, General use, 1 x 12 feet, Vinyl mesh
Non-skid matting, General use, 1 x 54 feet, not further specified
Non-skid matting, General use, 1 x 54 feet, Rubber coated mesh
Non-skid matting, General use, 12 x 120 inches, Slippery when wet
Non-skid matting, General use, 16 inches x 10 yards, High-tack soft plastic
Non-skid matting, General use, 16 inches x 10 yards, not further specified
Non-skid matting, General use, 16 x 36 inches, High-tack soft plastic
Non-skid matting, General use, 16 x 36 inches, High-tack soft plastic textured
Non-skid matting, General use, 16 x 36 inches, not further specified
Non-skid matting, General use, 16 x 72 inches, High-tack soft plastic
Non-skid matting, General use, 16 x 72 inches, not further specified
Non-skid matting, General use, 16 x 72 inches adhesive back, High-tack soft plastic
Non-skid matting, General use, 2 x 6 feet, High-tack soft plastic
Non-skid matting, General use, 2 x 6 feet, not further specified
Non-skid matting, General use, 23 x 78 inches, High-tack soft plastic
Non-skid matting, General use, 23 x 78 inches, not further specified
Non-skid matting, General use, 23.5 in x 6.5 yards, High-tack soft plastic
Non-skid matting, General use, 23.5 in x 6.5 yards, not further specified
Non-skid matting, General use, 8 in x 10 yards, High-tack soft plastic
Non-skid matting, General use, 8 in x 10 yards, not further specified
Non-skid matting, General use, 8 in x 72 inches, High-tack soft plastic
Non-skid matting, General use, 8 in x 72 inches, not further specified
Non-skid matting, General use, 8 inches x 10 yards, High-tack soft plastic
Non-skid matting, General use, 8 inches x 10 yards, not further specified
Non-skid matting, General use, 8 x 12 inches, High-tack soft plastic
Non-skid matting, General use, 8 x 12 inches, not further specified
Non-skid matting, General use, 8 x 72 inches, High-tack soft plastic
Non-skid matting, General use, 8 x 72 inches, not further specified
Non-skid matting, General use, 8 x 78 inches, High-tack soft plastic
Non-skid matting, General use, 8 x 78 inches, not further specified
Non-skid netting, see, Non-skid matting, ... mesh ...
Non-skid stair tread, Grit surface, Self adhesive, Indoor/outdoor
Non-skid stair tread, Grit surface, Self adhesive, not further specified
Non-skid stair tread, Textured surface, Self adhesive, Indoor/outdoor
Non-skid stair tread, Textured surface, Self adhesive, not further specified
Non-skid strips, Adhesive back, For bathtubs, not further specified
Non-skid strips, Adhesive back, For bathtubs, Textured surface
Non-skid strips, Adhesive back, For floors, not further specified
Non-skid strips, Adhesive back, For floors, Textured surface
Non-skid strips, Adhesive back, General use, not further specified
Non-skid strips, For rugs, Adhesive back, 6 inches x 25 feet
Non-skid strips, For rugs, Adhesive back, not further specified
Non-skid tape, Grit surface, Adhesive back, For indoor/outdoor steps
Non-skid tape, Grit surface, Adhesive back, not further specified
Non-slip strips, Adhesive back, For handles, High-tack soft plastic
Non-slip strips, Adhesive back, For handles, not further specified
Non-slip tabs, Adhesive back, 5/8 inch diameter, High-tack soft plastic
Non-slip tabs, Adhesive back, 5/8 inch diameter, not further specified
Non-slip tabs, Adhesive back, 7/8 inch diameter, High-tack soft plastic
Non-slip tabs, Adhesive back, 7/8 inch diameter, not further specified
Nose/ear hair trimmer, Straight blade, Cordless non-recharge, Battery powered
Nose/ear hair trimmer, Straight blade, Cordless non-recharge, not further specified
Nose/ear hair trimmer, Tubular blade, Cordless non-recharge, Battery powered
Nose/ear hair trimmer, Tubular blade, Cordless non-recharge, not further specified
Nose/ear hair trimmer, Tubular blade, Manually operated, not further specified
Nose/ear hair trimmer, Tubular blade, not further specified
Nosey cup, see, Tumbler with nose cut-out

Octopus, see, Suction disk, multi-cup general
Offset door hinge, Adds 2 inches to width, Use existing holes, not further specified
Offset door hinge, Adds 2 inches to width, Use existing holes, Pair
Opener ..., see, object to be opened

Organizer ..., see, Wire rack ...
Organizer for shoes, see, Shoe organizer
Organizer for ties, see, Tie organizer
Organizer pole, see, Garment rack on tension pole, floor to ceiling mount
Organizer system, see, Wire rack system
Ortho shoe lace, see, Shoe lace fastener, velcro tab closure
Outdoor clock, 18 inch diameter, Large numbers, not further specified
Oven, Free standing 24 inch, Electric, not further specified
Oven, Free standing 24 inch, Electric, Storage drawer below
Oven, Free standing 24 inch, Gas self cleaning, not further specified
Oven, Free standing 24 inch, Gas self cleaning, Storage drawer below
Oven, Wall mounted 24 inch, Electric, not further specified
Oven, Wall mounted 24 inch, not further specified
Oven mitt, 16 inches long, Flame resistant, not further specified
Oven mitt, 16 inches long, Flame resistant, Quilted
Oven rack stick, Notched for oven, 12 inches, not further specified
Oven rack stick, Notched for oven, 12 inches, To push and pull
Over-the-neck viewer, see, Magnifier, neck suspend reading
Overbed table, Floor base non-tilting top, Adjusts 28 to 42 inches, C-base for wheelchair
Overbed table, Floor base non-tilting top, Adjusts 28 to 42 inches, not further specified
Overbed table, Floor base split tilting top, Adjustable height, not further specified
Overbed table, Floor base split tilting top, Adjustable height, T-base
Overbed table, Floor base tilting top, Adjusts 26 to 39 in high, Crank adjustment
Overbed table, Floor base tilting top, Adjusts 26 to 39 in high, not further specified
Overbed table, Floor base tilting top, Adjusts 28 to 38 inches, Folds
Overbed table, Floor base tilting top, Adjusts 28 to 38 inches, not further specified
Overbed table, Floor base tilting top, Adjusts 28 to 38 inches, U-base folding
Overbed table, Floor base tilting top, Adjusts 28 to 39 inches, not further specified
Overbed table, Floor base tilting top, Adjusts 28 to 39 inches, T-base
Overbed table, Floor base tilting top, Adjusts 28 to 45 inches, C-base for wheelchair
Overbed table, Floor base tilting top, Adjusts 28 to 45 inches, not further specified
Overbed table, Floor base tilting top, Fixed height, 14 X 18 inch top
Overbed table, Floor base tilting top, Fixed height, 15 X 30 inch top
Overbed table, Floor base tilting top, Fixed height, not further specified
Overshoe, Unisex, With traction sole, High-Cut
Overshoe, Unisex, With traction sole, Low-Cut

Page turner, Book holder, Microswitch actuated, Battery powered
Page turner, Book holder, Microswitch actuated, Forward and backward
Page turner, Book holder, Microswitch actuated, Forward only
Page turner, Book holder, Microswitch actuated, not further specified
Page turning stick, Hand clip mount, Curved rubber tip, not further specified
Page turning stick, Hand clip mount, not further specified
Page turning stick, Mouthstick, Straight, 2 vacuum pickup ends
Page turning stick, Mouthstick, Straight, not further specified
Pajamas, Men's, Velcro closure, not further specified
Pajamas, Men's, Velcro closure, Various colors
Pan (cooking), see, Saucepan
Pant rack, Hangs on rod, Open end, 5-tier rack
Pant rack, Hangs on rod, Open end, not further specified
Pant rack, Hangs on rod, Open end, One pant per rack
Pant rack, Mounts on wall hook, Swinging arms, 5-arm
Pant rack, Mounts on wall hook, Swinging arms, not further specified
Pants, Men's, Full cut seat, not further specified
Pants, Men's, Full cut seat, Polyester
Pants, Men's, Velcro fly, Cotton/polyester twill
Pants, Men's, Velcro fly, not further specified
Pants, Men's dress pants, Velcro fly, not further specified
Pants, Men's dress pants, Velcro fly, Various colors
Pants, Men's drop seat, Velcro closure, Cotton/polyester
Pants, Men's drop seat, Velcro closure, not further specified
Pants, Men's elastic waist, Zipper fly, Casual cut
Pants, Men's elastic waist, Zipper fly, Cotton/polyester
Pants, Men's elastic waist, Zipper fly, not further specified
Pants, Men's sweat pants, 3/4 side zipper, not further specified
Pants, Men's sweat pants, Full side zipper, not further specified
Pants, Women's, Elastic waist, not further specified
Pants, Women's, not further specified
Pants, Women's drop front, Velcro closure, not further specified
Pants, Women's drop front, Velcro closure, Polyester
Pants pull, Loop webbing, Hooks into belt loop, not further specified
Pants pull, Loop webbing, Hooks into belt loop, Pull and roll body
Panty, see, Brief
Panty, Women's, Band leg brief, Acetate nylon
Panty, Women's, Band leg brief, Cotton/polyester
Panty, Women's, Band leg brief, not further specified
Panty, Women's, Bloomers, Cotton
Panty, Women's, Bloomers, not further specified
Panty, Women's, Elastic leg brief, Cotton/polyester
Panty, Women's, Elastic leg brief, not further specified
Panty, Women's, Elastic leg brief, Super size-cotton
Panty, Women's, Flare pant, Cotton/polyester
Panty, Women's, Flare pant, not further specified
Pantyhose aid, One-hand operated, Semi-rigid trough, No clips

Pantyhose aid, One-hand operated, Semi-rigid trough, not further specified
Pantyhose aid, Two hands needed to operate, Flexible trough, No clips
Pantyhose aid, Two hands needed to operate, Flexible trough, not further specified
Pantyhose aid, Two hands needed to operate, Flexible trough, not further specified
Pantyhose aid, Two hands needed to operate, Flexible trough, With clips
Pantyhose aid, Two hands needed to operate, Rigid trough, not further specified
Pantyhose aid, Two hands needed to operate, Rigid trough, With clips
Patio cover, 10 feet deep x 20 wide, Aluminum, Enamel finish
Patio cover, 10 feet deep x 20 wide, Aluminum, not further specified
Peeler for vegetables, see, Vegetable peeler
Pen, Built-up, Weighted, not further specified
Pen, Built-up, Weighted, Refillable ball point
Pen, Contoured, 19 degree curve, not further specified
Pen, Contoured, 19 degree curve, Smooth finish
Pen, Contoured, 19 degree curve, Suede finish
Pen, Contoured & built-up, Adjustable weight, Refillable ball point
Pen, Contoured & built-up, Weighted, not further specified
Pen, Contoured & built-up, Weighted, Refillable ball point
Pen, Hole for index finger, Uses modified pen grasp, Refillable ball point
Pen, Indented, built-up, 'arthritic' design, not further specified
Pen, Indented, built-up, not further specified
Pen, Straight, Writes bold black, Fiber tip
Pen, Straight, Writes bold black, not further specified
Pen, Straight & weighted, Adjustable weight, Large diameter
Pen, Straight & weighted, Adjustable weight, not further specified
Pen, Straight & weighted, not further specified
Pen grip, see, Pen-and-pencil grip
Pen holder, Cross dowel with set screw, Changeable pen, not further specified
Pen holder, Cross dowel with set screw, Changeable pen, Velcro strap attachment
Pen holder, Fits universal cuff, Rollers hold pen, Metal frame
Pen holder, Fits universal cuff, Rollers hold pen, not further specified
Pen holder, Molded palmar cuff, For Left hand use, Adjustable with heat gun
Pen holder, Molded palmar cuff, For Left hand use, not further specified
Pen holder, Molded palmar cuff, For Right hand use, Adjustable with heat gun
Pen holder, Molded palmar cuff, For Right hand use, not further specified
Pen holder, Palm clip/finger/wrist support, For Left hand use, For large hand
Pen holder, Palm clip/finger/wrist support, For Left hand use, For small hand
Pen holder, Palm clip/finger/wrist support, For Left hand use, not further specified
Pen holder, Palmar ball grip, Changeable pen, not further specified
Pen holder, Palmar ball grip, Changeable pen, Velcro strap attachment
Pen holder, Palmar cuff & finger support, For Right hand use, For large hand
Pen holder, Palmar cuff & finger support, For Right hand use, not further specified
Pen holder, Palmar cylinder grip, Changeable pen, not further specified
Pen holder, Palmar cylinder grip, Changeable pen, Velcro strap attachment
Pen holder, Spring wire frame, For use with either hand, 3 point paper contact
Pen holder, Spring wire frame, For use with either hand, not further specified
Pen holder, With palm clip, For Left hand use, For large hand
Pen holder, With palm clip, For Left hand use, For small hand
Pen holder, With palm clip, For Left hand use, not further specified
Pen holder, With palm clip, For Right hand use, For large hand
Pen holder, With palm clip, For Right hand use, For small hand
Pen holder, With palm clip, For Right hand use, not further specified
Pen holder, With palm clip & wrist support, For Left hand use, For large hand
Pen holder, With palm clip & wrist support, For Left hand use, For small hand
Pen holder, With palm clip & wrist support, For Left hand use, not further specified
Pen holder, With palm clip & wrist support, For Right hand use, For large hand
Pen holder, With palm clip & wrist support, For Right hand use, For small hand
Pen holder, With palm clip & wrist support, For Right hand use, not further specified
Pen holder, With palm clip & wrist support, For Right hand use, not further specified
Pen holder, With wrist support, Small, Left
Pen holder, With wrist support, Small, not further specified
Pen holder sliding, Angled base, Holds pen or pencil, not further specified
Pen holder sliding, Angled base, Holds pen or pencil, Solid plastic
Pen holder sliding, Angled base, Low-friction base pad, not further specified
Pen holder sliding, Angled base, Low-friction base pad, Pen permanently mounted
Pen holder sliding, Angled base, Solid plastic, not further specified
Pen holder sliding, Angled base, Solid plastic, Pen permanently mounted
Pen holder sliding, Palmar support, Bird shaped, Holds pen or pencil
Pen holder sliding, Palmar support, Bird shaped, not further specified
Pen holder sliding, Wide base, Base has a hand-rest, Clear plastic
Pen holder sliding, Wide base, Base has a hand-rest, not further specified

Pen-and-pencil grip, Ball-shaped, For standard pencil, Large enough to fill hand
Pen-and-pencil grip, Bulb-shaped, For standard pencil, Non-rolling
Pen-and-pencil grip, Bulb-shaped, For standard pencil, not further specified
Pen-and-pencil grip, Moldable material, For other items also, not further specified
Pen-and-pencil grip, Moldable material, not further specified
Pen-and-pencil grip, Rigid slip-on gripper, Thumbscrew attached, Adjustable position
Pen-and-pencil grip, Rigid slip-on gripper, Thumbscrew attached, not further specified
Pen-and-pencil grip, Slip-on gripper, not further specified
Pen-and-pencil grip, Slip-on gripper, Round, Large diameter
Pen-and-pencil grip, Slip-on gripper, Round, Medium diameter
Pen-and-pencil grip, Slip-on gripper, Round, not further specified
Pen-and-pencil grip, Slip-on gripper, Round, not further specified
Pen-and-pencil grip, Slip-on gripper, Round, not further specified
Pen-and-pencil grip, Slip-on gripper, Round, Small diameter
Pen-and-pencil grip, Slip-on gripper, Triangular, Assorted sizes in packet
Pen-and-pencil grip, Slip-on gripper, Triangular, Cut to length
Pen-and-pencil grip, Slip-on gripper, Triangular, Fixed length
Pen-and-pencil grip, Slip-on gripper, Triangular, Medium diameter
Pen-and-pencil grip, Slip-on gripper, Triangular, not further specified
Pen-and-pencil grip, Slip-on gripper, Triangular, Slim size
Pen-and-pencil grip, Wet-and-slip-on gripper, not further specified
Pen-and-pencil grip, Wet-and-slip-on gripper, Round, not further specified
Pen-and-pencil holder, Built up and weighted, Adjustable weights
Pen-and-pencil holder, Right angle holder block, Fits universal cuff pocket
Pencil, Large diameter, not further specified
Pencil, Large diameter, Soft black lead, not further specified
Pencil grip, see, Pen-and-pencil grip
Pencil holder sliding, Angled base, For use with either hand, Mechanical pencil permanent
Pencil holder sliding, Angled base, For use with either hand, not further specified
Pencil with holder, Spring wire frame, For use with either hand, Mechanical pencil permanent
Pencil with holder, Spring wire frame, For use with either hand, not further specified
Personal alarm, see also, Personal alerting device
Personal alerting device, Carried in hand or purse, 130 decibel siren, not further specified
Personal alerting device, Carried in hand or purse, 130 decibel siren, Pull pin activated
Personal alerting device, Carried on neck cord, not further specified
Personal alerting device, Carried on neck cord, Whistle, not further specified
Personal amplifier, see, Speech amplifier
Personal FM system, Transmit & receive, Wireless receiver, 3 frequencies
Personal FM system, Transmit & receive, Wireless receiver, not further specified
Personal sound amplifier, Headset, Microphone & amplifier, Battery powered
Personal sound amplifier, Headset, Microphone & amplifier, not further specified
Personal sound amplifier, Headset & pocket model, Mike & amplifier in pocket, Battery powered
Personal sound amplifier, Headset & pocket model, Mike & amplifier in pocket, not further specified
Personal sound amplifier, Table or pocket model, Mike-amplifier/cord/earphone, Battery powered
Personal sound amplifier, Table or pocket model, Mike-amplifier/cord/earphone, not further specified
Personal visibility light, Flashing strobe, To be seen at night, not further specified
Personal visibility light, Flashing strobe, To be seen at night, With belt clip
Phone ..., see, Telephone ...
Phone number organizer, Cards in case, Hand held, not further specified
Phone number organizer, Cards in case, not further specified
Pill bottle opener, Two hands needed to operate, Fits over cap, not further specified
Pill bottle opener, Two hands needed to operate, Fits over cap, Push and turn
Pill bottle opener, Two hands needed to operate, not further specified
Pill bottle opener, Two hands needed to operate, Wedge lever, not further specified
Pill box, see, Medication manager, manual compartments
Pill crusher, Durable plastic, not further specified
Pill crusher, Durable plastic, Twist operated, not further specified
Pill holder, For nitroglycerin, Waterproof, Brass screw cylinder
Pill holder, For nitroglycerin, Waterproof, not further specified
Pill planner, see, Medication manager
Pill splitter, Close lid to split, Does not crush pill, not further specified
Pill splitter, Close lid to split, not further specified
Pill splitter, For pills to 1/2 inch diameter, Cuts coated pills, not further specified
Pill splitter, For pills to 1/2 inch diameter, not further specified
Pillow, Adjustable position, Eggcrate, Hand washable
Pillow, Adjustable position, Eggcrate, not further specified
Pillow, King size, Polyester fill, Firm
Pillow, King size, Polyester fill, not further specified
Pillow, Queen size, Polyester fill, Firm
Pillow, Queen size, Polyester fill, not further specified
Pillow, Standard size, Eggcrate, Hand wash
Pillow, Standard size, Eggcrate, not further specified
Pillow, Standard size, Polyester fill, Firm
Pillow, Standard size, Polyester fill, not further specified
Pillow, With neck roll, Foam, Contoured
Pillow, With neck roll, Foam, Firm inner core

Pillow, With neck roll, Foam, not further specified
Pillow protector, Standard size, Zippered, not further specified
Pillow protector, Standard size, Zippered, Soft vinyl
Pizza cutter, see, Table knife, rolling blade
Pizza knife, see, Kitchen knife, rolling blade
Plant caddy, see, Floor cart
Plant hanger, Pulley operated, Holds 25 pounds, Lowers 3 feet
Plant hanger, Pulley operated, Holds 25 pounds, not further specified
Plant stand, Swivel casters, No handle, Brass
Plant stand, Swivel casters, No handle, not further specified
Planter, Fits on railing, Cedar, not further specified
Plastisol, see, Soft plastic coated ..., Hard plastic coated ...
Plate, Divided 3 section high sided, 10 inch round, No lid
Plate, Divided 3 section high sided, 10 inch round, not further specified
Plate, Divided 3 section high sided, 10 inch round, With lid
Plate, Divided 3 section scoop back, 10 inch round, Insulated no lid
Plate, Divided 3 section scoop back, 10 inch round, not further specified
Plate, Divided 3 section scoop back, 5-1/2 inch round, Insulated no lid
Plate, Divided 3 section scoop back, 5-1/2 inch round, not further specified
Plate, Divided 3 section scoop back, 9 inch round, not further specified
Plate, Divided 3 section scoop back, 9 inch round, Vertical back/side
Plate, Divided 3 section scoop back, 9-1/2 inch round, No lid
Plate, Divided 3 section scoop back, 9-1/2 inch round, not further specified
Plate, Divided 3 section slope sided, 10 inch round, not further specified
Plate, Divided 3 section slope sided, 10 inch round, With lid
Plate, Divided 3 section slope sided, 9.5 inch round, Insulated with lid
Plate, Divided 3 section slope sided, 9.5 inch round, No lid
Plate, Divided 3 section slope sided, 9.5 inch round, not further specified
Plate, High sided, 10 inch round, 1-1/4 to 1/2 inch sides
Plate, High sided, 10 inch round, not further specified
Plate, High sided, 7-3/4 inch round, not further specified
Plate, High sloping side, 8 inch round, not further specified
Plate, Inner well with platform lip, 10 inch round, not further specified
Plate, Inner well with platform lip, 10 inch round, With suction cup feet
Plate, Inner well with platform lip, 6-1/2 inch round, Ceramic
Plate, Inner well with platform lip, 6-1/2 inch round, not further specified
Plate, Inner well with platform lip, 9 inch round, not further specified
Plate, Inner well with platform lip, 9 inch round, Suction cup feet
Plate, Inner well with platform lip, 9-1/2 inch round, 1 inch deep well
Plate, Inner well with platform lip, 9-1/2 inch round, 1/2 inch deep well
Plate, Inner well with platform lip, 9-1/2 inch round, Non-skid bottom
Plate, Inner well with platform lip, 9-1/2 inch round, not further specified
Plate, Inner well with platform lip, 9-1/2 inch round, Polypropylene
Plate, Inner well with platform lip, 9-1/2 inch round, Scoop inner well
Plate, Inner well with platform lip, not further specified
Plate, Scoop back, 11 x 8 inch oval, not further specified
Plate, Scoop back, 8 x 10 inch oval, Non-skid bottom
Plate, Scoop back, 8 x 10 inch oval, not further specified
Plate, Scoop back, 9 x 6 inch oval, not further specified
Plate, Scoop back, not further specified
Plate, Scoop back or side, 6 x 8-1/2 inch oval, not further specified
Plate, Scoop back or side, 6-1/2 inch round, Non-skid bottom
Plate, Scoop back or side, 6-1/2 inch round, not further specified
Plate, Scoop back or side, 7-3/4 inch round, not further specified
Plate, Scoop back or side, 7-3/4 inch round, not further specified
Plate, Scoop back or side, 7-3/4 inch round, Rolled edges
Plate, Scoop back or side, 7-3/4 x 11 inch oval, not further specified
Plate, Scoop back or side, 8 inch round, Built-up edge
Plate, Scoop back or side, 8 inch round, Non-skid bottom
Plate, Scoop back or side, 8 inch round, not further specified
Plate, Scoop back or side, 9 inch round, not further specified
Plate, Scoop back or side, 9 inch round, not further specified
Plate, Scoop back or side, 9 inch round, Reinforced rim and base
Plate, Scoop back or side, 9 inch round, Suction cup feet
Plate, Scoop back or side, not further specified
Plate, Standard surface, Dinner plate size, Non-skid bottom
Plate, Standard surface, Dinner plate size, not further specified
Plate, Standard surface, Dinner plate size, Standard bottom
Plate, With inner lip, not further specified
Plate guard, see, Food guard for plate
Plate lid, For partitioned plate, Polycarbonate, Clear
Plate lid, For partitioned plate, Polycarbonate, not further specified
Plate lid, For partitioned plate, Polycarbonate, White
Playing card holder, Hand held fan clip holder, Holds fanned hand of cards, Can also stand on table
Playing card holder, Hand held fan clip holder, Holds fanned hand of cards, not further specified
Playing card holder, Hand held spring loaded disks, Foam-padded exterior, not further specified
Playing card holder, Hand held spring loaded disks, not further specified
Playing card holder, Hand held spring loaded disks, not further specified
Playing card holder, Hand held straight clip holder, Single slip-in clip, not further specified
Playing card holder, Hand held straight clip holder, Single slip-in clip, With finger loops
Playing card holder, not further specified
Playing card holder, Slotted block type, 1 slot, For use with mouthstick
Playing card holder, Slotted block type, 1 slot, not further specified
Playing card holder, Slotted block type, 1 slot, Wood 10 inches long

Playing card holder, Slotted block type, 1 slot 25 inches long, For use with mouthstick
Playing card holder, Slotted block type, 1 slot 25 inches long, not further specified
Playing card holder, Slotted block type, 3 slots, Elevated & tilted
Playing card holder, Slotted block type, 3 slots, not further specified
Playing card holder, Slotted block type, 3 slots, Wood
Playing card holder, Slotted block type, 4 angled slots, not further specified
Playing card holder, Slotted block type, 4 angled slots, Wood
Playing card holder, Slotted block type, 4 graduated slots, not further specified
Playing card holder, Slotted block type, 4 graduated slots, Wood
Playing card holder, Slotted type, 4 slots, Fiberboard
Playing card holder, Slotted type, 4 slots, Slanted frame
Playing card shuffler, One-deck, Battery powered, not further specified
Playing card shuffler, One-deck, Manually operated, not further specified
Playing card shuffler, One-deck, not further specified
Playing card shuffler, Two-deck, Battery powered, not further specified
Playing card shuffler, Two-deck, not further specified
Playing cards, 2-inch numbers, Poker sized cards, 4 color codes
Playing cards, 2-inch numbers, Poker sized cards, not further specified
Playing cards, Brailled & large print, not further specified
Playing cards, Brailled & large print, Poker sized cards, not further specified
Playing cards, Large print, Large cards, not further specified
Playing cards, Large print, not further specified
Playing cards, Large print, Poker sized cards, 4 color codes
Playing cards, Large print, Poker sized cards, not further specified
Playing cards, Large print, Poker sized cards, not further specified
Playing cards, Standard print, Magnetic, Metal board included
Playing cards, Standard print, Magnetic, not further specified
Playing cards, Standard print, Magnetic, not further specified
Playing cards, Standard print, not further specified
Playing cards set, Large print, not further specified
Playing cards set, Large print, Playing card shuffler included, not further specified
Pliers, Loop handle, not further specified
Pliers, Loop handle, Self-opening, not further specified
Plug puller, Electric cord, Push tab, Cam action
Plug puller, Electric cord, Push tab, not further specified
Plug puller, Electric cord, Straight pull, Loop handle
Plug puller, Electric cord, Straight pull, not further specified
Poncho, Side snap & drawstring, With hood, not further specified
Poncho, Side snap & drawstring, With hood, Water repellent nylon
Poncho, Zipper front, Velcro side closure, not further specified
Poncho, Zipper front, Velcro side closure, Short/black
Pool cue bridge, Bridge on wheels, not further specified
Pool cue bridge, Bridge on wheels, With fixed cue, not further specified
Pool cue cuff, Vinyl lined leather, not further specified
Pool cue cuff, Vinyl lined leather, With adjustable strap, not further specified
Pool transfer seat, Self-operated, Controls at deck & water level, Water pressure powered
Portable work desk, see, Book holder, portable work desk
Positioning cushion, Bolster type, Firm, not further specified
Positioning cushion, Bolster type, not further specified
Pot lid lifter, V-slot to insert under knob, not further specified
Pot lid lifter, V-slot to insert under knob, Plastic coated metal, not further specified
Pressure pad, Alternating, Bed, AC powered 110V pump
Pressure pad, Alternating, Bed, not further specified
Pressure pad, Alternating, Seat, AC powered 110V pump
Pressure pad, Alternating, Seat, AC powered 220V pump
Pressure pad, Alternating, Seat, not further specified
Pressure reduction mattress, see, Mattress, layered foam
Primer for plastic dip, Use with coatings, Increases bond, not further specified
Primer for plastic dip, Use with coatings, not further specified
Primer for rubber dip, Use with coatings, Increases bond, not further specified
Primer for rubber dip, Use with coatings, not further specified
Prism glasses, Not over regular glasses, not further specified
Prism glasses, Not over regular glasses, Up to 90 degree view, not further specified
Prism glasses, Over regular glasses, Shows 1/2 page, For reading supine
Prism glasses, Over regular glasses, Shows 1/2 page, not further specified
Prism glasses, Over regular glasses, With angle convergence device, For reading supine
Prism glasses, Over regular glasses, With angle convergence device, not further specified
Propane gas alarm, see, Gas detector alarm, natural and propane

Quad hair lift, see, Hair lift comb

Railing, For ramp, Aluminum, Custom fabricated
Railing, For ramp, Aluminum, not further specified
Railing panel, Steel indoor/outdoor, 48 inch long section, not further specified
Railing panel, Steel indoor/outdoor, 48 inch long section, Prime-coated
Railing panel, Steel indoor/outdoor, 72 inch long section, not further specified
Railing panel, Steel indoor/outdoor, 72 inch long section, Prime-coated
Railing post, Steel indoor/outdoor, 36 inches with base anchor, not further specified

Railing post, Steel indoor/outdoor, 36 inches with base anchor, Prime-coated
Rain gauge, Large print, Measures 5 inches rain, not further specified
Rain gauge, Large print, Measures 5 inches rain, Yellow plastic
Raised mark maker, Fluorescent colors, Dries in 3 to 4 hours, not further specified
Raised mark maker, Fluorescent colors, not further specified
Raised toilet seat, 2 inch height, No grips or rails, not further specified
Raised toilet seat, 2 inch height, No grips or rails, Standard seat
Raised toilet seat, 3-6 inch adjustable height, No grips or rails, not further specified
Raised toilet seat, 3-6 inch adjustable height, No grips or rails, Standard seat
Raised toilet seat, 4 inch height, No grips or rails, Contoured seat
Raised toilet seat, 4 inch height, No grips or rails, Doughnut seat
Raised toilet seat, 4 inch height, No grips or rails, Fits elongated bowls
Raised toilet seat, 4 inch height, No grips or rails, Left cut-out
Raised toilet seat, 4 inch height, No grips or rails, not further specified
Raised toilet seat, 4 inch height, No grips or rails, Open front
Raised toilet seat, 4 inch height, No grips or rails, Open front high back
Raised toilet seat, 4 inch height, No grips or rails, Right cut-out
Raised toilet seat, 4 inch height, No grips or rails, Standard seat
Raised toilet seat, 4 inch height, No grips or rails, With splash guard
Raised toilet seat, 4 inch height, With arm rests, Contoured seat
Raised toilet seat, 4 inch height, With arm rests, not further specified
Raised toilet seat, 4 inch height, With arm rests, Standard seat
Raised toilet seat, 4 inch height, With foam padded arm rests, For very heavy person
Raised toilet seat, 4 inch height, With foam padded arm rests, not further specified
Raised toilet seat, 4 inch height, With foam padded arm rests, Standard seat
Raised toilet seat, 4-6 inch adjustable height, No grips or rails, not further specified
Raised toilet seat, 4-6 inch adjustable height, No grips or rails, Slopes to front
Raised toilet seat, 4-6 inch adjustable height, No grips or rails, With splash guard
Raised toilet seat, 4.5 inch height, No grips or rails, not further specified
Raised toilet seat, 4.5 inch height, No grips or rails, Standard seat
Raised toilet seat, 4.5 inch height, Side handle grips, not further specified
Raised toilet seat, 4.5 inch height, Side handle grips, Standard seat
Raised toilet seat, 4.5-6.5 inch adjustable height, No grips or rails, not further specified
Raised toilet seat, 4.5-6.5 inch adjustable height, No grips or rails, Removable splash guard
Raised toilet seat, 4.5-6.5 inch adjustable height, No grips or rails, With splash guard
Raised toilet seat, 4.75 inch height, No grips or rails, not further specified
Raised toilet seat, 4.75 inch height, No grips or rails, Standard seat
Raised toilet seat, 4.75 inch height, Side handle grips, not further specified
Raised toilet seat, 4.75 inch height, Side handle grips, Standard seat
Raised toilet seat, 5 inch height, Armrests, Fits elongated bowls
Raised toilet seat, 5 inch height, No grips or rails, Fits elongated bowls
Raised toilet seat, 5 inch height, No grips or rails, not further specified
Raised toilet seat, 5 inch height, No grips or rails, Padded seat with splash guard
Raised toilet seat, 5 inch height, No grips or rails, Standard seat
Raised toilet seat, 5.5 inch height, Side handle grips, Contoured seat
Raised toilet seat, 5.5 inch height, Side handle grips, not further specified
Raised toilet seat, Adjustable height, No grips or rails, Adjustable slope to front
Raised toilet seat, Adjustable height, No grips or rails, For very heavy person
Raised toilet seat, Adjustable height, No grips or rails, not further specified
Raised toilet seat, Adjustable height, No grips or rails, Padded seat
Raised toilet seat, Adjustable height, With hand rails, Doughnut seat
Raised toilet seat, Adjustable height, With hand rails, not further specified
Raised toilet seat, Adjustable height, With hand rails, Swivel & with front opening
Raised toilet seat, Adjustable height, With hand rails, With splash guard
Raised toilet seat, Fixed height, No grips or rails, Left cut-out
Raised toilet seat, Fixed height, No grips or rails, not further specified
Raised toilet seat, Fixed height, No grips or rails, Open front sloped
Raised toilet seat, Fixed height, No grips or rails, Right cut-out
Razor, Men's, Triple head, not further specified
Razor, Men's, Triple head, Rechargeable battery powered
Razor, Men's, Wet/dry use, not further specified
Razor, Men's, Wet/dry use, Rechargeable battery powered
Razor holder, For Trac II razor, With palm cuff, not further specified
Razor holder, For Trac II razor, With palm cuff, Plastic coated
Razor holder, For using electric razor, Adjustable velcro strap, Foam padding on grip
Razor holder, For using electric razor, Adjustable velcro strap, Metal palm cuff
Razor holder, For using electric razor, Adjustable velcro strap, not further specified
Razor holder, For using electric razor, Adjustable velcro strap, Plastic coated handle
Reacher, D-grip, Squeeze operated, horizontal jaws
Reacher, D-grip, squeeze operated, horizontal jaws
Reacher, D-grip, squeeze operated, vertical jaw
Reacher, No grip, Trigger operated, Horizontal jaws
Reacher, No grip, Trigger operated, not further specified
Reacher, No grip with wrist support, Cord operated, Locking horizontal jaws
Reacher, No grip with wrist support, Cord operated, not further specified

Reacher, No grip with wrist support, Trigger operated, Horizontal jaws
Reacher, No grip with wrist support, Trigger operated, not further specified
Reacher, No grip with wrist support, Wrist extension operated, Horizontal jaws
Reacher, No grip with wrist support, Wrist extension operated, not further specified
Reacher, No grip with wrist support, Wrist flexion operated, Horizontal jaws
Reacher, Pistol grip, Battery operated, not further specified
Reacher, Pistol grip, Battery operated, Rotating jaw holds 3 pounds
Reacher, Pistol grip, Lever operated, Locking vertical jaw
Reacher, Pistol grip, Lever operated, not further specified
Reacher, Pistol grip, Squeeze operated, Horizontal jaws
Reacher, Pistol grip, Squeeze operated, Horizontal jaws hold 2 pounds
Reacher, Pistol grip, Squeeze operated, Horizontal jaws hold 6.5 pound
Reacher, Pistol grip, Squeeze operated, Horizontal jaws-26 inch
Reacher, Pistol grip, Squeeze operated, Horizontal jaws-30 inch
Reacher, Pistol grip, Squeeze operated, Locking horizontal jaws
Reacher, Pistol grip, Squeeze operated, not further specified
Reacher, Pistol grip, Squeeze operated, Rotating jaw
Reacher, Pistol grip, Squeeze operated, Rotating jaw - 18 inches long
Reacher, Pistol grip, Squeeze operated, Rotating jaw - 22 inches long
Reacher, Pistol grip, Squeeze operated, Rotating jaw - 28 inches long
Reacher, Pistol grip, Squeeze operated, Rotating jaw - 30 inches long
Reacher, Pistol grip, Squeeze operated, Vertical jaw
Reacher, Pistol grip, Squeeze operated, Vertical jaw - 32 inches long
Reacher, Pistol grip, Squeeze operated, With shoehorn
Reacher, Pistol grip, Trigger operated, Horizontal jaws
Reacher, Pistol grip, Trigger operated, Horizontal jaws - 30 inches
Reacher, Pistol grip, Trigger operated, not further specified
Reacher, Pistol grip, Trigger operated, Single jaw - 22 inches long
Reacher, Pistol grip, Trigger operated, Single jaw with magnetic tip
Reacher, Pistol grip, Trigger operated, Single jaw-32 inch
Reacher, Pistol grip, Trigger operated, Vertical jaw
Reacher, Pistol grip, Trigger operated, Vertical jaw-32 inch
Reacher, Pistol grip with wrist support, Squeeze operated, Horizontal jaws
Reacher, Pistol grip with wrist support, Squeeze operated, not further specified
Reacher, Pistol grip with wrist support, Trigger operated, Horizontal jaws
Reacher, Pistol grip with wrist support, Trigger operated, not further specified
Reacher, Scissor handle, Tongs, 2 hand required
Reacher, Scissor handle, Tongs, 2 hand-33 inch
Reacher, Straight handle, No operation, Cup hook on end
Reacher, Straight handle, No operation, not further specified
Reacher, Straight handle, No operation, Telescoping/hook/adhesive pad
Reacher, Straight handle, Squeeze operated, Horizontal jaws
Reacher, Straight handle, Squeeze operated, Horizontal jaws hold 5 pounds
Reacher, Straight handle, Squeeze operated, Horizontal jaws-32 inch
Reacher, Straight handle, Squeeze operated, not further specified
Reacher, Straight handle, Squeeze operated, Vertical jaw 20 inch
Reacher, Straight handle, Squeeze operated, Vertical jaw 32 inch
Reacher, Straight handle, Squeeze operated, Vertical jaw with peg hook
Reacher, Straight handle, Squeeze operated to open, Auto-closing horizontal jaws
Reacher, Straight handle, Squeeze operated to open, Auto-closing vertical jaw
Reacher holder, For wheelchair, Clamps to tubing, not further specified
Reacher holder, For wheelchair, not further specified
Reacher holder, Wheelchair/walker, Attached by bracket, not further specified
Reacher holder, Wheelchair/walker, not further specified
Reacher wrist support, For specific reacher, not further specified
Reacher wrist support, For various reachers, Adjustable fit, not further specified
Reacher wrist support, For various reachers, not further specified
Reacher wrist support, not further specified
Reading aid, Bars adhere to page, 4 sized bars, not further specified
Reading aid, Overlay adheres to page, 5 overlays, not further specified
Recreation belt, One-hand operated, not further specified
Recreation belt, One-hand operated, not further specified
Recreation belt, One-hand operated, Sockets at chest and waist, Holds any handled implement
Remote control, Appliance operation, Color coded buttons, not further specified
Remote control, Appliance operation, Color coded buttons, Runs 4 appliances
Remote control, TV and/or audio, Large buttons, Battery powered
Remote control, TV and/or audio, Large buttons, not further specified
Remote control, TV and/or audio, Wide angle or greater power, Battery powered
Remote control, TV and/or audio, Wide angle or greater power, not further specified
Remote wall switch, Controls lamp, Wall switch conversion, not further specified
Remote wall switch, Controls lamp, Wall switch conversion, Sending & receiving units
Rifle rest, For Recreation belt, not further specified
Robe, Women's, Ankle length, Front button chenille
Robe, Women's, Ankle length, not further specified
Rocker blade knife, see, Table/kitchen knife, crescent blade
Rocker knife, see, Table/kitchen knife, rocker blade

Rocker switch, see, Wall switch
Rocking chair, Arrowback, No arms, Hardwood
Rocking chair, Arrowback, No arms, not further specified
Rocking chair, Mission style, Straight arms, not further specified
Rocking chair, Mission style, Straight arms, Oak finish
Rocking chair stop, Button for under rocker front, Prevents over-rocking forward, not further specified
Rocking chair stop, Frame to limit rocking, Chair is set on frame, not further specified
Rocking chair stop, Frame to limit rocking, not further specified
Rocking-T knife, see, Table/kitchen knife, top palmar handle
Roho cushion, see, Seat cushion, cellular inflated
Roho cushion cover, not further specified
Roller knife, see, Kitchen knife, rolling blade
Rolling pin, One-hand operated, 1 roller, not further specified
Rolling pin, One-hand operated, 1 roller, Single handle
Rolling pin, One-hand operated, 2 rollers, not further specified
Rolling pin, One-hand operated, 2 rollers, Single handle
Rolling plant caddy, see, Floor cart
Rotating bathtub, see, Bathtub that rotates
Rubber dip coating, For utensils, not further specified
Rubber dip coating, For utensils, Use with primer, not further specified
Rug, Hearth, Fireproof, 22 x 40 inch half circle
Rug, Hearth, Fireproof, not further specified
Rug, Hearth, Fireproof, Rectangular

Safety strips, see, Non-skid strips, adhesive back
Sandwich board, One-handed, With corner guards, High-tack soft plastic
Sandwich board, One-handed, With corner guards, not further specified
Sandwich board, One-handed, With corner guards, Slanted with non-skid bottom
Sandwich board, see, Cutting board
Sandwich holder, One-hand operated, Fits universal cuff, not further specified
Sandwich holder, One-hand operated, Fits universal cuff, Rubber band clamp
Sandwich holder, One-hand operated, Fits universal cuff, Spring clamp
Saucepan, Curled handle grips, Allows two-hand lift, not otherwise specified
Saucepan, Locking drain lid, Allows two-hand lift, not further specified
Saucepan, Locking drain lid, Allows two-hand lift, Various sizes
Saucepan, Two hands needed to operate, Handle and handgrip, not further specified
Saucepan, Two hands needed to operate, Handle and handgrip, Various sizes
Saucepan pour stand, Holds common pans, Tilts saucepan, Low effort
Saucepan pour stand, Holds common pans, Tilts saucepan, not further specified
Saucepan stabilizer, Stovetop, Suction feet, Folds for storage
Saucepan stabilizer, Stovetop, Suction feet, For handles 5 inches high
Saucepan stabilizer, Stovetop, Suction feet, not further specified
Saucepan stabilizer, Stovetop, Suction feet, Open-top slot for pot handle
Scissor pick-up aid, Clear plastic shield, Scissors insert in slot, Holds handle above table
Scissors, Electric, Hand held, Battery powered
Scissors, Electric, Hand held, not further specified
Scissors, For Left hand, 7-1/2 inches, Bent handle
Scissors, For Left hand, 7-1/2 inches, not further specified
Scissors, Not self-opening, Large loop handles, not further specified
Scissors, Not self-opening, not further specified
Scissors, Not self-opening, Soft large finger loops, not further specified
Scissors, Self-opening, End loop, Finger loops
Scissors, Self-opening, End loop, not further specified
Scissors, Self-opening, End loop, Plier handles
Scissors, Self-opening, Spring opening, not further specified
Scissors, Self-opening, Spring opening, Plier handles
Scissors, Self-opening, Spring opening, Press down to cut
Scissors, Self-opening, T-handle, not further specified
Scissors, Self-opening, T-handle, Press down to cut
Scissors heavy duty, Angled cutting edge, Finger loop, 3.5 inch blade
Scissors heavy duty, Angled cutting edge, Finger loop, not further specified
Scissors heavy duty, Not self-opening, 9 inch, Finger loops
Scissors heavy duty, Not self-opening, 9 inch, not further specified
Scissors pointed tip, Self-opening, End loop, not further specified
Scissors pointed tip, Self-opening, End loop, Plier handles
Scissors round tip, Self-opening, End loop, not further specified
Scissors round tip, Self-opening, End loop, Plier handles
Scoop bowl, see, Bowl for eating, inner lip
Scoop dish, see, Bowl for eating, scoop
Scooter for limited mobility, Capacity up to 250 lbs, 30 inch turning radius, Indoor
Scooter for limited mobility, Capacity up to 250 lbs, 31 inch turning radius, Indoor-outdoor
Scooter for limited mobility, Capacity up to 300 pound, 31 inch turning radius, Indoor-outdoor
Scooter lift, For car rear end, 3 or 4 wheel up to 200 lbs, Requires Class III hitch
Scooter lift, For car rear end, 3 or4 wheel up to 200 lbs, Requires Class III hitch
Scooter lift, For motor home rear end, 3 or 4 wheel up to 200 lbs, Requires Class III hitch
Scrabble game, Large print, not further specified
Scrabble game, not further specified
Scrub brush/squeegee, Garden hose attachment, Extends 4 to 14 feet, not further specified
Scrub brush/squeegee, Garden hose attachment, Extends 4 to 14 feet, Soap reservoir

Sealer for plastic bags, For zip-type bags, Wall mounted, Pull-through operation
Seat & back cushion, Lateral support, Urethane foam, not further specified
Seat & back cushion, Lateral support, Urethane foam, Strap to wheelchair
Seat & back cushion, Lumbar support, Foam/gel, Contoured base
Seat & back cushion, Lumbar support, Foam/gel, not further specified
Seat cushion, Cellular inflated, Alternation cell inflation, AC powered
Seat cushion, Cellular inflated, Alternation cell inflation, Battery powered
Seat cushion, Cellular inflated, Motorized air alternating cell, 15 X 15 X 4 inches
Seat cushion, Cellular inflated, Motorized air alternating cell, High profile
Seat cushion, Cellular inflated, Motorized air alternating cell, Low profile
Seat cushion, Cellular inflated, Motorized air alternating cell, not further specified
Seat cushion, Chair seat, Eggcrate foam, Cutout slot in center
Seat cushion, Chair seat, Eggcrate foam, not further specified
Seat cushion, Chair seat, Foam wedge, 16 x 16 inch
Seat cushion, Chair seat, Foam wedge, 18 x 18 inch
Seat cushion, Chair seat, Foam wedge, Coccyx cutout
Seat cushion, Chair seat, Foam wedge, not further specified
Seat cushion, Chair seat, Polyester filled, For wicker armchair
Seat cushion, Chair seat, Polyester filled, not further specified
Seat cushion, Chair seat, Square foam, Coccyx cutout
Seat cushion, Chair seat, Square foam, not further specified
Seat cushion, Chair seat, Square foam, Sheepskin/cotton
Seat cushion, Chair seat, Square open-cell foam, 1 inch thick firm
Seat cushion, Chair seat, Square open-cell foam, not further specified
Seat cushion, Chair seat pad, Cotton/polyester, not further specified
Seat cushion, Chair seat pad, Cotton/polyester, Waterproof back
Seat cushion, Contoured, Foam, 3 section
Seat cushion, Contoured, Foam, not further specified
Seat cushion, Donut, 12 x 14 inches, Foam
Seat cushion, Donut, 12 x 14 inches, not further specified
Seat cushion, Donut, 14 x 16 inches, Foam
Seat cushion, Donut, 14 x 16 inches, not further specified
Seat cushion, Donut, Inflatable, not further specified
Seat cushion, Donut, Inflatable, Rubber
Seat cushion, For wheelchair, Foam & gel, 2 inches thick
Seat cushion, For wheelchair, Foam & gel, 3 inches thick
Seat cushion, For wheelchair, Foam & gel, Narrow adult
Seat cushion, For wheelchair, Foam & gel, not further specified
Seat cushion, For wheelchair, Foam & gel, Rear cutout/adult
Seat cushion, For wheelchair, Foam & gel, Rear cutout/narrow
Seat cushion, For wheelchair, Foam wedge, not further specified
Seat cushion, For wheelchair, Foam wedge, Vinyl covered
Seat cushion, For wheelchair, Foam with water core, not further specified
Seat cushion, For wheelchair, Gel, 2 inches thick
Seat cushion, For wheelchair, Gel, not further specified
Seat cushion, For wheelchair, Inflatable rubber, Denim cover
Seat cushion, For wheelchair, Inflatable rubber, Denim cover/small
Seat cushion, For wheelchair, Inflatable rubber, not further specified
Seat cushion, For wheelchair, not further specified
Seat cushion, For wheelchair, Square open-cell foam, 1 inch thick
Seat cushion, For wheelchair, Square open-cell foam, 2 in thick/soft
Seat cushion, For wheelchair, Square open-cell foam, 2 inches thick/firm
Seat cushion, For wheelchair, Square open-cell foam, 3 inch thick/firm
Seat cushion, For wheelchair, Square open-cell foam, 3 inch thick/soft
Seat cushion, For wheelchair, Square open-cell foam, not further specified
Seat cushion, see, Wheelchair pad
Seat cushion, Swiveling, Lazy susan type, not further specified
Seat cushion, Swiveling, not further specified
Seat cushion, Water filled, Air filled outer pad, not further specified
Seat cushion, Water filled, Air filled outer pad, Vinyl
Seat cushion cover, For cellular inflated cushion, For high profile cushion, not further specified
Seat cushion cover, For cellular inflated cushion, For low profile cushion, not further specified
Seat pad, see, Wheelchair pad
Sewing machine control, Hand lever, Uses regular plug, not further specified
Sewing machine control, Hand lever, Uses regular plug, Replaces foot control
Sewing machine control, Hand pressure, Uses regular plug, not further specified
Sewing machine control, Hand pressure, Uses regular plug, Replaces foot control
Sewing machine control, Knee lever, Uses regular plug, not further specified
Sewing machine control, Knee lever, Uses regular plug, Replaces foot control
Shampoo basin, Inflatable, With drain, 28 X 24 X 6 inches
Shampoo basin, Inflatable, With drain, Neck cut-out
Shampoo basin, Inflatable, With drain, not further specified
Shampoo basin, Inflatable, With drain, Round 24 inches
Shampoo basin, Tray, With drain, Holds 2 gallons
Shampoo basin, Tray, With drain, Neck cut-out
Shampoo basin, Tray, With drain, not further specified
Shampoo basin, Wheelchair tray, With drain, not further specified
Shampoo basin, Wheelchair tray, With drain, Person holds strap

Shaver, see, Razor
Shelf, For storage, Stackable 24 inches wide, not further specified
Shelf, For storage, Stackable 24 inches wide, Plastic with 12 inch legs
Shelf, For storage, Stackable 24 inches wide, Vinyl coated wire
Shelves on pole, Tension pole mount, 2 or more shelves, not further specified
Shelves on pole, Tension pole mount, 2 or more shelves, With closet rod
Shelves on pole, Tension pole mount, 2 swinging shelves, not further specified
Shelves on pole, Tension pole mount, not further specified
Shirt, Men's long sleeve, Velcro front closure, Cotton flannel
Shirt, Men's long sleeve, Velcro front closure, Cotton/polyester
Shirt, Men's long sleeve, Velcro front closure, not further specified
Shirt, Men's short sleeve, Velcro front closure, Cotton/polyester
Shirt, Men's short sleeve, Velcro front closure, not further specified
Shoe, Men's, Velcro front closure, Non-skid sole
Shoe, Men's, Velcro front closure, not further specified
Shoe, Men's, With no-slip sole, Grips oily and wet surfaces
Shoe, Men's dress leather, Tie closure, Non-skid sole
Shoe, Men's dress leather, Tie closure, not further specified
Shoe, Men's slip on, Canvas, Non-skid sole
Shoe, Men's slip on, Canvas, not further specified
Shoe, Men's slip on, Vinyl, Non-skid sole
Shoe, Men's slip on, Vinyl, not further specified
Shoe, Men's slip-on, Leather, Non-skid sole
Shoe, Men's slip-on, Leather, not further specified
Shoe, Men's sneaker, Velcro closure, Non-skid sole
Shoe, Men's sneaker, Velcro closure, not further specified
Shoe, Unisex, Adjustable width & length, Non-skid sole
Shoe, Unisex, Adjustable width & length, not further specified
Shoe, Women's, Slip-on, Non-skid sole
Shoe, Women's, Slip-on, not further specified
Shoe, Women's, With no-slip sole, Grips oily and wet surfaces
Shoe, Women's sneaker, Velcro closure, Non-skid sole
Shoe, Women's sneaker, Velcro closure, not further specified
Shoe, Women's wedge leather, Tie closure, Non-skid sole
Shoe, Women's wedge leather, Tie closure, not further specified
Shoe, Women's wedge/pump leather, Tie closure, Non-skid sole
Shoe, Women's wedge/pump leather, Tie closure, not further specified
Shoe donning aid, Frame over shoe back, 24 inch handle, not further specified
Shoe donning aid, Frame over shoe back, 24 inch handle, Smooth plastic
Shoe donning aid, Frame over shoe back, No handle, not further specified
Shoe donning aid, Frame over shoe back, No handle, Smooth plastic
Shoe donning aid, Shoe fitting stool type, not further specified
Shoe lace elastic, see, Elastic shoe lace
Shoe lace fastener, One-hand operated, Five eyelet, not further specified
Shoe lace fastener, One-hand operated, Five eyelet, Velcro tab closure
Shoe lace fastener, One-hand operated, Four eyelet, not further specified
Shoe lace fastener, One-hand operated, Four eyelet, Velcro closure
Shoe lace fastener, One-hand operated, not further specified
Shoe lace fastener, One-hand operated, Pinch operated, not further specified
Shoe lace fastener, One-hand operated, Pinch operated, Various colors
Shoe lace fastener, One-hand operated, Pull operated, not further specified
Shoe lace fastener, One-hand operated, Six eyelet, not further specified
Shoe lace fastener, One-hand operated, Six eyelet, Velcro closure
Shoe lace fastener, Screw button top lacing hole, Wrap slack tied lacing, not further specified
Shoe lace fastener, Sliding knob, not further specified
Shoe lace fastener, Sliding knob, Pull to release, not further specified
Shoe lace fastener, Wrap button, In top lacing hole, not further specified
Shoe lace fastener, Wrap button, In top lacing hole, Various colors
Shoe organizer, Drawer type, Stackable set of 6, not further specified
Shoe organizer, Drawer type, Stackable set of 6, One pair per drawer
Shoe organizer, Free standing, Expandable, For 17 pair shoes
Shoe organizer, Free standing, Expandable, not further specified
Shoe organizer, Free standing, Expanding on casters, For 14 pair shoes
Shoe organizer, Free standing, Expanding on casters, not further specified
Shoe organizer, Free standing, Expanding stackable, For 15 pair shoes
Shoe organizer, Free standing, Expanding stackable, not further specified
Shoe organizer, Free standing, Holds shoes vertical, For 15 pair shoes
Shoe organizer, Free standing, Holds shoes vertical, not further specified
Shoe organizer, Free standing, On casters, For 24 pair shoes
Shoe organizer, Free standing, On casters, not further specified
Shoe organizer, Free standing, Shelf sets on floor, For 5 pair shoes
Shoe organizer, Free standing, Shelf sets on floor, For 9 pair shoes
Shoe organizer, Free standing, Shelf sets on floor, not further specified
Shoe organizer, Free standing, Shoes held vertical, For 9 pair shoes
Shoe organizer, Free standing, Shoes held vertical, not further specified
Shoe organizer, Over-door mount, Shoes held vertical, For 15 pair shoes
Shoe organizer, Over-door mount, Shoes held vertical, For 18 pair shoes
Shoe organizer, Over-door mount, Shoes held vertical, For 21 pair shoes
Shoe organizer, Over-door mount, Shoes held vertical, not further specified
Shoe organizer, Tension pole mount, Manual rotating, For 24 pair shoes
Shoe organizer, Tension pole mount, Manual rotating, not further specified
Shoe organizer, Wall mounted, 4 foot long shelf, not further specified

Shoehorn, Long handle 36 inch, Adjustable hand loop on handle, Wooden handle and metal blade
Shoehorn, Long handle 36 inch, Textured handle, not further specified
Shoehorn, Long handle 36 inch, Textured handle, Plastic coated steel blade
Shoehorn, Long handle 12 inch, Handle with finger hook, not further specified
Shoehorn, Long handle 18 inch, Handle with finger hook, not further specified
Shoehorn, Long handle 25 1/2 inch, Handle with finger hook, not further specified
Shoehorn, Long handle 30 inch, Handle with finger hook, not further specified
Shoehorn, Long handle 36 inch, Rubber handle grip, not further specified
Shoelace elastic, see, Elastic shoe lace
Shopping cart, 2 wheel/folding, Rigid plastic grids, not further specified
Shopping cart, 2 wheel/folding, Rigid plastic grids, Single pole handle
Shopping cart, 2 wheel/folding, Wire basket frame, Canvas lining
Shopping cart, 2 wheel/folding, Wire basket frame, not further specified
Shopping cart, 4 wheel/folding, Wire basket frame, 10 inch rear wheels
Shopping cart, 4 wheel/folding, Wire basket frame, not further specified
Shower & tub spout, Hand held shower hose & head, Fitted to pipe plumber install, not further specified
Shower & tub spout, Hand held shower hose & head, Fitted to pipe plumber install, On-off at head
Shower arm and head, Adjustable, Attaches to shower arm, Adjustable 9 in pipe
Shower arm and head, Adjustable, Attaches to shower arm, not further specified
Shower arm and head, Adjustable angle, Fitted to pipe plumber install, 20 inch chromed
Shower arm and head, Adjustable angle, Fitted to pipe plumber install, not further specified
Shower caddy, 2 baskets 1 rack, Hangs on shower head, 2 wash cloth hangers
Shower caddy, 2 baskets 1 rack, Hangs on shower head, not further specified
Shower caddy, Four shelf, On vertical tension pole, not further specified
Shower caddy, Three shelf, Hangs on shower head, 2 wash cloth hangers
Shower caddy, Three shelf, Hangs on shower head, not further specified
Shower caddy, Two shelf, Hangs on shower head, 2 wash cloth hangers
Shower caddy, Two shelf, Hangs on shower head, not further specified
Shower chair, Casters with brakes, Mesh back, Aluminum tube frame
Shower chair, Casters with brakes, Mesh back, not further specified
Shower chair/commode, 4 inch casters, Backrest & arms, Aluminum tube frame
Shower chair/commode, 4 inch casters, Backrest & arms, not further specified
Shower chair/commode, Casters with brakes, Backrest & arms, Aluminum tube frame
Shower chair/commode, Casters with brakes, Backrest & arms, not further specified
Shower door for tub, Has upper track only, Folding, Non-shatter panels
Shower door for tub, Has upper track only, Folding, not further specified
Shower enclosure, No threshold, No molded-in seat, not further specified
Shower enclosure, No threshold, No molded-in seat, To roll into
Shower enclosure, With threshold, not further specified
Shower enclosure, With threshold, With molded-in seat, not further specified
Shower hose and head, Hand held, Attaches to faucet, not further specified
Shower hose and head, Hand held, Attaches to faucet, Suction cup bracket
Shower hose and head, Hand held, Attaches to shower arm, not further specified
Shower hose and head, Hand held, Attaches to shower arm, not further specified
Shower hose and head, Hand held, Attaches to shower arm, On-off at head
Shower hose and head, Hand held, Attaches to shower arm, Pulsating spray
Shower hose and head, Hand held, Attaches to shower arm, Restricted flow
Shower hose and head, Hand held, Attaches to shower arm, Wall brackets
Shower hose and head, Hand held, Attaches to tub spout, not further specified
Shower hose and head, Hand held, Fitted to pipe plumber install, not further specified
Shower hose and head, Hand held, Fitted to pipe plumber install, not further specified
Shower hose and head, Hand held, Fitted to pipe plumber install, On-off at head
Shower hose and head, Hand held, not further specified
Shower mat, 21 inch diameter, Terry top, not further specified
Shower mat, 21 inch diameter, Terry top, Suction cup back
Shower mat, 23 inch diameter, Vinyl top, not further specified
Shower mat, 23 inch diameter, Vinyl top, Suction cup back
Shower mat, 24 x 24 inch, Vinyl top, not further specified
Shower mat, 24 x 24 inch, Vinyl top, Suction cup back
Shower seat, see, Shower enclosure, molded seat
Shower seat, Wall mounted, Adjustable height folding, not further specified
Shower seat, Wall mounted, Adjustable height folding, Peri-anal cutout
Shower seat, Wall mounted, Adjustable height folding, Solid seat
Shower seat, Wall mounted, Fixed height, Back and armrests
Shower seat, Wall mounted, Fixed height, not further specified
Shower seat, Wall mounted, Folding, not further specified
Shower seat, Wall mounted, Folding, Padded solid seat
Shower seat, Wall mounted, Folding, Smooth seat
Shower seat, Wall mounted, With transfer extension, Non-skid coating
Shower seat, Wall mounted, With transfer extension, not further specified

Shower slippers, Men's, Large, not further specified
Shower slippers, Men's, Large, Nylon mesh uppers
Shower slippers, Men's, Medium, not further specified
Shower slippers, Men's, Medium, Nylon mesh uppers
Shower slippers, Men's, Small, not further specified
Shower slippers, Men's, Small, Nylon mesh uppers
Shower slippers, Unisex, Extra large, not further specified
Shower slippers, Unisex, Extra large, Nylon mesh uppers
Shower slippers, Unisex, Large, not further specified
Shower slippers, Unisex, Large, Nylon mesh uppers
Shower slippers, Unisex, Medium, not further specified
Shower slippers, Unisex, Medium, Nylon mesh uppers
Shower slippers, Unisex, Small, not further specified
Shower slippers, Unisex, Small, Nylon mesh uppers
Shower slippers, Women's, Large, not further specified
Shower slippers, Women's, Large, Nylon mesh uppers
Shower slippers, Women's, Medium, not further specified
Shower slippers, Women's, Medium, Nylon mesh uppers
Shower slippers, Women's, Small, not further specified
Shower slippers, Women's, Small, Nylon mesh uppers
Shower temperature controller, Inserted behind shower head, Auto shut off at 114 degrees, not further specified
Shower temperature controller, Inserted behind shower head, Auto shut off at 114 degrees, With restart button
Signaler, see, Alerting device
Sink-front tray, Inside sink front, 11-1/4 inches wide, not further specified
Sink-front tray, Inside sink front, 11-1/4 inches wide, Steel tray
Skirt, A-line, Velcro front closure, not further specified
Skirt, A-line, Velcro front closure, Polyester
Skirt, Drop front, Velcro front closure, Cotton/polyester
Skirt, Drop front, Velcro front closure, not further specified
Slacks, see, Pants
Sliding pen holder, see, Pen holder sliding
Slip, Adjustable straps, With shadow panel, Cotton/polyester
Slip, Adjustable straps, With shadow panel, not further specified
Slip, Adjustable straps, With shadow panel, Nylon
Slip, Built-up wide straps, not further specified
Slip, Cut-out seat, not further specified
Slip, Front & back opening, Lace trim, Cotton/polyester
Slip, Front & back opening, Lace trim, not further specified
Slip, Front & back opening, Without lace, Cotton/polyester
Slip, Front & back opening, Without lace, not further specified
Slip, Front-wrap, A-line, not further specified
Slip, Front-wrap, A-line, Polyester/cotton
Slip, Half-slip, Cling-free, not further specified
Slip, Half-slip, Cling-free, Nylon
Slip, Non-adjustable straps, Full cut, Cotton
Slip, Non-adjustable straps, Full cut, not further specified
Slip, Non-adjustable straps, Full cut, Short
Slip, Non-adjustable straps, Full-cut wide, Cotton
Slip, Non-adjustable straps, Full-cut wide, not further specified
Slip, not further specified
Slipper-socks, Unisex, Terry pull-on, not further specified
Slipper-socks, Unisex, Terry pull-on, Vinyl-button bottoms
Slipper-socks, Women's, Pull-on acrylic, not further specified
Slipper-socks, Women's, Pull-on acrylic, Soft vinyl sole
Slippers, Men's, Acrylic upper, not further specified
Slippers, Men's, Acrylic upper, Soft vinyl sole
Slippers, Men's, Brushed velour, not further specified
Slippers, Men's, Brushed velour, Vinyl sole
Slippers, Men's, Corduroy, Crepe sole
Slippers, Men's, Corduroy, not further specified
Slippers, Men's, Double-knit polyester upper, Crepe sole firm heel
Slippers, Men's, Double-knit polyester upper, not further specified
Slippers, Men's, Elastic sides, Hard sole
Slippers, Men's, Elastic sides, not further specified
Slippers, Men's, Pile lined, not further specified
Slippers, Men's, Pile lined, Soft vinyl sole
Slippers, Men's, Quilted fleece, Firm non-skid sole
Slippers, Men's, Quilted fleece, not further specified
Slippers, Men's, Terry uppers, Firm non-skid sole
Slippers, Men's, Terry uppers, not further specified
Slippers, Men's, Velour upper, not further specified
Slippers, Men's, Velour upper, Vinyl sole
Slippers, Men's, Vinyl uppers, Crepe sole
Slippers, Men's, Vinyl uppers, not further specified
Slippers, Women's, Corduroy, not further specified
Slippers, Women's, Corduroy, Rubber sole
Slippers, Women's, Elastic sides, Firm non-skid sole
Slippers, Women's, Elastic sides, not further specified
Slippers, Women's, Fleece lined, not further specified
Slippers, Women's, Fleece lined, Vinyl sole low heel
Slippers, Women's, Open heel and toe, not further specified
Slippers, Women's, Open heel and toe, Wedge heel
Slippers, Women's, Quilted fleece lined, not further specified
Slippers, Women's, Quilted fleece lined, Soft non-skid sole
Slippers, Women's, Satin lined, Firm non-skid sole
Slippers, Women's, Satin lined, not further specified
Slippers, Women's, Terry velour, Crepe sole
Slippers, Women's, Terry velour, not further specified
Slippers, Women's, Vinyl, not further specified

Slippers, Women's, Vinyl, Vinyl sole low heel
Slippers, Women's, Vinyl foam insole, Crepe sole
Slippers, Women's, Vinyl foam insole, not further specified
Slow cooker, Removable crock, 3-1/2 quart, not further specified
Slow cooker, Removable crock, 3-1/2 quart, With cookbook
Slow cooker, Removable crock, 5 quart, not further specified
Slow cooker, Removable crock, not further specified
Small appliance mechanism, Swing up, Up to 25 lbs, Mounts under drawer
Small appliance mechanism, Swing up, Up to 25 lbs, Mounts without drawer
Small appliance mechanism, Swing up, Up to 25 lbs, 13 Inches, not further specified
Smock, 5 pocket carryall, Adjustable neck strap, Large
Smock, 5 pocket carryall, Adjustable neck strap, not further specified
Smoke detector alarm, Flashes light, In light fixture, not further specified
Smoke detector alarm, Flashes light, In light fixture, Rechargeable battery powered
Smoke detector alarm, Horn & strobe light, Separate unit, AC powered hard wired
Smoke detector alarm, Horn & strobe light, Separate unit, AC powered portable
Smoke detector alarm, Horn & strobe light, Separate unit, Battery powered
Smoke detector alarm, Horn & strobe light, Separate unit, not further specified
Smoke detector alarm, Horn signal, Separate unit, AC powered hard wired
Smoke detector alarm, Horn signal, Separate unit, not further specified
Smoke detector alarm, Sound signal & light, Light indicates exit, Can be used as flashlight
Smoke grabber, see, Smokeless ashtray
Smokeless ashtray, Charcoal filter, Table model, Battery powered
Smokeless ashtray, Charcoal filter, Table model, not further specified
Smoker's aid, 36 in tube replacement, For smoker's robot, not further specified
Smoker's aid, 36 in tube replacement, not further specified
Smoker's aid, Cigarette holder, Palm clip grip, not further specified
Smoker's aid, Cigarette holder, Palm clip grip, Plastic mouth piece
Smoker's aid, Tube & mouthpiece & holder, 36 inch tube on tray, Holder for cigarette
Smoker's aid, Tube & mouthpiece & holder, 36 inch tube on tray, not further specified
Smoker's robot, see, Smoker's aid, tube & mouthpiece & holder
Soap dispenser, One-hand operated/wall mounted, 2 section, Dispenses pre-measured amounts
Soap dispenser, One-hand operated/wall mounted, 2 section, not further specified
Soap dispenser, One-hand operated/wall mounted, 4 section, Dispenses pre-measured amounts
Soap dispenser, One-hand operated/wall mounted, 4 section, not further specified
Sock aid, 2 hand use, Cord handle, Flexible trough
Sock aid, 2 hand use, Cord handle, Floppy trough
Sock aid, 2 hand use, Cord handle, not further specified
Sock aid, 2 hand use, Cord handle, Rigid trough
Sock aid, 2 hand use, Cord handle, Semi-rigid trough
Sock aid, 2 hand use, Cord handle, Terry semi-rigid trough
Sock aid, 2 hand use, Cord handle, Trough with clips
Sock aid, 2 hand use, Cord handles, Flexible trough
Sock aid, 2 hand use, Cord handles, not further specified
Sock aid, 2 hand use, Cord handles, Notched trough
Sock aid, 2 hand use, One cord handle, Flexible trough
Sock aid, 2 hand use, One cord handle, not further specified
Sock aid, 2 hand use, Strap handle, not further specified
Sock aid, 2 hand use, Strap handle, Terry semi-rigid trough
Sock aid, 2 hand use, Strap handle, Trough with clips
Sock aid, 2 hand use, Strap handles, not further specified
Sock aid, 2 hand use, Strap handles, Rigid trough
Sock aid, 2 hand use, Strap handles, Semi-rigid trough
Sock aid, 2 hands using 2 rods, Plastic handle 36 inches, Clips
Sock aid, 2 hands using 2 rods, Plastic handle 36 inches, not further specified
Sock aid, 2 hands using 2 rods, T-handle aluminum, Clips
Sock aid, 2 hands using 2 rods, T-handle aluminum, not further specified
Sock aid, One-hand operated, Angled rod handle, not further specified
Sock aid, One-hand operated, Angled rod handle, Rigid notched trough
Sock aid, One-hand operated, Cord handle, not further specified
Sock aid, One-hand operated, Cord handle, Terry semi-rigid trough
Sock aid, One-hand operated, One cord handle, Flexible trough
Sock aid, One-hand operated, One cord handle, Floppy trough
Sock aid, One-hand operated, One cord handle, not further specified
Sock aid, One-hand operated, One cord handle, not further specified
Sock aid, One-hand operated, Rod-tong handle, not further specified
Sock aid, One-hand operated, Rod-tong handle, Trough with velcro holder
Sock aid, One-hand operated, Strap handle, not further specified
Sock aid, One-hand operated, Strap handle, Terry semi-rigid trough
Sock aid, One-hand operated, Strap handles, Terry semi-flexible trough
Sock aid, Two hands to load, Frame-held, not further specified
Sock aid, Two hands to load, Frame-held, Push foot in
Sock aid, Two hands to load, Single rod 38 inch, Clips
Sock aid, Two hands to load, Single rod 38 inch, not further specified
Sock aid pad, Replacement, For sock aid, Adhesive back
Sock aid pad, Replacement, For sock aid, not further specified
Sock aid with shoehorn, 2 hands to load, 24 inch shaft, not further specified

Speech amplifier, Breast pocket model/handheld mike, Microphone/amplifier/speaker, Battery powered
Speech amplifier, Table-top model/handheld mike, Microphone/amplifier/speaker, Battery powered
Speech amplifier, Table-top model/handheld mike, Microphone/amplifier/speaker, not further specified
Speech amplifier, Wireless microphone, Table-top speaker, Battery powered
Speech amplifier, Wireless microphone, Table-top speaker, not further specified
Spice rack, Inside cabinet door, Wire rack, Four tier
Spice rack, Inside cabinet door, Wire rack, not further specified
Spice rack, Inside cabinet door, Wire rack, One tier
Spice rack, Under-cabinet mount, Spring hinge mount, Lowers into position
Spice rack, Under-cabinet mount, Spring hinge mount, not further specified
Spice rack, Wall mounted, Wire rack, not further specified
Spice rack, Wall mounted, Wire rack, Single tier
Spice rack, Wall mounted, Wire rack, Two tier
Sponges, Assortment, not further specified
Sponges, Assortment, Round & square, not further specified
Spoon, see also, Kitchen spoon
Spork, Built-up handle, Angled for Left hand, not further specified
Spork, Built-up handle, Angled for Left hand, Plastic handle cover
Spork, Built-up handle, Angled for Left hand, Polypropylene handle
Spork, Built-up handle, Angled for Right hand, Collar on handle
Spork, Built-up handle, Angled for Right hand, not further specified
Spork, Built-up handle, Angled for Right hand, Polypropylene handle
Spork, Built-up handle, Standard bowl angle, not further specified
Spork, Built-up handle, Standard bowl angle, Ridged handle
Spork, Built-up handle, Swivel head no stops, Foam handle cover
Spork, Built-up handle, Swivel head no stops, not further specified
Spork, Built-up handle, Swivel head no stops, not further specified
Spork, Built-up handle, Swivel with stops, not further specified
Spork, Built-up handle, Swivel with stops, Oval handle
Spork, Built-up handle, Swivel with stops, Plastic oval handle
Spork, Built-up weighted, Angled for Left hand, 8 ounce weight
Spork, Built-up weighted, Angled for Left hand, not further specified
Spork, Built-up weighted, Angled for Right hand, 8 ounce weight
Spork, Built-up weighted, Angled for Right hand, not further specified
Spork, Built-up weighted, Standard bowl angle, 8 ounce weight
Spork, Built-up weighted, Standard bowl angle, not further specified
Spork, Standard handle, Large bowl standard angle, 7 inch
Spork, Standard handle, Large bowl standard angle, not further specified
Spork, Standard handle, not further specified
Spork, Standard handle, Oval bowl & swivel with stops, not further specified
Spork, Standard handle, Standard bowl angle, 5 inch
Spork, Standard handle, Standard bowl angle, 6 inch
Spork, Standard handle, Standard bowl angle, not further specified
Spork, Standard handle, Swivel, not further specified
Spork, Standard handle, Swivel with adjustable stops, not further specified
Sport grasping cuff, Holds bat/paddle/racquet, Adjustable strap, Leather and velcro
Sport grasping cuff, Holds bat/paddle/racquet, Adjustable strap, not further specified
Spray can aid, Dispenser handle, Adjustable trigger operated, Large handle
Spray can aid, Dispenser handle, Adjustable trigger operated, not further specified
Spray can aid, Dispenser handle, For shaving cream, Adjustable can clamp
Spray can aid, Dispenser handle, For shaving cream, not further specified
Spray can dispenser handle, Adjustable push-down lever, not further specified
Spray can dispenser handle, Adjustable trigger operated, not further specified
Spray can dispenser handle, not further specified
Stair lift, Can fit curved staircases, Can have landing, AC powered
Stair lift, Can fit curved staircases, Can have landing, not further specified
Stair lift, Can fit curved staircases, Can have landing, With safety surround arms
Stair lift, Fits straight staircases, Cannot have landing, AC powered
Stair lift, Fits straight staircases, Cannot have landing, not further specified
Stair lift, Fits straight staircases, Cannot have landing, With safety surround arms
Stair rail extender, Folds out from wall, Narrows the span between rails, Provides second rail
Stair treads, Rubber, 10-1/4 x 24 inches, not further specified
Stair treads, Rubber, 10-1/4 x 24 inches, Various colors
Stairway lights, Small lights for each step, Electrician installed, not further specified
Stairway lights, Small lights for each step, not further specified
Standing aid, see, Chair rising aid
Standing aid, Swinging grab frame, Attaches to chair or bed, Assists in rising
Standing aid, Swinging grab frame, Attaches to chair or bed, not further specified
Steering wheel knob, Clamp-on, not further specified
Steering wheel knob, Clamp-on, Spinner knob grip, Can clamp to straight handle
Step ladder, With left handrail, 3 step, Casters retract when weighted
Step ladder, With top hand rail, 3 step, Aluminum
Step ladder, With top hand rail, 3 step, not further specified

Step ladder, With top hand rail, 3 step, Wood
Step ladder, Without handrail, 3 step, Casters retract when weighted
Step lights, see, Stairway lights
Step lights, see, Stairway lights
Step stool, With top hand rail, One step, 9 inch
Step stool, With top hand rail, One step, not further specified
Stereo enhancer, see, TV sound enhancer, filters frequencies
Stool, 12 to 15 inches high, not further specified
Stool, 12 to 15 inches high, With locking casters, not further specified
Stool, 25 to 27 inches high, not further specified
Stool, 25 to 27 inches high, With locking casters, not further specified
Stool, Chair height, not further specified
Stool, Chair height, With casters, not further specified
Stool, Chair height, With locking casters, not further specified
Stool, No backrest, 30 inches high, not further specified
Stool, With adjustable backrest, 30 inches high, not further specified
Stove element heat sensor, For electric stove, Breaks current if extreme heat, Works with RangeTimer
Stove element timer, For electric stove, Set time interval, With heat-guard, can deactivate
Stove knob turner, For knob with a fin, Push-and-turn operation, not further specified
Stove knob turner, For knob with a fin, Push-and-turn operation, Provides large handle
Strainer, Attaches to cooking pot, Adjustable to pot size, not further specified
Strainer, Attaches to cooking pot, Adjustable to pot size, Steel & aluminum
Strap, Replacement, not further specified
Strap, Replacement, Velcro & D-ring closure, not further specified
Suction cup foot, Replacement, For cutting board, not further specified
Suction cup foot, Replacement, For cutting board, On #8 wood screw
Suction cup foot, Replacement, For plate, not further specified
Suction cup foot, Replacement, For tub transfer bench, not further specified
Suction cup foot, Replacement, not further specified
Suction disk, Double sided, Multi-cup general, 2-1/2 inch
Suction disk, Double sided, Multi-cup general, 3 inch
Suction disk, Double sided, Multi-cup general, not further specified
Suction disk, Double sided, not further specified
Suction disk, Double sided, Rotating, not further specified
Sunglasses, Bifocal non-prescription, not further specified
Sunglasses, Bifocal non-prescription, Powers are 1.25 & 3 diopters, not further specified
Sunglasses, Shield fits behind glasses, Amber, 22 % light transmission
Sunglasses, Shield fits behind glasses, Amber, not further specified
Sunglasses, Shield fits behind glasses, Gray/green, 1 % light transmission
Sunglasses, Shield fits behind glasses, Gray/green, 18 % light transmission
Sunglasses, Shield fits behind glasses, Gray/green, 40 % light transmission
Sunglasses, Shield fits behind glasses, Gray/green, not further specified
Sunglasses, Shield fits behind glasses, Medium amber, 10 % light transmission
Sunglasses, Shield fits behind glasses, Medium amber, not further specified
Sunglasses, Shield fits behind glasses, Ultraviolet blocking amber, 16 % light transmission
Sunglasses, Shield fits behind glasses, Ultraviolet blocking amber, not further specified
Sunglasses, Shield fits behind glasses, Ultraviolet blocking gray, 13 % light transmission
Sunglasses, Shield fits behind glasses, Ultraviolet blocking gray, 32 % light transmission
Sunglasses, Shield fits behind glasses, Ultraviolet blocking gray, 4 % light transmission
Sunglasses, Shield fits behind glasses, Ultraviolet blocking gray, not further specified
Sunglasses, Shield fits behind glasses, Ultraviolet blocking green, 7 % light transmission
Sunglasses, Shield fits behind glasses, Ultraviolet blocking green, not further specified
Sunglasses, Shield fits behind glasses, Ultraviolet blocking orange, 49 % light transmission
Sunglasses, Shield fits behind glasses, Ultraviolet blocking orange, not further specified
Sunglasses, Shield fits behind glasses, Ultraviolet blocking yellow, 65 % light transmission
Sunglasses, Shield fits behind glasses, Ultraviolet blocking yellow, not further specified
Swedish knife, see, Kitchen knife, 120 degree handle
Switch, For battery operated items, Actuated by hand pressure, With cord and plug
Switch, For battery operated items, Actuated by thumb pressure, With cord and plug
Switch cover, see, Wall switch cover
Swivel seat, see, Seat cushion, Swiveling
Syringe holder, With magnifier, Insulin, not further specified
Syringe holder, With magnifier, Insulin, One-piece
Syringe stabilizer, Suction cup base, Holds bottle & guides syringe, Vertical or horizontal mount

Tab & twist-cap opener, Two hands needed to operate, not further specified
Table, Adjustable height & angle, Spring balance frame, 18 x 12 inch
Table, Adjustable height & angle, Spring balance frame, not further specified
Table, Adjustable height & angle, Spring balance frame, Supports 30 pounds
Table knife, 90 degree handle, Rocker blade, not further specified
Table knife, 90 degree handle, Rocker blade, Plastic handle
Table knife, 90 degree handle, Straight blade, not further specified
Table knife, 90 degree handle, Straight blade, Plastic handle
Table knife, Blade only, For removable handle system, not further specified
Table knife, Blade only, not further specified

Teaspoon, Built-up handle, Soft plastic coated bowl, Oval bowl
Teaspoon, Built-up handle, Soft plastic coated bowl, Weighted
Teaspoon, Built-up handle, Standard bowl, 1 inch diameter foam handle
Teaspoon, Built-up handle, Standard bowl, 1 inch diameter vinyl handle
Teaspoon, Built-up handle, Standard bowl, 1-1/2 inch removable handle
Teaspoon, Built-up handle, Standard bowl, 1-1/2 inch vinyl handle
Teaspoon, Built-up handle, Standard bowl, 1-1/4 inch diameter handle
Teaspoon, Built-up handle, Standard bowl, 1-1/4 inch tapered foam handle
Teaspoon, Built-up handle, Standard bowl, 1-5/16 inch diameter handle
Teaspoon, Built-up handle, Standard bowl, Bendable handle
Teaspoon, Built-up handle, Standard bowl, Collar on oval handle
Teaspoon, Built-up handle, Standard bowl, Light weight handle
Teaspoon, Built-up handle, Standard bowl, not further specified
Teaspoon, Built-up handle, Standard bowl, not further specified
Teaspoon, Built-up handle, Standard bowl, Ridged handle
Teaspoon, Built-up handle, Standard bowl, Tapered upward curve
Teaspoon, Built-up handle, Standard bowl, Ultralight tapered foam handle
Teaspoon, Built-up handle, Standard bowl, Upward curved handle
Teaspoon, Built-up handle, Standard bowl, Weighted
Teaspoon, Built-up handle, Standard bowl, Weighted 7 ounces
Teaspoon, Built-up handle, Standard bowl, Weighted 8 ounces
Teaspoon, Built-up handle, Standard bowl, Weighted with finger ridges
Teaspoon, Built-up handle, Swivel head adjustable stops
Teaspoon, Built-up handle, Swivel head no stops
Teaspoon, Built-up handle, Swivel head no stops, not further specified
Teaspoon, Built-up handle, Swivel head no stops, not further specified
Teaspoon, Built-up handle, Swivel head no stops, Ridged handle
Teaspoon, Built-up handle, Swivel with stops, not further specified
Teaspoon, Built-up handle, Swivel with stops, Oval handle
Teaspoon, Built-up handle finger rings, Angled for Left hand, Adjustable finger rings
Teaspoon, Built-up handle finger rings, Angled for Left hand, not further specified
Teaspoon, Built-up handle finger rings, Standard bowl, Adjustable finger rings
Teaspoon, Built-up handle finger rings, Standard bowl, not further specified
Teaspoon, Built-up long handle, Standard bowl, Collar on handle
Teaspoon, Built-up long handle, Standard bowl, not further specified
Teaspoon, Built-up tube handle, Hard plastic coated bowl, 1 inch diameter handle
Teaspoon, Built-up tube handle, Hard plastic coated bowl, 1 inch diameter long handle
Teaspoon, Built-up tube handle, Hard plastic coated bowl, 1-1/2 inch diameter handle
Teaspoon, Built-up tube handle, Hard plastic coated bowl, 1-1/4 inch diameter handle
Teaspoon, Built-up tube handle, Hard plastic coated bowl, not further specified
Teaspoon, Built-up tube handle, not further specified
Teaspoon, Built-up tube handle, Soft plastic coated bowl, 1 inch diameter handle
Teaspoon, Built-up tube handle, Soft plastic coated bowl, 1 inch diameter long handle
Teaspoon, Built-up tube handle, Soft plastic coated bowl, 1-1/2 inch diameter handle
Teaspoon, Built-up tube handle, Soft plastic coated bowl, 1-1/4 inch diameter handle
Teaspoon, Built-up tube handle, Soft plastic coated bowl, not further specified
Teaspoon, Built-up tube handle, Standard bowl
Teaspoon, Built-up tube handle, Standard bowl, 1-3/8 inch diameter handle
Teaspoon, Built-up tube handle, Standard bowl, not further specified
Teaspoon, Curved handle, Curved for Left hand
Teaspoon, Curved handle, Curved for Right hand
Teaspoon, Curved handle, not further specified
Teaspoon, Curved handle, Shallow bowl, For Left hand
Teaspoon, Curved handle, Shallow bowl, For Right hand
Teaspoon, Curved handle, Shallow bowl, not further specified
Teaspoon, Cut to shape, All nylon
Teaspoon, Cut to shape, not further specified
Teaspoon, Handle separable from head, Interchangeable heads
Teaspoon, Handle separable from head, not further specified
Teaspoon, Large, not further specified
Teaspoon, Large, Shallow bowl
Teaspoon, Long handle, Hard plastic coated bowl, not further specified
Teaspoon, Long handle, not further specified
Teaspoon, Long handle, Soft plastic coated bowl
Teaspoon, Long handle 10 inches, Adjustable angle
Teaspoon, Long handle 10 inches, not further specified
Teaspoon, Long handle 15 inches, Adjustable angle
Teaspoon, Long handle 15 inches, not further specified
Teaspoon, Moldable handle, not further specified
Teaspoon, Moldable handle, Standard bowl
Teaspoon, On horizontal palm clip, Hard plastic coated bowl, Adjustable clip
Teaspoon, On horizontal palm clip, Hard plastic coated bowl, Long adjustable clip
Teaspoon, On horizontal palm clip, Hard plastic coated bowl, not further specified
Teaspoon, On horizontal palm clip, Soft plastic coated bowl, Adjustable clip
Teaspoon, On horizontal palm clip, Soft plastic coated bowl, Long adjustable clip
Teaspoon, On horizontal palm clip, Soft plastic coated bowl, not further specified
Teaspoon, On horizontal palm clip, Standard bowl, Adjustable clip

Tumbler holder/handle, Hook handle, Adjustable diameter, not further specified
Tumbler holder/handle, Hook handle, Adjustable diameter, Thumb screw attached
Tumbler holder/handle, Hook handle, Fixed diameter, Non-skid feet
Tumbler holder/handle, Hook handle, Fixed diameter, not further specified
Tumbler with lid, No handle, Lid, Can be cut for nose
Tumbler with lid, No handle, Lid, not further specified
Tumbler with nose cut-out, No handle, No lid, 12 ounce capacity
Tumbler with nose cut-out, No handle, No lid, 4 ounce capacity
Tumbler with nose cut-out, No handle, No lid, 6 ounce capacity
Tumbler with nose cut-out, No handle, No lid, 8 ounce capacity
Tumbler with nose cut-out, No handle, No lid, not further specified
Tumbler with nose cut-out, No handle, No lid, Shatter resistant
Tumbler with vacuum control, No handle, Lid with hole, Flow control lid
Tumbler with vacuum control, No handle, Lid with hole, not further specified
Tumbler with vacuum control, No handle, Lid with spout, Flow control lid
Tumbler with vacuum control, No handle, Lid with spout, not further specified
Tumbler with vacuum control, No handle, Lid with spout, Uses separate base
Tumbler with wide base, No handle, No lid, Goblet-style
Tumbler with wide base, No handle, No lid, not further specified
TV and appliance turntable, 360 degree turning radius, Capacity up to 125 pounds, not further specified
TV and appliance turntable, 360 degree turning radius, Capacity up to 250 pounds, not further specified
TV and appliance turntable, 360 degree turning radius, Capacity up to 50 pounds, not further specified
TV and appliance turntable, 360 degree turning radius, Capacity up to 80 pounds, not further specified
TV magnifier, Fits 17-19 inch screens, Enlarges to 25 inch, Free standing frame
TV magnifier, Fits 17-19 inch screens, Enlarges to 25 inch, not further specified
TV magnifier, Fits 19-26 inch screens, Enlarges to 30 inch, Free standing frame
TV magnifier, Fits 19-26 inch screens, Enlarges to 30 inch, not further specified
TV magnifier, Projection type, For 13 inch TV, not further specified
TV magnifier, Projection type, For 13 inch TV, Sits atop control panel
TV magnifier, Projection type, For 19 inch TV, not further specified
TV magnifier, Projection type, For 19 inch TV, Sits atop control panel
TV sound enhancer, Filters frequencies, Cordless headset, Controls in headset
TV sound enhancer, Filters frequencies, Cordless headset, not further specified
TV/stereo headphones, Infrared transmitter, For independent volume control, AC powered
TV/stereo headphones, Infrared transmitter, For independent volume control, not further specified
TV/stereo headphones, Transmitter, Headset receiver, Battery powered
TV/stereo headphones, Transmitter, Headset receiver, not further specified
Tweezers, 10-inch, not further specified
Tweezers, With magnifying lens, not further specified
Twist-cap opener, Hand held, Fit cap to 1 inch
Twist-cap opener, Hand held, not further specified
Typing aid, Hand-held stick, Adjustable loop either hand, not further specified
Typing aid, Hand-held stick, Adjustable loop either hand, Plastic tip
Typing aid, Lever key-lockdown, Allows multiple key use, Adheres to keyboard
Typing aid, Lever key-lockdown, Allows multiple key use, not further specified
Typing aid, Mouth stick, Large small & curved tips
Typing aid, Stick on palmar cuff, For Left hand, Heat-moldable cuff
Typing aid, Stick on palmar cuff, For Left hand, not further specified
Typing aid, Stick on palmar cuff, For Right hand, Heat-moldable cuff
Typing aid, Stick on palmar cuff, For Right hand, not further specified
Typing aid, Stick on palmar loop, For Left hand, not further specified
Typing aid, Stick on palmar loop, For Left hand, Velcro adjustable hand loop
Typing aid, Stick on palmar loop, For Right hand, not further specified
Typing aid, Stick on palmar loop, For Right hand, Velcro adjustable hand loop

---

Ulu, see, Table/kitchen knife, top palmar handle
Umbrella, One-hand operated, Push button, Curved handle
Umbrella, One-hand operated, Push button, not further specified
Umbrella, Wheelchair clamp-on, 50 inch diameter
Umbrella, Wheelchair clamp-on, not further specified
Undershirt, Women's, Sleeveless, Cotton rib knit
Undershirt, Women's, Sleeveless, not further specified
Universal cuff, For broom or similar handle, With rod shaped holder, not further specified
Universal cuff, For broom or similar handle, With rod shaped holder, Replaces grasp
Universal cuff, For either hand, Horizontal pocket, Metal finger loops
Universal cuff, For either hand, Horizontal pocket, not further specified
Universal cuff, For either hand, Leather utensil pocket, Elastic band
Universal cuff, For either hand, Leather utensil pocket, not further specified
Universal cuff, For either hand, not further specified
Universal cuff, For either hand, Palmar block with pocket, D-ring velcro close
Universal cuff, For either hand, Palmar cuff 2 pocket
Universal cuff, For either hand, Palmar cuff 2 pocket, Heat-moldable clip

Universal cuff, For either hand, Palmar cuff 2 pocket, not further specified
Universal cuff, For either hand, Palmar cuff 2 pocket, Rotatable pocket
Universal cuff, For either hand, Palmar cuff w pocket, D-ring velcro close
Universal cuff, For either hand, Palmar cuff w pocket, not further specified
Universal cuff, For either hand, Palmar cuff with pocket, Elastic band
Universal cuff, For either hand, Palmar cuff with pocket, Heat-moldable clip
Universal cuff, For either hand, Palmar cuff with pocket, not further specified
Universal cuff, For either hand, Palmar cuff with pocket, Rotatable pocket
Universal cuff, For either hand, Palmar cuff with pocket, Wide pocket
Universal cuff, For either hand, Single pocket, Cotton fabric
Universal cuff, For either hand, Single pocket, not further specified
Universal cuff, For either hand, Vertical pocket, Metal finger loops
Universal cuff, For either hand, Vertical pocket, not further specified
Universal cuff, For either hand, With wrist support, Kit for fabrication
Universal cuff, For either hand, With wrist support, not further specified
Universal cuff, For either hand, With wrist support, Velcro closure
Universal cuff, For Left hand, Palmar cuff with pocket, Heat-moldable clip
Universal cuff, For Left hand, Palmar cuff with pocket, not further specified
Universal cuff, For Left hand, With wrist support, Holds thumb opposed
Universal cuff, For Left hand, With wrist support, not further specified
Universal cuff, For Left hand, With wrist support, Velcro closure
Universal cuff, For Right hand, With wrist support, Adjustable pocket
Universal cuff, For Right hand, With wrist support, Holds thumb opposed
Universal cuff, For Right hand, With wrist support, Moldable palm clip
Universal cuff, For Right hand, With wrist support, not further specified
Universal cuff, For Right hand, With wrist support, Velcro closure
Universal turner, see, Knob turner, spring loaded pins
Upholstered chair, Upholstered seat & back, Arms extend to front seat edge
Upholstered chair, Upholstered seat & back, not further specified
Urinal, Female, Bottle type, not further specified
Urinal, Female, Bottle type, Plastic
Urinal, Female, External catheter, not further specified
Urinal, Female, External catheter, Uses disposable bags
Urinal, Female, For wheelchair use
Urinal, Female, not further specified
Urinal, Female, Spill-proof, Handle allows hanging
Urinal, Female, Spill-proof, not further specified
Urinal, Female, Use in seated position, 600 cc capacity
Urinal, Female, Use in seated position, not further specified
Urinal, Female, Use in seated position, Volume-measuring end
Urinal, Male, Bottle type, not further specified
Urinal, Male, Bottle type, Spill-proof
Urinal, Male, For wheelchair use
Urinal, Male, not further specified
Urinal, Male, Spill-proof, Handle allows hanging
Urinal, Male, Spill-proof, not further specified
Urinal, Male, Use in seated position, not further specified
Urinal, Male, Use in seated position, Volume-measuring end
Urinal, Male sheath, Bag straps to leg, Non-return valve
Urinal, Male sheath, Bag straps to leg, not further specified
Urinal, Unisex, For wheelchair use
Urinal, Unisex, not further specified
Urinal, Unisex, With female adapter, not further specified
Urinal, Unisex, With female adapter, Plastic bottle
Urinal bag, Replacement, For Sheath urinal, not further specified
Urinal bag, Replacement, For Sheath urinal, With male sheath
Utensil grip, Palmar ball, Oval grip with palm clip, Fits handle of eating utensil
Utensil grip, Palmar ball, Oval grip with palm clip, not further specified
Utensil handle, Built-up handle, Leather pocket, Fits handle of eating utensil
Utensil handle, Built-up handle, Leather pocket, not further specified
Utensil handle, For any utensil, Soft triangular, Fits handle of eating utensil
Utensil handle, For any utensil, Soft triangular, not further specified
Utensil handle, For demountable-head system, Oval grip, For interchangeable heads
Utensil handle, For demountable-head system, Round grip, For interchangeable heads
Utensil handle, For removable handle system, Oval grip, not further specified
Utensil handle, For removable handle system, Round grip, not further specified
Utensil handle strap, For demountable-head system
Utensil handle strap, not further specified
Utensil holder, For either hand, Palmar cuff with pocket, Cotton fabric
Utensil holder, For either hand, Palmar cuff with pocket, not further specified
Utensil holder, For either hand, Palmar cuff with pocket, not further specified
Utensil holder, For either hand, Palmar cuff with pocket, Velcro closure
Utensil holder, On palmar cuff, Bendable clip, not further specified
Utensil holder, On palmar cuff, Bendable clip, Velcro closure
Utensil holder, Palm & thumb loops, With pocket, not further specified
Utensil holder, Palm & thumb loops, With pocket, Velcro closure
Utensil holder, Palmar block, With pocket, not further specified
Utensil holder, Palmar block, With pocket, Velcro closure
Utensil holder, Palmar block with finger loops, Horizontal pocket
Utensil holder, Palmar clip, Utensil held by spring clip, not further specified
Utensil holder, Palmar clip, Utensil held by spring clip, Plastic
Utensil holder, Palmar cuff, With pocket, not further specified
Utensil holder, Palmar cuff, With pocket, Velcro closure

Utensil holder, Palmar cuff & loop, Pocket, not further specified
Utensil holder, Palmar cuff & loop, Pocket, Velcro closure
Utensil holder, Palmar pocket, Washable fabric, not further specified
Utensil holder, Palmar pocket, Washable fabric, Velcro closure
Utensil holder, Plastic hand loop, not further specified
Utensil holder, Plastic hand loop, With pocket
Utensil pocket, For universal cuff, not further specified
Utensil pocket, For universal cuff, Single pocket, not further specified
Utensil pocket, For universal cuff, Single pocket, Right angle pocket
Utensil pocket, For universal cuff, Two pockets
Utensil pocket, For universal cuff, Two pockets, Fits wide utensils
Utensil pocket, For universal cuff, Two pockets, not further specified
Utensil pocket, For universal cuff, Two pockets, Right angle pocket
Utensil/pen holder, Palmar ball 3 inches, Spherical grip, Hold any similar implement
Utensil/pen holder, Palmar ball 3 inches, Spherical grip, not further specified
Utility cart, 4 inch casters, 3 shelves, Light duty
Utility cart, 4 inch rubber tread casters, Metal posts & plastic shelves, 150 pound capacity per shelf
Utility cart, Rolling/folding, 30 inches high, Folds for storage
Utility cart, Rolling/folding, 30 inches high, not further specified
Utility cart, Rolling/folding, Accepts 2 baskets, Folds for storage
Utility cart, Rolling/folding, Accepts 2 baskets, not further specified
Utility cart, Rolling/folding, Large casters, Folds for storage
Utility cart, Rolling/folding, Large casters, not further specified
Utility cart & desk, Rolling/folding, 27 inches high, Bottom tray folds
Utility cart & desk, Rolling/folding, 27 inches high, not further specified

---

Vacuum cleaner, Canister, Portable, not further specified
Vacuum cleaner, Canister, Portable, With shoulder strap
Vacuum cleaner, Electric broom, Rug/floor nozzle, Hand carry
Vacuum cleaner, Electric broom, Rug/floor nozzle, not further specified
Vacuum cleaner, Upright, Top fill bag, Edge cleaner
Vacuum cleaner, Upright, Top fill bag, not further specified
Vacuum cleaner system, Central canister, Wall model/built-in, not further specified
Vacuum cleaner system, Central canister, Wall model/built-in, Professional install
Vacuum cup button, For lid with flow control, For vacuum control cup, not further specified
Vacuum cup button, For lid with flow control, For vacuum control cup, Valve button only
Vacuum cup lid, Replacement, For vacuum control cup
Vacuum cup lid, Replacement, not further specified
Vegetable brush, One-hand operated, Suction cup base, Kitchen/bathroom use
Vegetable brush, One-hand operated, Suction cup base, not further specified
Vegetable peeler, Hand held, D-handle, not further specified
Vegetable peeler, Hand held, Long loop handle, not further specified
Vegetable peeler, Hand held, Manual, Cushion grip handle
Vegetable peeler, Hand held, not further specified
Vegetable peeler, One-hand operated, Manual, Clamps to counter
Vegetable peeler, One-hand operated, Manual, not further specified
Vegetable peeler, One-hand operated, Manual, Suction mounted
Vegetable peeler, Vibrating blade, Electric/portable, Hand held
Vegetable peeler, Vibrating blade, Electric/portable, Sets on table
Vegetable peeler and brush, Hand held, Long handle, not further specified
Venetian blind brush, For vacuum cleaner, 5 brushes, Fits standard hoses
Venetian blind brush, For vacuum cleaner, 5 brushes, not further specified
Vent extension, Heating, Adjust length to 36 inches, Directs heated air
Vent extension, Heating, Adjust length to 36 inches, not further specified
Vest, Sleeveless, Long arm opening, not further specified
Vest, Sleeveless, Long arm opening, Short back
Videotape rack, Over-door mount, 6-shelf vinyl coated, Holds 78 VHS tapes
Videotape rack, Over-door mount, 6-shelf vinyl coated, not further specified

---

Walker, Four wheels, With hand brake, not further specified
Walker, Four wheels, With hand brake, With seat
Walker, Four wheels, With hand brake, With tray
Walker, No wheels but rubber feet, Folding, With seat
Walker, No wheels but rubber feet, Folding, With tray
Walker, No wheels but rubber feet, not further specified
Walker, not further specified
Walker, With 2 wheels, With hand brake, not further specified
Walker, With 2 wheels, With hand brake, With seat
Walker, With 2 wheels, With hand brake, With tray
Walker, With two wheels, No hand brake, not further specified
Walker bag, Front pouch, 13 X 11 inches, not further specified
Walker bag, Front pouch, 13 X 11 inches, Velcro over crossbar
Walker bag, Front pouch, 2 large & 2 small pouches, not further specified
Walker bag, Front pouch, 2 large & 2 small pouches, Sling over crossbar
Walker bag, Front pouch, Double sided, not further specified
Walker bag, Front pouch, Double sided, Velcro over crossbar
Walker bag, Front pouch, Large with zipper, not further specified
Walker bag, Front pouch, Large with zipper, Velcro over crossbar
Walker bag, Front pouch, Separate pockets, not further specified
Walker bag, Front pouch, Separate pockets, Velcro over crossbar
Walker bag, Front pouch, Single pocket, not further specified

Walker bag, Front pouch, Single pocket, Velcro over crossbar
Walker bag, Front pouch, Spring frame holds it open, Attaches with straps
Walker bag, Front pouch, Spring frame holds it open, not further specified
Walker bag, Front pouch, Velcro closure, not further specified
Walker bag, Front pouch, Velcro closure, Velcro over crossbar
Walker bag, Front/side pouch, 12 x 10 x 4 inches, Fold-over flap
Walker bag, see also, Wheelchair/walker bag
Walker bag, Side pouch, Single pocket, not further specified
Walker bag, Side pouch, Single pocket, Velcro over top bar
Walker bag, Wraps around top, 4 pockets, Attaches with velcro
Walker bag, Wraps around top, 4 pockets, not further specified
Walker basket, Wire, 13 X 7-14 X 8-1/2 inches, Folds flat
Walker basket, Wire, 18 X 7 X 7 inches, not further specified
Walker basket, Wire, 18 X 7 X 7 inches, Wire bend to attach
Walker basket, Wire, With cup-holder tray, Attaches to front
Walker basket, Wire, With cup-holder tray, not further specified
Walker basket liner, Clear acrylic, See-through, Fits into basket
Walker basket liner, Clear acrylic, See-through, not further specified
Walker caddy, see, Walker carrying box
Walker carrying box, Solid walls and floor, With compartments, not further specified
Walker carrying box, Solid walls and floor, With compartments, Ring holder for beverage can
Walker carrying box adapter, Attaches box to crutch
Walker carrying box adapter, Attaches box to walker frame
Walker carrying box adapter, not further specified
Walker handgrips, Imitation lamb's-wool, Attaches with velcro, not further specified
Walker handgrips, Imitation lamb's-wool, Attaches with velcro, Washable
Walker handgrips, Terry-covered foam, Attaches with velcro, not further specified
Walker handgrips, Terry-covered foam, Attaches with velcro, Washable
Walker pouch, see, Walker bag
Walker seat, Denim sling, Folds aside, not further specified
Walker seat, Denim sling, Folds aside, Supports 250 pounds
Walker standing-assist handle, Clamps to walker frame, Rests on chair for support, Folds against walker
Walker tray, Attaches to crossbar, not further specified
Walker tray, Clips into place, Wells for plate & cup, not further specified
Walker tray, Sectional, Folds down, not further specified
Walker tray, Sectional, Folds down, Rimmed edge
Walker tray, Snaps into place, Spring clips above crossbar, Flat
Walker tray, Snaps into place, Spring clips above crossbar, not further specified
Walker tray, With 2 cup wells, Flips forward to store, not further specified
Walker tray, With cup & utensil holder, Slides away forward, not further specified
Walker tray, With cup & utensil holder, Slides away forward, With non-skid mat
Walker tray, With side pouches, Folds down, not further specified
Walker tray, With side pouches, Folds down, Rigid plastic
Walker tray straps, Replacement, For attachment of some trays
Walker tray straps, Replacement, not further specified
Wall clock, Large face & hands, Black on white, AC powered
Wall clock, Large face & hands, Black on white, Battery powered
Wall clock, Large face & hands, Black on white, not further specified
Wall switch, Large rocker, Replacement, not further specified
Wall switch, Large rocker, Replacement, Owner or professional install
Wall switch, Toggle, Replacement, not further specified
Wall switch, Toggle, Replacement, Owner or professional install
Wall switch cover, 1 switch 2 outlets, Porcelain, Cover only
Wall switch cover, 1 switch 2 outlets, Porcelain, not further specified
Wall switch cover, Double light switch, not further specified
Wall switch cover, Double light switch, Porcelain
Wall switch cover, Double outlet, not further specified
Wall switch cover, Double outlet, Porcelain
Wall switch cover, For rocker switch, not further specified
Wall switch cover, For rocker switch, Porcelain
Wall switch cover, Single light switch, not further specified
Wall switch cover, Single light switch, Porcelain
Wall switch cover, Triple light switch, not further specified
Wall switch cover, Triple light switch, Porcelain
Wall switch dropper, see, Light switch dropper
Wall switch guard, Prevents shut-off, Snaps open for use, Fits over switch
Wall switch guard, Prevents shut-off, Snaps open for use, not further specified
Washcloth, Disposable
Washcloth, not further specified
Watch, Ladies' wrist large LCD, For low vision, not further specified
Watch, Ladies' wrist large LCD, For low vision, Water resistant
Watch, Ladies' wrist with hands, For low vision, not further specified
Watch, Ladies' wrist with hands, For low vision, Water resistant
Watch, Men's wrist with hands, For low vision, Large print white on black
Watch, Men's wrist with hands, For low vision, not further specified
Watch, Men's wrist with hands, For low vision, Water resistant
Watch, Men's wrist with hands, For low vision, With large second hand
Watch, Talking digital, Voice gives time, English
Watch, Talking digital, Voice gives time, English & Spanish
Watch, Talking digital, Voice gives time, not further specified
Watch, Unisex wrist with hands, Low vision, Large numbers
Watch, Unisex wrist with hands, Low vision, not further specified
Water heater, Point-of-use, Limits water temperature, not further specified

Wheelchair cup holder, For standard arm, Fixed diameter, not further specified
Wheelchair cup holder, For standard arm, Fixed diameter, With non-spill cup
Wheelchair cushion, For arms, Desk length
Wheelchair cushion, For arms, not further specified
Wheelchair cushion, For arms, Standard length
Wheelchair cushion, For back, Built-forward sides, For lateral support
Wheelchair cushion, For back, Built-forward sides, not further specified
Wheelchair cushion, For back, With sections for cut-out, not further specified
Wheelchair cushion, For back, With sections for cut-out, To be individually fitted
Wheelchair cushion, For seat, 1 inch latex foam, not further specified
Wheelchair cushion, For seat, 1 inch latex foam, Vinyl covered
Wheelchair cushion, For seat, 1 inch water & gel, Adjustable density
Wheelchair cushion, For seat, 1 inch water & gel, not further specified
Wheelchair cushion, For seat, 2 inch latex foam, not further specified
Wheelchair cushion, For seat, 2 inch latex foam, Removable cover
Wheelchair cushion, For seat, 3 inch latex foam, not further specified
Wheelchair cushion, For seat, 3 inch latex foam, Removable cover
Wheelchair cushion, For seat, 4 inch latex foam, not further specified
Wheelchair cushion, For seat, 4 inch latex foam, Removable cover
Wheelchair cushion, For seat, Extended for left thigh, For BKA amputee
Wheelchair cushion, For seat, Extended for left thigh, not further specified
Wheelchair cushion, For seat, Extended for right thigh, For BKA amputee
Wheelchair cushion, For seat, Extended for right thigh, not further specified
Wheelchair cushion, For seat, not further specified
Wheelchair cushion, For seat, With coccyx cut-out
Wheelchair cushion, For seat, With ischial cut-out
Wheelchair cushion, For seat/back/arms, Fiber pad, Cotton/latex
Wheelchair cushion, For seat/back/arms, Fiber pad, not further specified
Wheelchair cushion, For side and arm padding, Folds over arms, Does not require seat cushion
Wheelchair cushion, For side and arm padding, Folds over arms, not further specified
Wheelchair cushion, For sides, Extends above arms, For use with seat cushion
Wheelchair cushion, For sides, Extends above arms, not further specified
Wheelchair cushion, For sides, Extends up to arms, For use with seat cushion
Wheelchair cushion, For sides, Extends up to arms, not further specified
Wheelchair elevator, Closet type, Cable mount, 700 pound test
Wheelchair elevator, see, Elevator, For wheelchair
Wheelchair elevator, Wall mounted, Platform style, 250 pound capacity
Wheelchair elevator, Wall mounted, Platform style, 500 pound capacity
Wheelchair elevator, Wall mounted, Platform style, not further specified
Wheelchair footrest cushion, Non-slip surface, not further specified
Wheelchair gloves fingerless, Gel-backed palm, Closed back cowhide, Fitted slip-on
Wheelchair gloves fingerless, Gel-backed palm, Closed back cowhide, not further specified
Wheelchair gloves fingerless, High-tack soft plastic palm, Closed back cowhide, D-ring velcro closure
Wheelchair gloves fingerless, High-tack soft plastic palm, Closed back cowhide, not further specified
Wheelchair gloves fingerless, Padded leather palm, Mesh backed goatskin, Fitted slip-on
Wheelchair gloves fingerless, Padded leather palm, Mesh backed goatskin, not further specified
Wheelchair gloves fingerless, Padded palm with thumb cover, Closed back cowhide, D-ring velcro closure
Wheelchair gloves fingerless, Padded palm with thumb cover, Closed back cowhide, not further specified
Wheelchair gloves fingerless, Smooth leather palm, Mesh backed goatskin, Fitted slip-on
Wheelchair gloves fingerless, Smooth leather palm, Mesh backed goatskin, not further specified
Wheelchair gloves fingerless, Suede leather palm, Closed back, D-ring strap closure
Wheelchair gloves fingerless, Suede leather palm, Closed back, not further specified
Wheelchair gloves with fingers, High-tack soft plastic palm, Closed back cowhide, D-ring velcro closure
Wheelchair gloves with fingers, High-tack soft plastic palm, Closed back cowhide, not further specified
Wheelchair gloves with fingers, Padded leather palm, Closed back cowhide, D-ring velcro closure
Wheelchair gloves with fingers, Padded leather palm, Closed back cowhide, not further specified
Wheelchair gloves with fingers, Smooth leather palm, Closed back cowhide, Fitted slip-on
Wheelchair gloves with fingers, Smooth leather palm, Closed back cowhide, not further specified
Wheelchair gloves with fingers, Suede leather palm, Closed back cowhide, Fitted slip-on
Wheelchair gloves with fingers, Suede leather palm, Closed back cowhide, not further specified
Wheelchair lap tray, see, Wheelchair tray
Wheelchair lift, For car rear end, Lifts folded chair, Car battery powered
Wheelchair lifter, For car trunk, Lifts & turns horizontally, Car battery powered
Wheelchair lifter, For van or mini-van, Lifts vertically, Car battery powered
Wheelchair ramp, Portable tracks, 28 w x 36 long, Fiberglas
Wheelchair ramp, Portable tracks, 28 w x 36 long, not further specified
Wheelchair ramp, Portable tracks, 28 w x 60 long, Fiberglas
Wheelchair ramp, Portable tracks, 28 w x 60 long, not further specified
Wheelchair ramp, Portable tracks, 28 wide x 48 long, Fiberglas
Wheelchair ramp, Portable tracks, 28 wide x 48 long, not further specified

Wheelchair ramp, Portable tracks, 30 w x 72 long, Holds 700 pounds
Wheelchair ramp, Portable tracks, 30 w x 72 long, not further specified
Wheelchair ramp, Portable tracks, 30 w x 84 long, Holds 700 pounds
Wheelchair ramp, Portable tracks, 30 w x 84 long, not further specified
Wheelchair ramp, Portable tracks, 30w x 48 long, Aluminum
Wheelchair ramp, Portable tracks, 30w x 60 long, Holds 600 pounds
Wheelchair ramp, Portable tracks, 36 inches, Holds 600 pounds
Wheelchair ramp, Portable tracks, 36 inches, not further specified
Wheelchair ramp, Portable tracks, Folds to 5 feet, not further specified
Wheelchair ramp, Portable tracks, Folds to 5 feet, Weighs 7 pounds
Wheelchair ramp, Portable tracks, Telescopes from 120 to 75 inch, Holds 300 pounds
Wheelchair ramp, Portable tracks, Telescopes from 120 to 75 inch, not further specified
Wheelchair ramp, Portable tracks, Telescopes from 60 to 28 inch, Holds 340 pounds
Wheelchair ramp, Portable tracks, Telescopes from 60 to 28 inch, Holds 600 pounds
Wheelchair ramp, Portable tracks, Telescopes from 60 to 28 inch, not further specified
Wheelchair ramp, Portable tracks, Telescopes from 64 to 24 inch, Holds 340 pounds
Wheelchair ramp, Portable tracks, Telescopes from 64 to 24 inch, not further specified
Wheelchair ramp, Portable tracks, Telescopes from 64 to 26 inch, Holds 350 pounds
Wheelchair ramp, Portable tracks, Telescopes from 64 to 26 inch, not further specified
Wheelchair ramp, Portable tracks, Telescopes from 72 to 45 inch, Holds 300 pounds
Wheelchair ramp, Portable tracks, Telescopes from 72 to 45 inch, not further specified
Wheelchair ramp, Portable tracks, Telescopes from 96 inches, Holds 340 pounds
Wheelchair ramp, Portable tracks, Telescopes from 96 inches, not further specified
Wheelchair seat, see, Wheelchair board
Wheelchair shelf, Under seat, 12 x 10 x 4-1/2 inches, not further specified
Wheelchair shelf, Under seat, 12 x 10 x 4-1/2 inches, Velcro straps attach
Wheelchair table, Rolling, 20 x 40 inch top, not further specified
Wheelchair table, Rolling, 20 x 40 inch top, White laminate
Wheelchair table, Rolling with brakes, 48 inches W x 30D x 35H inches, Metal frame
Wheelchair table, Rolling with brakes, Height adjusts 30 to 35 inches, Metal frame
Wheelchair tray, Bracket for padded left arm, Folds aside, Half tray
Wheelchair tray, Bracket for padded left arm, Folds aside, not further specified
Wheelchair tray, Bracket for padded right arm, Flips upward, Half tray
Wheelchair tray, Bracket for padded right arm, Flips upward, not further specified
Wheelchair tray, Clamps to padded right arm, Slides on, Half tray
Wheelchair tray, Clamps to padded right arm, Slides on, not further specified
Wheelchair tray, For desk arm, Adjustable height, Arm bracket
Wheelchair tray, For desk arm, Adjustable height, not further specified
Wheelchair tray, For left regular arm, Full tray, not further specified
Wheelchair tray, For left regular arm, Full tray, Slides away
Wheelchair tray, For regular arm, Arm rest protectors, D-ring velcro straps
Wheelchair tray, For regular arm, Arm rest protectors, not further specified
Wheelchair tray, For regular arm, Clear, D-ring velcro straps
Wheelchair tray, For regular arm, Clear, not further specified
Wheelchair tray, For regular arm, Clear plastic, D-ring velcro straps
Wheelchair tray, For regular arm, Clear plastic, Elastic fastening
Wheelchair tray, For regular arm, Clear plastic, not further specified
Wheelchair tray, For regular arm, Clear plastic, Velcro attachment
Wheelchair tray, For regular arm, Formica, D-ring velcro straps
Wheelchair tray, For regular arm, Formica, not further specified
Wheelchair tray, For regular arm, Hinged clear overlay, not further specified
Wheelchair tray, For regular arm, Hinged clear overlay, Velcro attachment
Wheelchair tray, For regular arm, Masonite, D-ring velcro straps
Wheelchair tray, For regular arm, Masonite, Elastic fastening
Wheelchair tray, For regular arm, Masonite, Long straps
Wheelchair tray, For regular arm, Masonite, not further specified
Wheelchair tray, For regular arm, Masonite, Velcro strap attach
Wheelchair tray, For regular arm, Plastic rimmed, D-ring velcro straps
Wheelchair tray, For regular arm, Plastic rimmed, not further specified
Wheelchair tray, For regular arm, Plastic rimmed, Velcro straps
Wheelchair tray, For regular arm, Slide-on, not further specified
Wheelchair tray, For regular arm, Slide-on, With velcro attached base
Wheelchair tray, For regular arm, Vinyl top masonite, D-ring velcro straps
Wheelchair tray, For regular arm, Vinyl top masonite, not further specified
Wheelchair tray, For regular arm, With non-skid arm pads, D-ring velcro straps
Wheelchair tray, For regular arm, With non-skid arm pads, not further specified
Wheelchair tray, For regular arm, With non-skid arm pads, Velcro attach
Wheelchair tray, For regular arm, Woodgrain formica, D-ring velcro straps
Wheelchair tray, For regular arm, Woodgrain formica, not further specified
Wheelchair tray, For right or left arm, Half tray, not further specified
Wheelchair tray, For right or left arm, Half tray, With elbow support
Wheelchair tray, Full tray, Clear, Velcro straps to armrests
Wheelchair tray, Full tray, Melamine impregnated, Velcro straps to armrests

Wire rack basket, For drawer frame, Single depth, Vinyl coated wire
Wire rack basket, For drawer frame, Triple depth, not further specified
Wire rack basket, For drawer frame, Triple depth, Vinyl coated wire
Wire rack basket, In-cabinet base, Sliding, 1 basket removable
Wire rack basket, In-cabinet base, Sliding, not further specified
Wire rack basket, In-cabinet mount, not further specified
Wire rack basket, In-cabinet mount, Sliding 14 inches wide, not further specified
Wire rack basket, In-cabinet mount, Sliding 20 inches wide, not further specified
Wire rack basket, Under-cabinet mount, Sliding, 2 removable baskets
Wire rack basket, Under-cabinet mount, Sliding, Half basket on top
Wire rack basket, Under-cabinet mount, Sliding, not further specified
Wire rack basket, Under-cabinet mount, Sliding, not further specified
Wire rack basket, Under-cabinet mount, Sliding, Removable
Wire rack basket, Under-sink mount, Sliding, 2 removable baskets
Wire rack basket, Under-sink mount, Sliding, Half basket on top
Wire rack basket, Under-sink mount, Sliding, not further specified
Wire rack basket, Under-sink mount, Sliding, not further specified
Wire rack drawer top, For wire rack drawer, not further specified
Wire rack drawer top, For wire rack drawer, White laminate surface, not further specified
Wire rack hooks, Over-door, Multiple double hooks, For clothes and similar
Wire rack hooks, Over-door, Multiple double hooks, not further specified
Wire rack hooks, Wall-mounted, 4 double hooks, For clothes and similar
Wire rack hooks, Wall-mounted, 4 double hooks, not further specified
Wire rack shelf, Cabinet door mounted, 4 adjustable shelves, For inside kitchen cabinet
Wire rack shelf, Cabinet door mounted, 4 adjustable shelves, not further specified
Wire rack shelf, Door-mounted, Four 18 x 34 inch, not further specified
Wire rack shelf, Door-mounted, Four 18 x 34 inch, Vinyl coated steel
Wire rack shelf, Door-mounted, Three 12 x 17 inch, not further specified
Wire rack shelf, Door-mounted, Three 12 x 17 inch, Vinyl coated steel
Wire rack shelf, Door-mounted, Three 18 x 17 inch, not further specified
Wire rack shelf, Door-mounted, Three 18 x 17 inch, Vinyl coated steel
Wire rack shelf, Door-mounted, Two 12 x 10 inch, not further specified
Wire rack shelf, Door-mounted, Two 12 x 10 inch, Vinyl coated steel
Wire rack shelf, Free standing, Expands from 14 to 27 inches, 3 tier
Wire rack shelf, Free standing, Expands from 14 to 27 inches, not further specified
Wire rack shelf with hooks, Over-door mount, not further specified
Wire rack shelf with hooks, Over-door mount, Single tier, not further specified
Wire rack storage, see, Wire rack system
Wire rack system, Wall-mounted, 10 feet wide, For closet
Wire rack system, Wall-mounted, 10 feet wide, not further specified
Wire rack system, Wall-mounted, 5 feet wide, For closet
Wire rack system, Wall-mounted, 5 feet wide, not further specified
Wire rack system, Wall-mounted, 7 feet wide, For closet
Wire rack system, Wall-mounted, 7 feet wide, not further specified
Wire rack system, Wall-mounted, 8 feet wide, For closet
Wire rack system, Wall-mounted, 8 feet wide, For walk-in storage
Wire rack system, Wall-mounted, 8 feet wide, not further specified
Wireless doorbell, Mechanical chime, Portable receiver, Battery powered
Wireless doorbell, Mechanical chime, Portable receiver, not further specified
Wireless doorbell, Musical electronic, Plug-in receiver, Battery powered
Wireless doorbell, Musical electronic, Plug-in receiver, not further specified
Wireless FM receiver, see, Personal FM system
Wireless speaker, see, Personal FM system
Work clamp, With 2 alligator clips, Jointed arms, not further specified
Work clamp, With 2 alligator clips, Jointed arms, On stand
Wrist splint, see, Wrist support
Wrist support, Adult Left, Cuff at palm, not further specified
Wrist support, Adult Left, Cuff at palm, Velcro closure
Wrist support, Adult Right, Cuff at palm, not further specified
Wrist support, Adult Right, Cuff at palm, Velcro closure
Writing aid, Guide slot, 1/2 inch opening, not further specified
Writing aid, Guide slot, 1/2 inch opening, Plastic template
Writing aid, Guide slot, For #10 envelopes, not further specified
Writing aid, Guide slot, For #10 envelopes, Plastic template
Writing aid, Guide slot, For checks, not further specified
Writing aid, Guide slot, For checks, Plastic template
Writing aid, Guide slot, Letter writing, not further specified
Writing aid, Guide slot, Letter writing, Plastic template
Writing aid, Guide slot, Signature, not further specified
Writing aid, Guide slot, Signature, Plastic template
Writing aid, Magnetic wrist hold-down, With metal writing panel, not further specified
Writing aid, Magnetic wrist hold-down, With metal writing panel, Velcro strap closure
Writing aid, Paper holder board, Ruled lines, Magnetic strip paper holder
Writing aid, Paper holder board, Ruled lines, not further specified
Writing aid, Paper holder board, Suction cup feet, not further specified
Writing aid, Paper holder board, Suction cup feet, Paper clamp on left
Writing aid, Paper holder board, Suction cup feet, Paper clamp on right
Writing aid, Paper holder board, Suction cup feet, Paper clamp top & side
Writing paper, not further specified
Writing paper, Raised lines, Narrow rule, not further specified

GLOSSARY

Glossary of Terms Used in Nomenclature

The following terms are used in the nomenclature of generic names of products. The terms that are defined here are those that may not be self-explanatory or that may be confused with each other or with terms in other listings. An example of products with unusually confusing trade names is found among products that deal with incontinence; this glossary is intended to make clear distinctions among them and among similarly confusing products.

AC POWERED: describes a device that is operated by house current or alternating current (AC). In North America, AC is 110 volts, 60 cycles per second.

[ALARM CLOCK] ... AC WITH AC OUTLET: an [alarm clock that has an] AC electrical outlet that is made "live" by the alarm, and that can then power an electrical appliance such as a lamp or a bed shaker or a radio.

[ALARM CLOCK] ... ELECTRONIC BEEP ALARM: [an alarm clock in which] the alarm signal is a relatively pure tone, an electrically-generated "beep." Unlike the sound of a mechanical device like a bell, this beep has no auxiliary tones at lower frequencies. It is helpful for the description of an alarm clock to specify whether the tone is above or below about 4000 cycles per second; tones higher than that are difficult for most older people to hear, even at fairly high volume.

ALERTING DEVICE: a device, such as a lamp or a horn or bell, that is used to alert the user to some such event as a knock on the door, the ringing of a telephone, or a hazardous condition in the environment.

BATH BENCH: a seat with legs, but with no back, that is designed for use in the bath tub or shower. It has no wheels or casters; see "Shower bench" for wheeled equivalents.

BATH CHAIR: a seat with legs and with a back that is designed for use in the bath tub or shower. It has no wheels or casters; see "Bath bench" for backless equivalents, and "Shower chair" for wheeled equivalents.

BATH TRANSFER BENCH: a particular kind of "Bath bench" that has a seat extension to or over the tub edge and that facilitates seated transfer across the tub edge.

BATH TRANSFER CHAIR: a particular kind of "Bath chair" that has a seat extension to or over the tub edge and that facilitates transfer over the tub edge.

CLIP [as in "palmar clip"]: a firm clip of metal or plastic, usually in the form of a "C," that is fitted across the person's palm and that clasps the hand with some degree of firmness. It does not enclose the back of the hand (see "Cuff" for contrast). It may be padded or unpadded and may or may not be extended beyond the hand. It usually serves as the base for some implement that the person cannot otherwise readily grasp.

CUFF [as in "universal cuff"]: a firm or flexible device that encloses the person's hand, not including the fingers or (usually) the thumb. It may be permanently closed and to be slipped on, or it may have a fastening device to complete its closure on the hand. It may or may not have a clip (which see) embedded in it for stability. It usually serves as the base for some implement that the person cannot otherwise readily grasp.

CUP: a drinking vessel that has a relatively small, single handle that is designed for the insertion of one or two fingers. See, for contrast, "Goblet," "Mug," and "Tumbler." Note that many vessels sometimes called "cup" in the trade are more properly called by other Generic Names.

CUTTING BOARD: a flat, smooth or grooved surface, usually of wood or plastic, on which a knife may be used without dulling the edge. It may or may not be fitted with spikes or edges or corner guards to hold the object being cut. See also "Sandwich board."

CUTTING FRAME: a holding device used to secure an object so that it may be cut with a knife. It usually has slots to guide the knife blade. It may or may not be fastened to a base.

EMERGENCY RESPONSE DEVICE: a device by which the user can send a message or an alerting signal to a receiving person or organization that will then activate some response: contact or emergency assistance or action to check the status of sender. It is normally not used for ordinary communication, it is designed for emergency response only. It may be worn on the person or placed in some location where the user can activate it.

FAUCET TURNER: a device that may be placed on a faucet handle, or fastened to it, and that makes turning the faucet easier for a person with some functional limitation. It differs from a "Knob turner" in that its design is specific to the shape and action of the faucet.

GOBLET: a drinking vessel that has no handles as such, but does not have straight sides and may have a constriction to the sides into a stem (which may be thick, even as thick as half the vessel), and has a base that is usually the same diameter as the top portion of the vessel. See "Tumbler, pedestal base" for contrast.

HEADPHONE: a hearing device worn on the head and projecting sound into both ears. It may hold only the ear speakers or it may also incorporate additional components such as an amplifier and/or a radio or infra-red receiver.

[INCONTINENCE]... LIGHT, MEDIUM, HEAVY: absorbency characteristics of incontinence devices. "Light" indicates the ability to absorb minor discharges of urine. "Medium" indicates the ability to absorb a full bladder discharge. "Heavy" indicates the ability to absorb or contain both bladder and bowel discharges.

INCONTINENCE BRIEF MEN'S: an incontinence garment consisting of jockey-style underpants with vertical or horizontal fly, but of absorbent fabric capable of absorbing minor discharges of urine. It is intended to be washed and re-used.

INCONTINENCE PAD DISPOSABLE, USE IN INCONTINENCE GARMENT: an absorbent pad for use in "Incontinence pants with pouch" (which see), and that is intended for a single use, after which it is discarded. The pad has no fastening device other than being fitted into a special pouch or pocket in the pants.

INCONTINENCE PAD DISPOSABLE, USE IN REGULAR UNDERWEAR: an absorbent pad for use in regular, nonspecial underwear, intended for single use, after which it is discarded. The pad has adhesive backing that adheres to the underwear.

INCONTINENCE PANTS OPEN NET ... WITH PAD HOLDER: a type of "Incontinence pants with pouch" in which the sides are of mesh material; other parts of the pants may also be made of mesh.

INCONTINENCE PANTS WASHABLE: a type of incontinence pants that is for minor discharge of urine, that has no fly, that has its absorbency built in by absorbent and/or layered fabric, and that with washing may be used many times. It is distinguished from "Incontinence shield" by having fully-enclosing pants structure, with the side panels of lighter fabric than the absorbency panel. It is usually of the pull-on type, and it may resemble ordinary underpants.

INCONTINENCE PANTS WITH POUCH: a type of incontinence pants that is for minor to medium discharge of urine. With the use of "Incontinence pad, heavy absorbent" it may accommodate bowel discharge as well, though this may require it to have a larger pouch. It is distinguished from "Incontinence shield" by having a fully-closed pants construction. It is usually of the pull-on type, though it may open at the sides with an adhesive pad or another device, and it may resemble ordinary underpants except for the bulking of the pad.

INCONTINENCE SEATPAD: a seatpad for use by an incontinent person, absorbent of light urine discharges, and usually with a waterproof bottom panel.

INCONTINENCE SHIELD DISPOSABLE, ADHESIVE TAB SIDE CLOSURE: an absorbent garment that resembles a diaper more than it does underpants. It is generally of medium to heavy absorbency. It usually fully encloses the sides, but is designed to be opened and closed at the sides with adhesive tabs. It is designed to be discarded after one use.

INCONTINENCE SHIELD DISPOSABLE, WAIST BAND NO SIDES: an absorbent garment that resembles a loincloth more than it does underpants. It is generally of medium to heavy absorbency, and it is designed to be pulled on rather than to be opened and closed at the sides. It may be worn under regular underpants. It is designed to be discarded after one use.

INCONTINENCE SHIELD WASHABLE, PIN CLOSURE (or, SNAP CLOSURE), FULL SIDE COVERAGE: an absorbent garment that resembles a diaper more than it does underpants. It is generally of medium to heavy absorbency. It is fully enclosed at the sides, and is opened and closed at the sides with safety pins (PIN CLOSURE) or by snaps (SNAP CLOSURE). It is designed to be used more than once, and to be washed.

KITCHEN KNIFE, TOP PALMAR HANDLE, CRESCENT BLADE: a sharp knife with its blade of crescent shape (usually about a quarter circle) with an edge that is parallel to and below the user's hand. Its handle is grasped with a palmar grip. It may be used to slice, to cut with a rocking motion, or to chop. It is sometimes called an "ulu" or a "rocking-T knife."

KNOB TURNER: a device designed to grasp either a knob with a flat face and a flange, or a knob with an edge that is not smoothly round, and to transmit the user's twisting motion to the knob. It provides a substantial handle for the user to grasp.

LAMP: a light that can be moved, and that is usually plugged into an electrical outlet. It may also be battery powered. It may be designed for table-top or floor placement, or it may be clamped or otherwise fastened.

LIGHT FIXTURE: a light that is fixed in place, as by a ceiling mount. It is usually operated by a switch that is fixed as some distance such as a wall switch.

MAGNIFIER ... FOR DETAIL VIEWING 4.1 TO 8X: a magnifying lens or lenses that enlarge visual detail by a power of from 4 to 8. It usually is too small in diameter to be used for general reading.

MAGNIFIER ... FOR VERY FINE DETAIL 8.1 TO 20X: a magnifying lens or lenses that enlarges very small visual detail at a power ranging from 8 to 20. Its focal distance is usually very short and shallow. It is designed for use with small items such as the eye of a needle or a sliver, or for scientific field use.

MAGNIFIER ... READING TO 4X: a magnifying lens or lenses that enlarge visual matter in the range from 1.5 to 4 power. It is usually large enough to show a significant, readable amount of text, and its focal distance is usually not critical.

MEDICATIONS MANAGER: any device or object that is used to make daily or time-of-day doses of medication available as sets. It may be passive, requiring the user to remember when to open it, like a set of snap-lidded compartments. It may be active, like a loaded mechanism that makes and audible or visible signal on schedule and that may even dispense doses.

MIRROR SELF INSPECTION: any mirror that is designed for the user to inspect parts of the body that are not readily seen directly. The self-inspection may be accompanied by action upon the body, such as inserting a catheter, but not necessarily. This name includes "cathing mirrors."

MUG: a drinking vessel with one or more handles that are large enough for the insertion of several fingers, or handles that are gripped by the whole hand. See, for contrast, "Cup" and "Tumbler."

NON-SKID MAT: a flat section of material that resists skidding of objects on it by increasing surface friction; a mat is of fixed size.

NON-SKID MATTING: flat material that resists skidding of objects on it by increasing surface friction; matting is usually furnished in rolls or sheets that are to be cut to size.

NON-SKID STRIPS: flat material that resists skidding, usually of a person, by increasing surface friction; it usually has an adhesive backing to apply it to the surface to be made skid-resistant, such as a bathtub; it is furnished in strips.

NON-SKID TAPE: flat material that resists skidding, usually of a person, by increasing surface friction; it usually has an adhesive backing to apply it to the surface to be made skid-resistant; it is furnished in rolls, to be cut to length.

NON-SLIP ...: character of a material (tape, coating, sleeve, etc.) that is applied to an object such as a handle, to increase its surface friction so that the user's hand does not slip.

ONE-HAND OPERATION: description of a device that can be, or is claimed to be, capable of being operated by a person using only one hand. (In the Nomenclature, such items can be retrieved by the search for the term "one-hand.")

PEN HOLDER: a device that holds a pen, enlarging the user's grip or stabilizing it, in order to facilitate the pen's use in writing by a person with functional limitations.

PEN-AND-PENCIL GRIP: a device, usually a sleeve, that may be applied to a pen or pencil in order to bulk up the gripping area or in order to give a more secure or comfortable grip.

PERSONAL SOUND AMPLIFIER: a device that picks up sound in the environment, amplifies it, and relays it to the ear or ears of the user; it is usually two or more elements connected by an electrical cord. It differs from a body or table hearing aid in that it is not a medical device and is not individually fitted; it may have a frequency filter.

PLATE ... SLOPED SIDES: a plate for eating that has a raised edge (or raised dividers) that is more than a rim and less than vertical. PLATE, HIGH SIDED: a plate with one or more sides that are higher than a regular plate rim and lower than those of a bowl.

PLATE, INNER WELL WITH PLATFORM LIP: a plate with a central portion that is at least a half inch lower than the platform lip, and with a slightly sloping platform lip that surrounds the well and is wide enough for the placement of some kinds of food.

PLATE, SCOOP BACK OR SIDE: a plate with one side turned up and curled back beyond the vertical.

REACHER ... any device for extending the reach of a person. (In this nomenclature, "Reacher" is further specified in the second term by the kind of handle or grip, in the third term by the mechanism by which it is operated, and in the fourth term by the kind of grasping mechanism.)

ROCKER BLADE: a table knife that has a curved or rocker-shaped edge, and with the blade positioned ahead of the handle, not beneath the handle; it is designed to cut food with a rocking motion that concentrates the force. Distinguished from "Table/kitchen knife, Palmar handle, Crescent blade," which has different functional characteristics.

SANDWICH BOARD: a particular kind of "Cutting board" that has a holding device that is designed to hold a slice of bread in place while the bread is being spread.

SHOWER CHAIR: a seat with legs and back, and with wheels or casters, that is designed for use in a shower, and that may be rolled into the shower if there is not a significant threshold. See "Bath chair" for the seat that may also be used in the shower, but that has no wheels or casters.

SHOWER SEAT: a seat that is affixed to, or is a part of, a shower enclosure.

TABLE/KITCHEN KNIFE, TOP PALMAR HANDLE, CRESCENT BLADE: a dull-edged or semi-sharp knife with a blade of crescent shape (usually about a quarter circle), the edge of which is parallel to and below the user's hand, and the handle of which is designed to be held in a palmar grasp. It may be used to cut with a rocking motion on a plate. It is sometimes called an "ulu" or a "rocking-T" knife.

HIGH-TACK PLASTIC: a soft plastic with a surface that retains a very high coefficient of friction (feels "tacky") during use and after cleaning, but does not adhere to hands or objects. The trade name of one such product is Dicem.

TELEPHONE, TRANSMITS TO HEARING AID: a telephone that has an earpiece that emits electromagnetic fields that may be picked up by a hearing aid that is capable of this kind of pick-up. (Note: a telephone that is merely "hearing aid compatible" may only avoid feed-back squeal in a hearing aid, but does not emit the electromagnetic field.

TWO HANDS NEEDED TO OPERATE: a term applied to a device that obviously, or by claim, requires the simultaneous use of both the user's hands. (In this nomenclature, these devices may be retrieved by search for "two hands.")

SPEECH AMPLIFIER: a device that picks up the user's voice, amplifies it, and drives a speaker so that others can hear the user.

TELEPHONE AMPLIFIER: a device that causes a telephone earpiece to sound at amplified volume, or that may be attached to the earpiece and produced amplified output. It is designed to be either inserted in the telephone line or to be clipped over the earpiece; the former type requires a particular telephone design.

TELEPHONE SIGNALER: any device that receives the input or the sound of the telephone ringer, and that then produces a signal (amplified sound, flashing light, etc.) that signals that the phone is ringing.

TELEPHONE WITH AMPLIFIER: a telephone with an integral amplifier to drive the earpiece.

TELEPHONE WITH AMPLIFIER, AMPLIFIES HIGH FREQUENCIES: a "Telephone with amplifier" that selectively amplifies higher frequencies in the speech range but above the frequency that is easily heard by elderly people and by people with some kinds of hearing loss.

TUMBLER: a drinking vessel with no handles. It is usually a cylinder or tapered cylinder. It may or may not have a lid, and if it does the lid may or may not have a device to control drinking. (One type of this last is commonly called a "feeding cup," but it does not meet the definition of a cup. See, for functional differences, "Cup," "Mug," and "Goblet.")

UNIVERSAL CUFF: a cuff that goes around the hand, leaving the thumb and fingers free, and that may be slipped on or may be closed with hook-and-loop or Velcro, AND that has a holder into which various implements may be inserted and fastened, so that the implement may be used by a person without functional grasp.

WIRE RACK .... rack made of heavy wires or rods, usually set parallel and close enough together to support objects stored on the rack. It is fabricated into shelves and baskets, and usually the wires or rods are coated with soft but durable rubber-like plastic.

WIRE RACK SYSTEM: a set of "Wire rack shelves" and related storage surfaces and hooks, united into a single unit that may be mounted on a wall or floor; may be several feet in size.

WRIST SUPPORT: a device, or the extension of a device, that extends back beyond the user's wrist onto the forearm, and that compensates for functional weakness of the wrist. It is to be distinguished from a brace, which is a medical device that is independent of an implement.